Philosophy and Psychiatry

Philosophy and Psychiatry

Edited by

Thomas Schramme
Johannes Thome

Walter de Gruyter · Berlin · New York

Printed with the kind support of Merz Pharmaceuticals GmbH

♾ Printed on acid-free paper which falls within
the guidelines of the ANSI to ensure permanence and durability.

ISBN 3-11-017800-1

Library of Congress – Cataloging-in-Publication Data

A CIP catalogue record for this book is available from
the Library of Congress.

Bibliographic information published by Die Deutsche Bibliothek

Die Deutsche Bibliothek lists this publication in the Deutsche Nationalbibliografie;
detailed bibliographic data is available in the Internet at <http://dnb.ddb.de>.

Printed in Germany

Disk conversion: DTB Johanna Boy, Brennberg
Cover design: Christopher Schneider, Berlin
Picture: "Numerisches Feld", Karl Schwarzenberg, 1996, oil on canvas, 141 × 119 cm
Photo: © Dorothea Burkhardt

Preface

Philosophy and psychiatry not only have a common history but also share several concepts such as consciousness, self, identity, psyche and, of great significance, mind or mental. Plato was concerned with the harmony of the human soul. Aristotle's ethics developed an account of *eudaimonia*, or the good life. How should one live? This is one of the oldest questions of philosophy – and, similarly, the whole point of psychiatric treatment is to help people live their lives to the best of their ability. But despite their common roots, psychiatry and philosophy have become individual disciplines, philosophy being a human science (*Geisteswissenschaft*) and psychiatry being a medical discipline, identifying more and more with the principles of the natural sciences. This anthology is an attempt to bring back together what came apart. We are convinced that both psychiatry and philosophy can benefit from one another; that a fruitful interaction between the two disciplines will help to solve some common problems.

We asked several distinguished scholars, psychiatrists and philosophers to write on their preferred topic in order to give a comprehensive picture of the multiplicity of shared themes. During the preparation of this collection we were happy to notice a huge enthusiasm regarding these themes. It seems that the interest in the subject is much more pervasive and deeper than we expected. Maybe the time is ripe for launching a new philosophy of psychiatry, as recently suggested in the first issue of a book series on international perspectives in philosophy and psychiatry (Bill Fulford et al., *Nature and narrative. An introduction to the new philosophy of psychiatry*, Oxford U.P. 2003). Although we are aware of the problematic nature and inconveniences of interdisciplinary work and multi-author books, we believe that the collected essays are accessible both from a philosophical and a psychiatric perspective, thus demonstrating how philosophy and psychiatry may benefit from each other.

When conceptionalizing this book, the question arose whether it should be written in our native tongue or if the "lingua franca" of present times should be used. After intense discussions, we decided to publish this anthology in the English language. This made the task for several of our contributors, many of them non native-speakers, rather difficult (including ourselves), but will hopefully propagate a wide reception, enable a cross-national discussion and contribute to the international discourse about the conditions of the possibility of a philosophy of psychiatry.

We would like to thank all co-authors for their highly interesting and in many ways pioneering contributions.

Also, we are very thankful to Dr. Gertrud Grünkorn of our publisher de Gruyter, Berlin, for her encouraging support right from the beginning of the planning and throughout the publication process of this anthology. Last but not least, we would like to express our gratitude to Kerrin Jacobs and Nicola van Dornick for their reliable and indispensable help with editorial and linguistical issues.

Mannheim, March 2004

Johannes Thome
Thomas Schramme

Contents

The Relation of Philosophy and Psychiatry

Classification and Conceptual Considerations

Methodology and Philosophy of Science

Epistemology

Compulsion, Volitional Disorder, and Freedom of the Will

Personal Identity

Psychiatric Ethics

Contributors

Hans-Jörg Assion, MD, is Physician of Neurology, Psychiatry and Psychotherapy; residencies at the Universities of Bonn and Bochum; Assistant Medical Director of the emergency and the rehabilitation wards at the Centre for Psychiatry, Ruhr-University, Bochum; his scientific work focuses on schizophrenia, psychopharmacological topics and crosscultural psychiatry.

Aisling Campbell, MRCPsych, MMedSc, is Consultant Psychiatrist in Cork University Hospital and Senior Lecturer in the Department of Psychiatry, University College, Cork. She also works as a psychoanalyst. Her interests include the application of Lacanian theory to psychiatric practice, trauma and the nosology of traumatic stress syndromes, and Freudian and Lacanian perspectives on subjective space. She is a member of the Association of Psychoanalysts and Psychotherapists in Ireland (APPI).

Detlef E. Dietrich studied medicine at the Medizinische Hochschule Hannover (MHH); holding the title of MD since 1990, he worked in different neurological clinics before becoming a specialist in psychiatry and psychotherapy at the MHH. Since 1995 he is Consultant Psychiatrist at the Department of Clinical Psychiatry and Psychotherapy and received his Habilitation in 2001. Main fields of research include cognition, especially neurophysiology of emotion-cognitive bonding as well as neurobiology and treatment of affective illnesses.

Harald Raimund Dreßing, MD, is Consultant Psychiatrist at the Central Institute of Mental Health, Mannheim and Director of CIMH's Day Hospital and the Department of Forensic Psychiatry, Ludwigshafen. From 1983 to 1990 he was engaged in postgraduate training in psychiatry. His recent interests in scientific research include neurobiology, sexual offenders, forensic psychiatry in the European Union and stalking.

Hinderk M. Emrich is Chair of the Department of Psychiatry at the Hannover Medical School. He holds an MD (University of Bern) and a PhD (University of Munich); In 1972 he received his Habilitation in Molecular Neurobiology (Technical University of Berlin), from 1973-1974 he undertook patho-physiological studies at the Pediatric Hospital, University of Munich in collaboration with the Department of Physiology; from 1975-1978 he was engaged in postgraduate training in psychiatry, neurology and clinical psychopharmacology; 1979-1987 he became Group and later Department Leader of Clinical Psychopharmacology at the Max-Planck-Institute for Psychiatry; 1991-1992 he was Fellow of the Wissenschaftskolleg Berlin; Visiting Professor at several universities, e.g. at the Universität Witten-Herdecke and the Deutsche Film- und Fernsehakademie Berlin.

Thomas Fuchs, MD, PhD, is psychiatrist and philosopher, Assistant Professor, Head of the Section "Phenomenological Psychopathology and Psychotherapy", Senior Psychiatrist at the Department of Psychiatry, University of Heidelberg. His major areas of research are psychopathology, phenomenology, theory of psychiatry, and medical ethics; his empirical research focuses on depression and on mother-child interaction in postpartum disorders.

Bill (K.W.M.) Fulford is Professor of Philosophy and Mental Health in the Department of Philosophy, University of Warwick, where he runs Masters, PhD, and research programmes in Philosophy, Ethics and Mental Health Practice. He is also an Honorary Consultant Psychiatrist in the Department of Psychiatry, University of Oxford; Visiting Professor in Psychology, The Institute of Psychiatry and King's College, London University; Visiting Professor in Philosophy and Professional Practice Skills in the Centre for Professional Ethics, University of Lancashire; and Visiting Professor, Kent Institute of Medicine and Health Sciences, University of Kent. He is the Founder Chair of the Philosophy Special Interest Group in The Royal College of Psychiatrists. He is a fellow of both the Royal College of Psychiatrists and the Royal College of Physicians (London). He is the Editor of the first international journal for philosophy and mental health, *PPP – Philosophy, Psychiatry and Psychology*. He has published widely on philosophical and ethical aspects of mental health, in particular *Moral theory and medical practice* (1989, paperback 1995, reprinted 1999, second edition forthcoming from Cambridge University Press).

Andreas Heinz, MD, is Director and Chair of the Department of Psychiatry and Psychotherapy, Charité University Medicine Berlin, Campus Charité Mitte. He was previously Associate Professor for addiction research at the University of Heidelberg, ZI Mannheim. He studied medicine, philosophy and anthropology in Bochum, Berlin and at Howard University, Washington DC and received his clinical education at the Department of Neurology, Ruhr-Universität, Bochum, the Department of Psychiatry of the Free University Berlin and the National Institute of Mental Health. His research focuses on monoaminergic dysfunction in psychiatric disorders and on anthropology in psychiatry.

Hanfried Helmchen is Emeritus Professor of Psychiatry at the Free University Berlin. He was Head of the Department of Psychiatry from 1971–1999. From 1979-1980 he was President of the German Society for Psychiatry and Neuroscience. He has published 25 books and around 400 articles. His research interests are, among others, psychiatric therapy, methodology of clinical trials, criteria of evaluation, psychiatric diagnostics and classification (methodology), mental disorders in old age, dementia, subthreshold psychiatric disorders and ethical questions in psychiatry.

Georg Juckel, MD, PhD, is Consultant Psychiatrist and Deputy Head of the Department of Psychiatry and Psychotherapy, Charité University Medicine Berlin, Campus Charité Mitte. He was previously Senior Researcher and Consultant at the Department of Psychiatry, Ludwig-Maximilians-University (LMU), Munich. He studied medicine and philosophy at the Free University Berlin and received his clinical education at the Department of Psychiatry, Free University Berlin and LMU Munich. He has been engaged in research at the Hungarian Academy of Sciences in Budapest (Department of Psychophysiology) and in the Program in Neuroscience of Princeton University. He is the recipient of various research awards in the field of psychiatry, e.g. the DGPPN-Duphar/Solvay-Award. His main research interests are the monoaminergic modulation of neurophysiological parameters, motor functions in psychiatry, the combination of EEG and fMRI, and animal models of psychiatric disorders.

Martin Löw-Beer, PhD, is now working at the Institute of Social Research in Frankfurt. He studied philosophy in Berlin and Frankfurt am Main and has written a book on self-deception. He taught philosophy in Frankfurt and in Berlin.

Rainer Luthe is former Director and Emeritus Professor of the Institute of Forensic Psychology and Psychiatry at Saarland University. Holding a Dr. jur. h.c., he, in addition, serves as forensic psychiatric expert who testifies before criminal courts on matters of mental health, penal responsibility and prognosis of delinquents. His former and current research includes the history, epistemological background and principles of psychopathology and structural psychopathology.

Lou Marinoff has been affiliated with University College London, the Hebrew University of Jerusalem, the University of British Columbia, and the City College of New York, where he is currently a Professor of Philosophy. Lou Marinoff is author of *Plato Not Prozac* (published in 24 languages), is founding President of the American Philosophical Practitioners Association (www.appa.edu), and is a Fellow of the World Economic Forum (Geneva & Davos).

Thomas Metzinger is Professor of Philosophy at the Johannes Gutenberg-University in Mainz, where he is Head of the Department for Theoretical Philosophy. He is a Member of the Board of Directors of the "Association for the Scientific Study of Consciousness". He is author of the recent book *Being No One – The Self-Model Theory of Subjectivity* and has edited the anthologies *Neural Correlates of Consciousness* and *Bewusstsein – Beiträge aus der Gegenwartsphilosophie.*

Hans-Jürgen Möller, MD, has been working in the field of psychiatry for 30 years. After obtaining his Doctor of Medical Science in 1972 from the Universities of Göttingen and Hamburg, Germany, he then specialised in psychiatry and postgraduate training at the Max-Planck-Institute of Psychiatry in Munich. Hans-Jürgen Möller completed a postdoctoral thesis in psychiatry and has held academic positions at Munich Technical University and the University of Bonn. He is currently Professor of Psychiatry and Chairman of the Psychiatric Department at the Ludwig-Maximilians-University in Munich. Professor Möller's main scientific contributions include clinical research into psychiatry, schizophrenia and depression, clinical psychopharmacology and psychogeriatrics. He sits on numerous national and international psychiatric societies and is currently Past-President of the World Federation of Societies of Biological Psychiatry and Co-Chairman of the Section on Pharmacopsychiatry of the World Psychiatric Association. In addition to authoring and co-authoring over 400 international publications and several books, he is also the Chief Editor of *The World Journal of Biological Psychiatry*, Main Editor of *European Archives of Psychiatry and Clinical Neuroscience*, and editor of both *Nervenarzt* and *Psychopharmakotherapie*, and holds positions on numerous other editorial boards for national and international psychiatric journals.

Georg Northoff is a psychiatrist, holds an MD in psychiatry/medicine and a PhD in philosophy. His research focuses on psychomotor syndromes (catatonia) and affective disturbances, imaging in emotions (fMRI), and neurophilosophical questions like personal identity, qualia, consciousness, neuroethics, and mind-body relation. In addition to numerous publications in the fields of psychiatry, imaging and neurophilosophy, his research includes major work on personal identity and surgical procedures in the brain and most recently a book about the *Philosophy of the Brain – the Brain Problem*. He is currently engaged as Associate Professor at the Department of Psychiatry, University of Magdeburg.

Markus R. Pawelzik, MD, is a psychiatrist, neurologist, psychotherapist and philosopher. He runs the EOS-Clinic for Psychotherapy in Münster. His philosophical work focuses on the ethics of psychotherapy and psychiatry and adjacent fields. The last important philosophical publication is the book *Krankheit, das gute Leben und die Krise der Medizin* (Münster 1999).

Pierre Pichot, MD, is a member of the French National Academy of Medicine. He is Professor of Psychiatry and until 1986 was Head of the Department of Psychiatry at the Paris Medical School, he also taught psychology at the Sorbonne. His work concerns mostly the application of quantitative psychological techniques to research in the clinical, nosological, psychopathological and therapeutic fields, and the history of psychiatry.

Aloys L. Prinz, Dr. rer. pol., is Professor of Economics at Westfälische Wilhelms-University Münster, Institute of Public Economics. His work focuses *inter alia* on health economics and the economics of social security. The last important publication in health economics is the book *E-Commerce im Arzneimittelhandel* (with Alexander Vogel), Gütersloh 2003.

Michael Rösler is Professor of Psychiatry at the Institute of Forensic Psychology and Psychiatry, Saarland University. He is a forensic psychiatric expert who testifies before criminal courts on matters of mental health, penal responsibility and prognosis of delinquents. His former research focused on clinical aspects, genetics and treatment of Alzheimer`s disease. His current research interests include epidemiology, clinical aspects, comorbidity and treatment of adult attention deficit- /hyperactivity disorder (ADHD), impact of ADHD on social deviance and crime.

Jann Schlimme, MD, works clinically and scientifically at the Department of Clinical Psychiatry and Psychotherapy, Hannover Medical School. His major interests of research are psychiatric anthropology and philosophical psychology.

Thomas Schramme is Lecturer at the Department of Philosophy, University of Mannheim. Prior to receiving a PhD from the Free University Berlin, he read philosophy in Frankfurt, Berlin and Oxford. For a couple of years he worked part-time in an out-patient centre for mentally ill adults. His book on the concept of mental illness has recently been reissued as *Psychische Krankheit aus philosophischer Sicht* (Gießen 2003).

Dieter Sigmund, MD, is a psychiatrist and neurologist. He studied medicine at the University of Tübingen. Since 1988, he has been working as Consultant at the Department of Psychiatry, University of Heidelberg. His research focuses on psychopathology.

Johannes Thome is Professor of Psychiatry at the University of Wales in Swansea. He received his MD and PhD degrees from Saarland University, Germany. After completing his residency training in psychiatry at the University of Würzburg, he became Postdoctoral Associate at the Division of Molecular Psychiatry, Yale University School of Medicine. Subsequently, he worked as Consultant Psychiatrist and Senior Lecturer at the University of Heidelberg, ZI Mannheim. His research interests focus on molecular psychiatry, psychopharmacology, psychopathology and interdisciplinary aspects of psychiatry.

Henrik Walter, MD, PhD, studied medicine, psychology and philosophy in Marburg, Gießen and Boston. He was trained in neurology and psychiatry, worked for two years in the Department of Philosophy in Braunschweig and is currently Vice-Director of the Department of Psychiatry at the University Clinic in Ulm, Germany, where he also leads a neuroimaging research group. His current empirical research interests are in working memory, emotions and their impact on cognition, as well as social cognitive neuroscience, both in basic research as well as in clinical applications in schizophrenia and depression. Furthermore, he is working in the field of neurophilosophy and the philosophy of mind, in particular, on the problem of free will and responsibility. He has published extensively in the fields of philosophy, neuroimaging and psychiatry and is author of the book *Neurophilosophy of Free Will* (MIT Press, 2001). Recently, he has edited, together with Achim Stephan, two books on emotions, *Natur und Theorie der Emotion*, mentis, Paderborn 2003 and *Moralität, Rationalität und die Emotionen*, Humboldt Universitätsverlag 2004.

Introduction: The Many Potentials for Philosophy of Psychiatry

Thomas Schramme and Johannes Thome

Psychiatry is a philosophical discipline. This might come as a surprising and even provocative claim. But it is obvious that in psychiatry many theoretical and practical issues have a philosophical connotation. What probably comes to mind first are ethical issues in the treatment of psychiatric patients. Confidentiality, informed consent and the criteria of competence, coercive treatment, the insanity defence, psychopathy and some other problems must be dealt with in medical ethics and law. Although they may raise specific questions in psychiatry, it is widely accepted that efforts to deal with these problems may benefit from a philosophical point of view, since ethics is, of course, one of the main and traditional subjects of philosophy.

But there are several other, more theoretical topics relevant to psychiatry which could also take advantage of philosophical expertise, but where, surprisingly, collaborations are hardly to be found. Examples include the mind-body-problem, freedom of the will, the concepts of rationality, of causation, of classification, the debate on the dichotomy of science and humanities (or natural and social sciences), personal identity, consciousness, the problem of other minds. These are common themes in theoretical philosophy, more specific in metaphysics, epistemology, action theory, philosophy of science, and philosophy of mind with the utmost relevance for psychiatry.

What about philosophy being a psychiatric discipline? Since not only could psychiatry gain by philosophical knowledge, but philosophical debates could be enriched by psychiatric expertise, too. Philosophy used to be regarded as a therapeutic discipline. Although this idea has declined in the past few centuries, especially in academic philosophy, it is still of some relevance. Many people today search for a meaning in their life, several still look for answers in philosophical books and some try to solve their problems by philosophical assistance. Admittedly, psychiatric illness is different from spiritual deficiency. But nevertheless, philosophy should be aware of its long history concerning the question of how we should live because there is a demand for "therapy" which overlaps with psychiatry.

Theoretical philosophy, too, can be enriched by considering psychiatric issues. For example, there is a common objection to certain theories in the philosophy of mind that have not been developed on the basis of empirical data, but mainly by means of thought experiments (Wilkes 1988). Psychiatry, in contrast, deals with real, not "possible" people, and certain philosophical accounts can, thus, gain support or opposition by their cases. For example, consider the philosophical problem of the unity of consciousness. How is it possible that sense-data and attitudes are integrated into one perspective, in the point of view of a self? Usually, philosophers – and not only them – tend to think of a person as consisting of just one self. They like to believe that there is only "one self to a customer" (Dennett 1991, p. 422). But what about patients with split brains, patients suffering from paranoid-hallucinatoric schizophrenic psychoses or persons experiencing multiple personalities? These real-life cases can put into doubt some philosophical theories about the unity of the self.

Because they are of obvious interest for philosophers, the so-called dissociative identity disorder, cases of patients with split corpus callosum and the phenomenon of schizophrenic psychoses have already caught the attention of some philosophers (Flanagan 1996, Glover 1988, Metzinger 1993, Metzinger 2003, Nagel 1971, Wilkes 1988). It should be mentioned that there are some other examples of already existing interdisciplinary discussions but these are still few considering the potentials (Baron-Cohen 1995, Bolton and Hill 1996, Graham and Stephens 1994, Löw-Beer 1990, Northoff 1997, Emrich et al. 2002, Heginbotham 2000, Heinze and Priebe 1996, Heinze et al. 1996, Hundert 1989, Fulford 1989, Fulford et al. 2003, Phillips Griffiths 1994, Reznek 1987, 1991, Sadler et al. 1994, Sadler 2002, Schramme 2000, Spitzer et al. 1988, 1990, Stephens and Graham 2000, Straus et al. 1969, Theunissen 1991).

In summary, psychiatry is neither a philosophical discipline nor philosophy a psychiatric discipline. However, philosophy as a fundamental reflection of the *conditio humana* can make significant contributions to the elucidation of the theoretical background which drives psychiatric research and practice. Vice versa, psychiatry as a rational science of the human mind and brain may enrich the philosophical discourse about several issues by pragmatism, rationalism, empirism and relevance.

Philosophy of psychiatry: Recent and past

Although philosophy of psychiatry is an emerging discipline, it already has a history even if there is admittedly more interdisciplinary work done in the related field of philosophy of psychology. Up to now, a considerable number of anthologies, authored books and articles has already been published. Several networks of scholars have been installed, at least one academic journal dedicated to this subject has been founded (*Philosophy, Psychiatry & Psychology*), and several conferences have taken place and enhanced the international collaboration of scholars in this field. A special masters degree in the "philosophy and ethics of mental health" is now available at the University of Warwick/England and the International Network for Philosophy and Psychiatry (INPP) has been launched. So it seems that philosophy of psychiatry today has at least a preliminary standing.

Arguably, the first modern classic of philosophy of psychiatry proper is Karl Jaspers's *General Psychopathology*, published in the first edition in 1913. In addition, Jaspers is one of its champions *in persona*, since he was trained both as psychiatrist and philosopher. Although in his work he was already concerned with almost all the main philosophical topics in psychiatry – whether or not psychiatry belongs to the natural sciences, the concept of mental illness, diagnosis and classification etc. – he is most of all remembered for his account of the subjective side of mental illness. A psychiatric patient not merely has a disease but is ill. Therefore, he or she develops a certain point of view which needs to be understood by the psychiatrist. Consequently, the task in psychiatry does not only consist in finding explanations of disorders but also in understanding patients as persons who take a subjective perspective.

Phenomenology is one of the traditional methods in philosophy dealing with the issue of understanding other minds and developing an account of subjectivity or the 'lived-world'. Jaspers is one main reference for phenomenological theories in psychiatry today. In addition, there is a recent interest in the work of Edmund Husserl, who was the founder of the phenomenological movement in Europe.

Although the common distinction between continental and analytical philosophy rightly became under attack in recent years, it is clear that Husserl and Jaspers stand for a certain tradition of philosophy. There is another tradition in philosophy of psychiatry which is connected to so-called analytical philosophy and is fuelled by an adherence to a scientific worldview. This philosophical account is potentially in conflict with the tradition of phenomenology. Gilbert Ryle may be named as one of its modern advocates. In his seminal book *The Concept of Mind*, published in 1949, Ryle tried to overcome Cartesian dualism – the dichotomy between *res extensa* and *res cogitans*, which was introduced by the French scholar René Descartes in 1641 and still is influential today – by analysing the language we use to refer to mental states and mental acts. Thereby, Ryle became one of the leading figures of 'ordinary language philosophy'. He maintained that the common distinction between mind and body rests on a certain linguistic error that could be labelled as 'category mistake'. He rejected Cartesianism as 'the dogma of the ghost in the machine' and developed his own theory of mind by defining mental terms in behavioural language, i.e. by reference to observable events.

Another strain of this philosophical tradition can be found in the proponents of Logical Positivism. In its early years, Rudolf Carnap, Friedrich Schlick, Otto Neurath, Alfred Ayer and their collaborators developed an account which focused on the reduction of all mental terms, thus psychology, to physics. They were highly critical of all metaphysical, i.e. non-verifiable statements which they especially ascribed to Martin Heidegger. Although their highly ambitious research program failed and reductionism in the philosophy of mind is widely abandoned today, their scientific and naturalistic worldview still lives on. Some recent publications in philosophy of psychiatry are clearly influenced by this tradition.

Last but not least, one can find some references to the early Greek philosophical tradition, especially regarding ethical questions in psychiatry. This interest can be seen in relation to the recent developments in virtue ethics, which, of course, mainly goes back to Aristotle's *Nichomachean Ethics*. But other theoretical issues, such as teleology, are also to be found in this context. Furthermore, it has been shown that Plato anticipated several modern concepts of the human psyche and developed a philosophy with considerable psychotherapeutic aspects (Thome 1995).

Certainly, none of what has been said so far should suggest one or another preferred way of seeing things in philosophy of psychiatry. On the contrary, we would like to point out the variety of philosophical traditions which may underlie different viewpoints. In this anthology, we have tried to show the potential of different philosophical perspectives for psychiatry in its multiplicity.

Up to this point, we have focused on establishing that there is a real potential for fruitful collaboration between philosophy and psychiatry which could aid both disciplines. In the next two sections we would like to give some evidence supporting our claim by discussing in greater depth two philosophical problems of psychiatry: Firstly, the mind-body-problem, which is one of the oldest topics of philosophy and also the most basic conundrum in psychiatry. Secondly, the philosophical debate on the concept of mental illness.

Mind, brain, and mental disorder

Some years ago, on the occasion of the annual "Festival of Science" of the British Association for the Advancement of Science, *The Guardian* published several short articles to inform the public about recent developments in different academic disciplines. The author who wrote about schizophrenic psychoses reported: "Now that it is generally accepted that schizophrenia is a disease of the brain, the next question is: how does it come about? There is little evidence of active degenerative changes in the brain, and it seems more likely that what goes wrong reflects an abnormality in brain development occurring early in life, perhaps even in the womb." (Iverson 1997)

These sentences represent a common opinion about mental illness, especially schizophrenic psychoses. Although there are no clear, generally accepted and in every single case demonstrable correlative disorders of the brain, i.e. neurobiological and morphological correlatives, yet known, there is no question that such mental illness is a brain disease. Usually this belief is fuelled by the efficacy of certain drugs which affect neurophysiological processes. Surely this fact should be seen as a hint at the general dependency of mental phenomena on brain processes. But does it imply that disorders which are identified on the level of the mental can be explained by respective disorders of neurophysiological processes? Can we abandon the reference to genuine mental processes? On the other hand, if we want to save the unity of body and mind, do we not need to search for mental illness in the brain?

There is an apparent dilemma in using the concept of mental illness. Thomas Szasz questioned its validity by rejecting the view that there can be a substance, called 'mind' or the 'mental', which can be affected by a disease in the way the body is. If we tried to counter this argument by explaining mental illness as manifesting itself in the brain, as the author of *The Guardian* article did, then we might question why we should still regard it as *mental* illness.

"Psychiatry is left with two seeming alternatives: either to say that personal, psychological and emotional disorders are really states of the body, objective features of brain-tissue, the organism-under-stress, the genes or what have you; or else to deny that such disorders are illnesses at all." (Sedgwick 1973, p. 127.) Peter Sedgwick describes a common opinion which leaves us only two options: either to somatize mental illness or else to question its medical status in principle. Many psychiatrists focus on biological accounts. When the concept of mental illness is based on physiological disorder like somatic illness then nothing counts against upholding medical terminology for psychiatric phenomena. But again, according to Szasz's opinion, this argument leads to a new problem. Why should one call diseases of the brain, hence somatically manifested illnesses, *mental* illnesses (Szasz 1987, p. 49)?

Thus adherents of the concept of mental illness may find themselves in an awkward dilemma: either they stress the bodily realization of mental illness and thereby perpetuate the analogy with somatic illness, and hence bio-medical terminology, but at the prize of losing the specific quality of mental illness, since it is reduced to bodily illness. Or they try to maintain the term of mental illness *sui generis*; but then it seems that they will have to postulate a mental realm which is distinct from the body. So this strategy, on the other hand, seems to lead to a mind-body dualism, which is no longer fashionable in philosophy. Thus the dilemma for adherents of the concept of mental illness seems to consist of the choice between the Scylla of reductionism and the Charybdis of dualism.

There are authors, especially psychiatrists, who are willing to dissolve the dilemma by consequently going the way of somatization (in the sense of physicalization) and thus actually abandoning the concept of mental illness. A prominent example is Robert Kendell: "[...] it follows that there is, strictly speaking, no such thing as disease of the mind or mental disorder and that

Griesinger was right – mental illnesses are diseases of the brain, or at least involve disordered brain function – because all mental events are accompanied by and dependent on events in the brain. (Thomas Szasz was also right; mental illness is a myth, though not for the reasons he believed.)" (Kendell 1993, p. 3.) Surprisingly, a downright grotesque alliance between so-called biological psychiatrists and sceptics like Szasz seems to be at hand: both are prepared to drop the concept of mental illness.

The task therefore consists of finding convincing arguments in favour of a concept of mental illness in its own right. From what we have said so far it might be already obvious that the dilemmatical structure can be put into doubt. There are possible positions between the extremes of the dilemma. For some (mainly philosophers who are interested in the modern debate on the mind-body problem), this will not come as a surprise, but many others (among them psychiatrists) are quite impressed by the critique of Cartesian dualism and believe the only alternative consists in biological accounts of mental disorder. Even the authors of the DSM-IV come up with the same argument: "Although this volume is titled the *Diagnostic and Statistical Manual of Mental Disorders*, the term *mental disorder* unfortunately implies a distinction between 'mental' disorders and 'physical' disorders that is a reductionistic [!] anachronism of mind/body dualism." (APA 1994, p. XXI)

There are many more alternatives to Cartesian dualism which do not seem to be widely known in present-day psychiatry (cf. Hannan 1994, Kim 1996). Anti-Dualism or Materialism about the mind does not necessarily commit to a reductionistic account. As mentioned above, theories about the relation of mind and body, which could result in the questioning of the concept of mental disorder, are *reductive*, i.e. they reduce the explanation of mental phenomena to statements about physical processes and therefore arrive at one extreme of the dilemma mentioned above.

This is not the place to discuss the relevant theories at length but it may suffice to allude to the fact that for a reductive account it would not be sufficient to demonstrate merely a *correlation* of some types of mental illness with particular neurophysiological states or processes. Rather, it would be necessary to prove an *identification* of mental with neurophysiological states which, in turn, would imply that every property of a mental phenomenon also has to be a property of a neurophysiological state, which was explicitly stated by the so-called type-identity theory (Smart 1959, Place 1956).

In the present-day philosophy of mind, reductionism is considerably less favoured than it used to be. Even if the problem of explaining consciousness and subjectivity in neurophysiological terms is disregarded – an awkward problem for every (even non-reductive) physicalist theory – the philosophical debate has demonstrated so far that there is a tall order for the reductionists. For example, Hilary Putnam's objection to the type-identity theory states that it is all too likely that the same type of mental state could be realized by multiple different brain states (Putnam 1967). Furthermore, it is known that, in some cases, the opposite can be true, too: The same pathological brain processes may result in different mental states. In order to explain what a certain mental illness is, generalizations would be needed rather than the description of singular brain-states of particular individuals with mental problems. Since the same mental disturbance may be connected to different neurophysiological processes in various individuals, the possibility of a reduction of mental illnesses (at least as defined in today's international classification criteria) to certain brain diseases is quite unlikely.

Further to this, it seems that the particular property of a mental state being pathological could hardly be comprehended, understood and explained solely on a neurophysiological level. After all, to assert that a brain process is pathological depends on its tallying with *mental* problems. If it did not, we should have no reason to regard it as pathological. The identification and explanation of mental disorder *as disorder* needs to be done on a mental level.

So psychiatrists could learn from the philosophical debate that there is no need to give up talk about the mental realm in its own right, even if they have good reasons not to postulate a non-material "mind stuff". "The concept of mental disorder is just the concept that something has gone wrong with the way the organism's mind is designed to function. In suggesting that such disorders exist, there need be no deep metaphysical assumptions about the nature of the mind, any more than there need be deep metaphysical assumptions about the nature of kidneys in saying that kidney disorders exist. Whatever the mind is made of, as long as the mind encompasses an identifiable realm of phenomena (e.g., perception, thought, feeling), then disorders within that realm are mental disorders." (Wakefield 1994, p. 11)

Altogether, this implies that biological accounts of mental disease cannot suffice for a proper explanation of psychiatric phenomena. This, however, does not mean that one should disregard somatic accounts in psychiatry altogether, but points out only their limitations. Psychiatry, after all, should be neither 'mindless' nor 'brainless' (Sullivan 1990, p. 271).

The concept of mental illness

Thomas Szasz claimed that mental illness is a myth. He reached this conclusion by arguing that the concept of mental illness is not a proper one. His argument works on two premises. Premise one: Physical illness is defined as a "*structural or functional abnormality of cells, tissues, organs, or bodies*" (Szasz 1987, p. 12). This, for him, states a scientific norm. We merely need anatomical or physiological terms in order to define what somatic illness is. Premise two: We can say that mental illness is a brain disease, it is then recognized as a proper concept – because it relies on a scientific norm – but then we lose a concept of *mental* illness in its own right. Alternatively, we need to argue for a different norm but by doing this we are necessarily bound to give up the scientific status of the concept: "The concept of illness, whether bodily or mental, implies *deviation from some clearly defined norm*. In the case of physical illness, the norm is the structural and functional integrity of the body. Thus, although the desirability of physical health as such is an ethical value, what health *is* can be stated in anatomical and physiological terms. What is the norm deviation for us to classify it as mental illness? This question cannot be easily answered, but whatever this norm might be, we can be certain of one thing: namely, that it is a norm that must be stated in terms of *psychosocial, ethical, and legal* concepts." (Szasz 1960, p. 21)

Since the norm consequently cannot be scientific, according to Szasz, the concept of mental illness merely feigns its proper medical status. We just hide our normative ideas of what we do not like, what we regard as bad or evil behind the mask of medical science. So the picture we get from Szasz can be summarized as follows: Mental illness is a myth because there is no proper scientific norm for its ascription. Unsurprisingly, the responses to his claim focus on his premises. Normativists argue against premise one, namely, that somatic illness is a scientific term. They assert that a definition both of the concept of somatic and mental illness involves a value-judgement. Naturalists, on the other hand, question Szasz's second premise. They claim that mental disease can be defined as a deviation from a natural norm.

We introduced the second premise as comprising two parts: Either you lose a concept of mental illness in its own right or, alternatively, you will end up with an unscientific term. Biological psychiatrists usually bite the bullet and talk in the tradition of Griesinger only about brain disorders. We already stated that it is very difficult to reduce the explanation of mental phenomena to the level of neurological events. But not all naturalists are reductionists. A naturalistic defender of the concept of mental illness accepts that there are scientific *psychological* norms and a deviation from those would be the criterion for the psychopathological. We will come back to this crucial issue but first we should say more about normativism.

At first sight, normativism is a very compelling theory. It seems perfectly clear that illness is *unpleasant*, *undesired* etc. In short, illness is harmful. Health, on the other hand, is a condition in which we feel well. Both concepts can only be defined by reference to our evaluations. This is the basic intuition of the normativists: illness always is a negatively evaluated condition (Engelhardt 1974, Nordenfelt 1987, Fulford 1989, Culver and Gert 1982).

Normativism can easily explain historical and cultural differences in the ascription of illness. For example, masturbation and homosexuality were regarded as mental illness for a long time because they were negatively valued. Today our values have changed in so far that only very few would see it as a medically relevant problem. Depending on how the involved value-judgement is interpreted, that is, whether universal values are believed to be possible, the normativistic theory is also relativistic.

Many normativists additionally infer from the so-called disvaluation-thesis that illness is always a condition which should be cured. The very fact that illness is unpleasant leads to the desire to become healthy again: "Judging that some condition is a disease commits one to stamping it out. And judging that a condition is not a disease commits one to preventing its medical treatment." (Reznek 1987, p. 171) From this stance the practice of medicine is legitimized, because it eliminates – if successful – undesired conditions and restores health. This may be called the "intervention-thesis" of normativism. However, formulated in this way the first difficulties for the normativistic theory present themselves, since we do not usually think that medicine should deal with *all* undesirable conditions, but only the medically relevant ones, or there is the danger of medicalizing several disvalued phenomena, from poverty to lovesickness to rebellious behaviour. With respect to psychiatry, the provocative question would obviously be: Do psychiatrists really treat medically relevant phenomena or do they merely adjust "undesired" people to a social standard? Thus, the normativists need additional criteria in order to distinguish illnesses from other unpleasant conditions. In short, not every disvalued condition represents an illness even if illness might be necessarily disvalued.

The other side of this problem is to explain our intuition that there can be a pathological condition even if there is *no* negative evaluation. There are many examples of this: the crippled feet of women in traditional Asian societies corresponding to the ideal of beauty; the iodine-deficiency goitre in remote Alpine communities, worship of mentally ill people as "gurus" etc. Should we not regard these conditions as pathological even if they are not disvalued in the respective society or by the affected individual? Or should we say instead that the people in question are mistaken about the "correct" values?

We will now turn our attention to naturalism and come back to the question of the role of psychological norms and psychopathology. Naturalists start their account from the fact that humans are part of nature just as other organisms are (Boorse 1976, Scadding 1988, Guze 1992, Klein 1978, Spitzer and Endicott 1978, Flew 1973, Kendell 1975). Their basic intuition is that there are certain mental and bodily processes which may not work in the way they naturally do. If this is so, we speak of a pathological condition. That does not mean that disease is "unnatural" or that every unnatural condition is an illness. Naturalists merely assert that the *criteria* for the distinction of health and disease are to be found in nature and are not determined by social or individual values. It may be that we disvalue the condition but this is not the defining characteristic of a disease. Even if every disease were disvalued, it would not be up to us to determine the respective underlying norm. Thus, the concept of disease is value-neutral according to the naturalists.

From the naturalists' perspective, it can be explained why there should be universal disease judgements. Since human beings (just as other organisms of a respective species) are similar in their structure, they are affected in the same way by a disease if deviations from a natural norm occur. Nevertheless, there remains the possibility of variety regarding disease in the naturalistic interpretation. Although nature delivers the standard of medical normality it may have a different content in different environments. For example, supposing conditions of severe anxiety were universally regarded as illness then it may nevertheless express itself in different ways in different cultures. So there may be culturally impregnated diseases despite universal disease-judgements, e.g. the syndrome called "Koro" that occurs only in South- and East-Asia.

What naturalism does rule out though, is the possibility of an ascription of disease where there is no deviation from a natural norm. If there is such an ascription, like in the example of masturbation, then the disease-judgement is simply *wrong*, rather than "outdated" or "not adequate today" as some normativists need to assert. So the benefit of the naturalistic position is to reject interest-laden illness-judgements. If the criteria for the ascription of disease are determined by human nature then arguments about whether particular conditions are pathological – e.g. whether dissidents in totalitarian regimes are mentally ill – can be decided empirically.

Much more needs to be said about the plausibility of a naturalistic account concerning *mental* disease. After all, mental phenomena seem more detached from a naturalistic explanation than do bodily mechanisms and it might seem hopeless to try and find a natural *psychological* norm. But it is common to talk about mental functions, for example, in cognitive sciences or in the most interesting research program of evolutionary psychology. In evolutionary psychology mental functions are explained as universal features of the human mind which evolved through evolutionary processes, hence mental functions are explained naturalistically (Tooby and Cosmides 1992, Mithen 1996, Nesse and Williams 1994, Stevens and Price 1996, Gray Hardcastle 1999).

"Evolutionary psychology is the application of the adaptionist program to the study of the human brain/mind. Evolutionary psychologists assume that the brain/mind has many functions – i.e., that it has been designed by selection to solve many different kinds of problems, each of which is likely to require its own distinctive kind of solution – and, therefore, that the brain/mind comprises many domain-specific specialized mechanisms." (Symons 1992, p. 155f.) So this account interprets particular mental abilities as adaptations, i.e. as complex mechanisms which were designed by natural selection. Here is not the place to scrutinize this theory thoroughly, of course, but it shall suffice to point out that evolutionary psychology represents at least one interesting naturalistic model of mental functions and, hence, that a naturalistic account of mental disease needs to be taken seriously.

Usually, normativism and naturalism are regarded as mutually exclusive positions. But both accounts seem to be important in their own right, since they reflect two different perspectives on medical phenomena. One may even say that they are using different concepts, i.e. a theoretical and a practical. The different terms or notions "illness" and "disease" clearly contain these different perspectives: 'Disease' refers to the bodily or mental condition of a person irrespective of his or her situation otherwise. So naturalism is focused on the living organism and its functioning or dysfunctioning – the internal mechanisms an individual is or is not able to perform. Call this the *scientific* perspective. It disregards the meaning of a condition for the *person* – to use a common philosophical term. 'Illness', on the other hand, reflects the specific situation of and the evaluation by the person in question. So normativists concentrate on the evaluation of a specific condition, that is, what it means for a person to be suffering from an illness and why an illness should be eliminated. Call this the *evaluative* perspective.[1]

According to this interpretation of the philosophical debate on the concept of mental disorder, naturalists talk about disease as a form of pathological condition, normativists about illness as an impairment of well-being. There is nothing incompatible in these theories. We are interested in *explanation* as well as *evaluation*. There are many examples of these different but compatible perspectives. For instance, we usually talk in an objective way about artefacts but also from an evaluative perspective about works of art.

Now one might ask why we need the objective point of view at all. Is it not so that the evaluative perspective is the only significant one? It is true that naturalism cannot explain why we may have different and even conflicting evaluative views on deviations from a natural norm. The evaluative perspective is essential in order to reflect the individually different situations of the various people in question and thereby to generate a judgement as to what is the best way to deal with a psychiatric disorder. Normativists have expressed the idea that an ascription of illness necessarily implies the value-judgement that it is harmful affliction and the wish to eliminate it. If one takes the naturalistic perspective instead, nothing is said about the evaluation of a condition. So if the disvaluation of an illness forms the starting-point for the justification of a medical treatment then the naturalistic perspective needs to be *supplemented* by the evaluative perspective of the normativists. It does not need to be supplemented in order to determine what is pathological but it does in order to judge when an impairment of well-being is present and

---

1 Our conceptualization of these two perspectives is similar to the distinction between *nature* and *narrative*, which is introduced in Fulford et al. 2003. 'Nature' in this anthology stands for 'causes' and generally sciences, while 'narrative' stands for 'meanings' and generally humanities.

consequently needs treatment. For the patient concerned this is the relevant perspective on the phenomena of illness. So the answer to the question why we need an objective – or scientific – point of view is that we need it in order to distinguish the pathological from the normal without relying on subjective value-judgements. This is an important distinction which is necessary to bring to a halt the problem of medicalization. We already pointed out that normativists usually find themselves in trouble when explaining the distinction between illness proper and disvalued conditions in general.

In passing, we would like to make a minor point about the debate of naturalists and normativists: It is sometimes assumed that if a naturalistic account involves – contrary to its own assertions – reference to values of any kind, for example, because there is no value-free explication of the concept of function or because there is no value-free science, then the superiority of normativism over naturalism becomes evident. But this argument seems to miss a very crucial point concerning the kind of values involved: it is not obvious at all that in a scientific perspective these would be values *of the kind* that normativism puts forward. For example, it may be that a scientific perspective is *externally* value-laden – because it relies on scientific values concerning hypotheses giving the best explanation – without being *internally* value-laden, that is, without making value-judgements in the definition of the pathological. The distinction between a scientific and an evaluative perspective can be made independently of the issue whether the scientific account is altogether value-free or not.

To summarize the point of view we introduced: Mental disease is both a genuine *disease* – contrary to Szasz's assertion – and a genuine *mental* disease – contrary to the reductionistic thesis. It can be defined as an impairment of mental functional ability. Mental functions are natural abilities which evolve and can probably be determined according to the evolutionary perspective. In addition, the concept of mental illness is defined as a disvalued mental disease.

The scientific perspective leads to a distinction between pathological and normal phenomena. The pathological can be defined as a deviation from a natural norm. It determines the core of medical phenomena, i.e. only pathological conditions may indeed be called illnesses in an evaluative perspective. This is not to assert that medicine is not justified in helping people with problems other than illnesses. The claim is about the concept of illness – namely, that the extension of illness is determined by the extension of the pathological –, not on the proper scope of medicine.

But to say that a certain condition is pathological does not establish whether and why this situation might be harmful. This needs to be clarified from an evaluative perspective. From this perspective we must address, for example, the important question: who is to evaluate? The person himself or herself, the doctor or the society? Can a person be wrong about his or her own well-being? Is a person in a specific psychopathological condition able to evaluate his or her condition? These questions need to be asked and answered from an evaluative perspective. Normativists usually differ in their accounts on the question whether the disvaluation is due to society, to the doctor or to the individual. But there is often a clash between evaluations of pathological conditions from the subjective point of view and an "outside" view.

One might think that there is no problem with evaluation at all because to be in a pathological condition is enough to justify the claim that there is a harm which should be eliminated. But this assertion certainly does not convince everyone. There are people who do not accept that they are ill despite the fact that they have a disease. Several psychiatric patients reject the evaluation of psychiatrists or relatives and say that they do not see themselves as impaired in any way. That constituted one of the points of antipsychiatry: what many people regard as harmful does not necessarily agree with what the person in question himself or herself thinks. Consider, for example, the following statement of a psychiatric patient: "Gee, you know, they're telling me this is a disease. If it's a disease this is the one I want to have" (Farber 1993, p. 95). What should we say in a case like this? Should we say that the patient's own judgement does not count by definition because he or she suffers from an impairment of his or her mental faculties?

What we need, seen from an evaluative perspective, is a convincing argument why these people might be wrong in the judgement of their own well-being. This is a tall order since it seems to demand an objective account of human welfare. One might argue that some normativists do not take their normativism seriously enough on that particular point because they usually define 'harm' relative to the standards of the culture the person lives in (Wakefield 1992). But an account of why a pathological condition is harmful to the person in question should start from the evaluative perspective of a particular individual. It may be that there are convincing arguments against the subjective evaluation of the patient. But, after all, the concept of harm is as much in need of clarification as the concept of disease. It points to another genuine philosophical problem of psychiatry.

The essays

The first two essays, although focusing on different topics, both reflect on the relation of psychiatry and philosophy. According to these essays, neither discipline is taking over the role of the other but is standing in a relation of complementation.

Lou Marinoff, author of the highly-acclaimed books *Plato, not Prozac!* and *The Big Questions: How Philosophy Can Change Your Life* reminds us of one of the oldest possible uses of philosophy, namely, to help us to lead our own life in a meaningful way. Philosophical counselling is the fairly new term for this traditional way of seeking guidance in wisdom. Often, people do not only have problems in life which demand medical treatment but they also ask for moral or – generally speaking – spiritual advice. Being engaged in philosophy is practising wisdom; it is to exercise reason. In "Thus Spake Settembrini: A Meta-Dialogue on Philosophy and Psychiatry", Marinoff introduces the potentials of philosophical counselling. But he also delineates it from psychiatric treatment and defends it against a particular reproach by a psychiatrist in which he was likened to a character based in the novel *The Magic Mountain* by Thomas Mann: Lodovico Settembrini.

In "Ten Principles of Values-Based Medicine", Bill Fulford shows how philosophical reflection on values, i.e. the theory of ethics, may contribute to a better understanding of psychiatric theory and practice. Medicine is value-based, not merely in its task to deal with patients in a way which accounts for their particular ideals and interests and, of course, moral norms. In addition, the most basic theoretical terms like 'mental illness' are value-laden. That does not imply that there is no use for scientific research on facts in psychiatry, but evidence-based medicine is not sufficient if it is not complemented by its values-based counterpart, since "all decisions stand on two feet, on values as well as on facts". Fulford here draws on a former analysis in his book *Moral Theory and Medical Practice* and several further publications in which he developed an influential and wide-ranging theory. In his essay, he sums up his account in ten principles and helpfully illustrates them with a psychiatric case.

The second section deals with conceptual problems and questions of classification in psychiatry, thereby touching on issues dealt with in theoretical philosophy. The article by Pierre Pichot, "The Concept of Psychiatric Nosology", gives a historical introduction to psychiatric classification of mental disorders from Sydenham to the DSMs. He also focuses on the main theoretical problems of nosology. First of all, there is the question which has already developed a long tradition, whether mental disorders are natural kinds. Then, there are several possibilities of setting the elements in a classificatory system, e.g. one may focus on symptoms or on aetiology. As is well known in psychiatric diagnostics, the problem of multiple diagnoses is also prevalent. Hence, in recent years an alternative to the categorical approaches has been discussed, namely, dimensional models. This may also be related to the different possible aims of nosology, whether it should guide research, ensure reliable and internationally valid diagnoses or else to gain predictive value in giving hints on possible developments and outcomes of diseases.

Next, in "The Legacy of Antipsychiatry", Thomas Schramme scrutinizes the most common objections to the very concept of mental disorder by the so-called Antipsychiatrists – or, as he prefers, "sceptics" –, in particular by Michel Foucault, Ronald Laing, Thomas Scheff, Ronald Laing and Thomas

Szasz. Although they were mainly influential during the seventies, their arguments against the use of supposedly objective, medical language in psychiatry still finds its supporters today. Schramme has developed a topology of the objections in five categories and finds all of them wanting. Nevertheless, he demonstrates why the sceptical point of view is still of use today in order to question an all too easy conceptual complacency and help increase the awareness of the need for a more theoretically minded approach in psychiatry.

Sceptical psychiatry emphasized the fact that many alleged mental disorders are actually positively evaluated signs of distinctions in several cultures. Much seems to depend on cultural influences whether or not a person is diagnosed as mentally ill.

Hans-Jörg Assion deals with this topic by discussing several examples of culturally–laden categories. In most Western countries, common beliefs in possession by demons, witchcraft and magic ideas have now been replaced by medical and scientific language, but in several territories these seemingly naïve beliefs are still popular today. Nevertheless, as Assion argues in "Archaic Concepts for Explaining Disorders", they may serve a function by providing alternative healing practices in certain cases.

Although human beings are obviously similar in being biological organisms of a certain kind, they also differ from each other in developing several ways of describing the world they live in. This has some impact on psychiatry, too, because different cultures find alternative conceptualizations of mental problems. Johannes Thome, in his essay "The Problem of Universalism in Psychiatry", challenges the problem of culture dependent accounts on a more general level. In what way may psychiatry claim to be a universalist discipline? A common way to secure universalism is to focus on our common nature, i.e. to develop scientific, especially biological models of mental illness. However, as Thome makes clear, this approach may suffer from serious shortcomings in the practice of psychiatric medicine. He states that "the daily clinical work and interaction with patients require a sensitivity to the cultural background and personal beliefs of each patient". Hence, psychiatry needs to be aware of possible conflicts between universalism and individualism. Probably the best way is to accept a moderate dualism between theory and practice.

Aisling Campbell, in "Lacan and Psychiatry" introduces the reflection of French psychoanalyst Jacques Lacan. His considerations are especially interesting, as Campbell vividly shows, because he formed a theory which may account for a theoretical background to be used in psychiatric theory and practice by providing a concept which secures against too hasty a reductionism as well as being adjustable to neuroscience. The combination of neuroscientific findings and psychoanalysis has long been off the agenda, although Freud himself tried to develop his theory – at least at the beginning of his career – in that very direction. In recent years there has been a revival of interest in neuropsychoanalysis. Lacan is particularly important because he focused on the "symbolic order", i.e. the distinctive ability of human beings to use language and hence provided a way of connecting conscious and unconscious processes.

The third part concentrates on methodological issues in psychiatry and philosophical questions related to philosophy of science. Hans-Jürgen Möller in his "Methodological Issues in Psychiatry: Psychiatry as an Empirical Science" tackles in depth the main theoretical problems concerning the scientific status of psychiatry. Are psychiatric findings to be presented in a law-like or nomothetic fashion? The same problems are to be found again on the more practical side: As already mentioned, different scientific methods and models make for alternative nosological systems. For example, the recent attempt to harmonize ICD and DSM has provided a better reliability at the expense of scientific validity. But Möller's treatise relates to almost all of the contexts discussed so far. The prospects of sceptical objections to psychiatry as well as of reductionism are influenced by its scientific status. He aims at an account of empirical psychiatry in the tradition of *Realwissenschaften* which tries to explain individual events by covering laws and to test theories by exposing them to possible falsification.

Interpreting psychiatry in a scientific fashion might be seen to close the way for the humanities. But, as Johannes Thome states in "Humanities and Molecular Psychiatry", this would paint an artless picture. In recent years, the discipline of "medical humanities" has paved its way and has also a saying in psychiatry. There are many topics in psychiatric theory and practice which cannot be adequately dealt with in merely focusing on biological or even molecular models, especially ethical problems. Again, this does not add up to a demonization of biological psychiatry but points to its possible limitations. Karl Jaspers, the founding father of a humanistic point of view in psychiatry, may well be the suitable classic to turn to.

The tradition of Jasper's *General Psychopathology* today lives on chiefly in phenomenological accounts. But, according to Thomas Fuchs, it would not do justice to its goals if one sees phenomenology merely as way of focusing on first-person data or the subjective point of view. In "The Challenge of Neuroscience: Psychiatry and Phenomenology Today", Fuchs elucidates the possible functions phenomenology may serve in modern psychiatry. One of the main important findings in brain science, namely, neuronal plasticity, calls for a systemic view which sees the whole person in relation to the world. "The brain is essentially a historical and social organ", says Fuchs. By using the examples of embodiment, time-consciousness and interpersonality he facilitates his viewpoint that a scientific outlook need not disregard subjectivity. Hence, cognitive neuroscience is comprehensive only when it has accounted for its alleged adversary.

Dieter Sigmund builds up on the phenomenological approach in "Diagnosis of Core Schizophrenia as an Example of Applied Phenomenological Methodology". His article also refers back to the problem of nosology by taking as its starting point the famous assertion of Kraepelin that he has identified a certain disease entity, namely, "Dementia Praecox" – or schizophrenia, as it was later baptized. Sigmund pursues the ambitious task of introducing a much more differentiated way of modelling types of schizophrenia by the method of phenomenology. He consequently introduces several axial syndromes which comprise "core schizophrenia".

The next two essays focus on epistemological issues. Georg Juckel and Andreas Heinz engage with a traditional philosophical question, namely, the problem of other minds. Historically, the fact that we cannot be sure of the thoughts of others has even led to solipsism, i.e. the conviction that only oneself is a conscious subject while the rest of the world may be a phantasm. Although we cannot directly see what is going on in the head of others, we may become acquainted with their feelings by means of communication. In "Can We Know What Others Feel? Anthropological and Epistemological Considerations in Emotional Neuroscience", Juckel and Heinz deal in particular with the role of emotions in trying to understand other people. We often attempt to use emotions for "symptoms" of the inner state of a person. But their outer signs might be based on a "private language" – an assertion the philosopher Ludwig Wittgenstein dealt with. Another question to arise is whether we are indeed able to interpret correctly the emotional reactions of people from other cultures. More precarious for psychiatry, the deductions from emotional attitudes seem to fail with people who are afflicted by certain mental disorders. So when people are emotionally disturbed this "road" to their mind seems to be blocked.

In their essay "On Time Experience in Depression – Dominance of the Past", Hinderk Emrich and Detlef E. Dietrich deal with a peculiar phenomenon in depressive illness, namely, the disturbance of inner time. Time obviously has a subjective side which we experience every day. With the help of philosophy in persona of Michael Theunissen and the neurophysiologist Christoph von der Malsburg, Emrich and Dietrich state the hypothesis that the subjective experience in depression is dominated by the past. They were able to validate their theory by experimental data. Drawing on these findings, they are also able to propose "active forgetting" as therapeutic device in depression. Following Theunissen, they call this the "Proustian method".

Whether we are free to do what we want to do is not only a philosophical question which, till today, is under heated debate but also a very important problem in psychiatry. Whether people are responsible for their doings may also be of interest in juridical trials. Many mental disorders are taken to be paradigm cases of heteronomy, hence philosophers who are interested in the metaphysical and ethical question of freedom of the will tend to use psychiatric examples in order to support their theories by empirical facts. The fifth section on compulsion, volitional disorders and freedom of the will sheds light on these issues.

In his essay "Rigidity: The Strange Preference for Compulsion", Martin Löw-Beer acquaints us with a peculiar way of dealing with common challenges of daily life. It seems as if rigid persons explicitly try to reduce their freedom by reducing their alternatives to act. They avoid to choose consciously between options and usually find reasons – even alleged necessities – why they must act in a certain way. Most distinctive in rigid people is that they identify with this behaviour; that they are not alienated at all, hence they are not merely compulsive characters. Nevertheless, Löw-Beer argues their way of living is to be criticized because they totally neglect personal and idiosyncratic values. By seeing himself as executor of what everybody would do in his place, a rigid person loses his individuality and the ability to find orientation in his own life. He does not take a stance of a participant but only an observational point of view.

Addiction may be the most familiar example of compulsive behaviour. In "Towards a Philosophical Anthropology of Addiction", Jann Schlimme tries to give an account of the "inner side" of addiction. The wish to add the subjective perspective of phenomena to the usual medical gaze relates him back to the phenomenological method. After introducing the historical background of our common model of addiction, culminating in Brühl-Cramer's account at the beginning of the 19th century, Schlimme goes on to make use of the famous novel *Naked Lunch* by William Burroughs in order to find an answer to the question: What it is like to be addicted? With Burroughs he maintains that "the algebra of addiction is total need".

The philosophical debate on freedom of the will usually concentrates on the alternatives of determinism and libertarianism. In the last few years, scientists have made a case for determinism which does not seem to allow for human freedom or responsibility. Although the scientific argumentation thereby seems to abandon any significant distinction between compulsion and being "normally" determined, it made a serious impact. Nevertheless, there are already a couple of so-called compatibilists who claim to make good sense of both freedom and responsibility on the one side and determinism on the other. In "Neurophilosophical Perspectives on Conservative Compatibilism", Henrik Walter, who recently published a book on *Neurophilosophy of Free Will*, deals with this debate. He pays attention to the philosophical debate as well as the neurological findings, hence he develops a perspective of "neurophilosophy". In particular, Walter argues for a revised account of moral responsibility, thereby challenging "conservative compatibilism".

Rainer Luthe and Michael Rösler, in "Freedom of Will, Freedom of Action and Psychiatry" transfer the metaphysical problem of freedom of the will to forensic psychiatry where it obviously has its most important applications.

Of consequence to a useful model of criminal liability is the reference to the ability of a person to reason and control. Nevertheless, criminal liability and freedom to act are not the same. What is at issue is the freedom to *will*. The usual slogan that I would be free if I could have done otherwise, is too simple, when the question whether I could have wanted to do otherwise is disregarded. According to Luthe and Rösler, spontaneity is the distinctive mark of the will. Because and insofar "it happens by itself", the will is free.

As mentioned before, many psychiatric disorders have caught the interest of philosophers because they seem to put into doubt widely accepted beliefs about personal identity. Identity disorders therefore form the sixth part of the anthology. First, Thomas Metzinger answers the question "Why Are Identity Disorders Interesting for Philosophers?" They are mostly noteworthy because they may be regarded as empirical test-cases of philosophical theories. Metzinger's own theory of the self, which he developed more thoroughly in his recent book *Being No One*, can account for many psychiatric phenomena. According to him, scientific findings suggest that there is no substantive Ego, a centre in the brain, a ghost in the machine or the like. Rather, the self is a useful fiction, which has evolved by evolution. Since there is no indivisible substance called the self, personal identity is very precarious. Hence, for example, Dissociative Identity Disorder does not pose severe metaphysical problems but is a probable consequence of disturbances in the development of a "self model". In his essay, Metzinger focuses on other psychiatric cases, namely, delusional misidentification syndrome and Cotard delusion, which he uses to put into doubt certain philosophical theses about self-reference, subjectivity and rationality.

Next, Georg Northoff uses empirical material he gained from a survey on people with Parkinson after having been treated by fetal tissue or electrodal brain implants. In "The Influence of Brain Implants on Personal Identity and Personality – a Combined Theoretical and Empirical Investigation in 'Neuroethics'" he also engages with some philosophical accounts on personal identity brought forward by Thomas Nagel and Derek Parfit. The traditional philosophical debate is mainly focused on the question whether diachronic personal identity is constituted by steady relations of conscious experiences or of bodily continuity. Philosophers engaged in this debate tend to use outlandish thought-experiments, so empirical findings on brain implants certainly have an impact by putting philosophy back on a solid empirical basis. Northoff's results do not establish a change in personal identity after transplantation, although there were some alterations in personality, i.e. in individual psychological characteristics. In closing, Northoff suggests anthropological criteria for the impact of brain surgery on personality and personal identity in order to guide ethical questions concerning neurological treatment.

The last section on psychiatric ethics is opened by Hanfried Helmchen, who considers "Ethics as a Focus of Controversy in Postmodern Antagonisms". Acknowledging that modern societies are commonly characterized by a profound value pluralism, the prospects for generally binding moral norms or even trans-cultural, universal human rights seem bleak. But globalization, which directly affects ethical questions in research and treatment, puts the sufficiency of mere regional or national regulations into doubt. In his essay, Helmchen touches on the already mentioned issue of universalism in psychiatry, which, in his context, generates a particular problem of ethics. What we need is a well-founded balance between communal traditions and universal norms. The recent Convention on Human Rights and Biomedicine (CHRB) of the Council of Europe may serve as an example. However, ethics remains in the centre of antagonisms.

One of the main ethical problems in psychiatry is the treatment of patients against their will. Compulsion, coercion and the use of force seem to necessarily accompany psychiatric practice while they often lead to outright opposition to medical interventions. Harald Dreßing begins with an outline of the history of compulsory psychiatric treatment in "Compulsory Admission and Compulsory Treatment in Psychiatry". The growing prominence of patients' rights and the reverence for informed consent led to scrupulous legislative norms for dealing with psychiatric patients. However, according to Dreßing, there remains an inherent conflict between the focus on individual autonomy and the medical impulse to help patients in need and to avoid harm.

In "Coercive Threats and Offers in Psychiatry", Thomas Schramme focuses on instances of possible coercion in psychiatry which are seldom acknowledged because patients have formally acquiesced with a certain treatment. But, he argues, the formation of the stated will might have been influenced by coercive measures which put the validity of the consent into doubt. Most common examples involve threats which are carefully differentiated from morally neutral warnings. He then goes on to consider whether offers can ever be coercive. This seems unlikely because they involve a promise to better the situation of a person without proposing to worsen his or her situation in case of non-compliance. However, Schramme argues that especially in psychiatric contexts there may be cases of coercive offers, in particular, when a dependency of a patient is exploited.

Markus Pawelzik and Aloys Prinz transfer the ethical consideration on a social level. In "The Moral Economics of Psychotherapy" they scrutinize the often stated conflict between economical considerations in medicine and the just distribution of goods according to medical needs. But they argue that this way of constructing a conflict between ethics and economics is ill-considered because medical treatment ought to be efficient in order to be justified. Ethics alone will not do but needs complementation by economic rationality. They go on to apply their thesis to the realm of psychotherapy. Since there is a social interest in effective treatment, incentives and regulations which influence the conduct of both patients and therapists need to be taken into account.

Altogether, from our point of view, the essays in this anthology show the full potentials of philosophy of psychiatry. They may be regarded as contributions to ongoing discussions but also as starting-points of new debates. Being engaged in philosophy is a never-ending practice. But this is the fun of it.

References

American Psychiatric Association (APA) 1994. *Diagnostic and Statistical Manual of Mental Disorders IV* (DSM-IV). Washington, DC: American Psychiatric Press.

Baron-Cohen, S. 1995. *Mindblindness. An Essay on Autism and Theory of Mind.* Cambridge, Mass.: MIT Press.

Bolton, D., Hill, J. 1996. *Mind, Meaning and Mental Disorder. The Nature of Causal Explanation in Psychology and Psychiatry.* Oxford: Oxford U.P.

Boorse, C. 1976. "What a Theory of Mental Health Should Be", *Journal for the Theory of Social Behaviour*, 6: 61-84.

Culver, C.M., Gert, B. 1982. *Philosophy in Medicine. Conceptual and Ethical Issues in Medicine and Psychiatry.* Oxford: Oxford University Press.

Dennett, D.C. 1991. *Consciousness Explained.* London: Penguin.

Engelhardt, H.T. 1974. "The Disease of Masturbation: Values and the Concept of Disease", *Bulletin of the History of Medicine*, 48(2): 234-248.

Emrich, H.M., Schlimme, J., Paetzold, W. (eds.) 2002. *Psyche und Transzendenz.* Würzburg: Königshausen & Neumann.

Farber, S. 1993. *Madness, Heresy, and the Rumour of Angels. The Revolt Against the Mental Health System.* Chicago and La Salle, Ill.: Open Court Publ. Co.

Flanagan, O. 1996. *Self Expressions. Mind, Morals, and the Meaning of Life.* Oxford: Oxford U.P.

Flew, A. 1973. *Crime or Disease?* London and Basingstroke: MacMillan Press.

Fulford, K.W.M. 1989. *Moral Theory and Medical Practice.* Cambridge: Cambridge U.P.

Fulford, K.W.M., Morris, K., Sadler, J., Stanghellini, G. (eds.) 2003. *Nature and narrative. An introduction to the new philosophy of psychiatry.* Oxford: Oxford U.P.

Glover, J. 1988. *I: The Philosophy and Psychology of Personal Identity.* London: Penguin.

Graham, G.; Stephens, L.G. (eds.) 1994. *Philosophical Psychopathology.* Cambridge, Mass.: MIT Press.

Guze, S.B. 1992. *Why Psychiatry is a Branch of Medicine.* Oxford: Oxford U.P.

Gray Hardcastle, V. (ed.) 1999. *Where Biology Meets Psychology. Philosophical Essays.* Cambridge, Mass.: MIT Press.

Hannan, B. 1994. *Subjectivity and Reduction. An Introduction to the Mind-Body Problem*, Boulder: Westview Press.

Heginbotham, C. (ed.) 2000. *Philosophy, Psychiatry and Psychopathy. Personal identity in mental disorder.* Aldershot: Ashgate.

Heinze, M., Priebe, S. (eds.) 1996. *Störenfried "Subjektivität". Subjektivität und Objektivität als Begriffe psychiatrischen Denkens.* Würzburg: Königshausen & Neumann.

Heinze, M., Kupke, C., Pflanz, S.V., Vogeley, K. (eds.) 1996. *Psyche im Streit der Theorien*. Würzburg: Königshausen & Neumann.
Hundert, E.M. 1989. *Philosophy, Psychiatry and Neuroscience. Three Approaches to the Mind*. Oxford: Clarendon Press.
Iverson, S. 1997. "Time out of Mind", *The Guardian*, September 4th: 2.
Kendell, R.E. 1975. "The Concept of Disease and Its Implications for Psychiatry", *British Journal of Psychiatry*, 127: 305-315.
Kendell, R.E. 1993. "The Nature of Psychiatric Disorders", in: Kendell, R.E., Zealley, A.K. (eds.) *Companion to Psychiatric Studies*, 5th Edition, Edinburgh etc.: Churchill Livingstone, 1-7.
Kim, J. 1996. *Philosophy of Mind*, Boulder: Westview Press.
Klein, D.F. 1978. "A Proposed Definition of Mental Illness", in: Spitzer, R.L., Klein, D.F. (eds.) *Current Issues in Psychiatric Diagnosis*, New York: Raven Press, 41-71.
Löw-Beer, M. 1990. *Selbsttäuschung. Philosophische Analyse eines psychischen Phänomens*. Freiburg: Alber.
Metzinger, T. 1993. *Subjekt und Selbstmodell. Die Perspektivität phänomenalen Bewusstseins vor dem Hintergrund einer naturalistischen Theorie mentaler Repräsentation*. Paderborn: Schöningh.
Metzinger, T. 2003. *Being No One: The Self-Model Theory of Subjectivity*. Cambridge, Mass.: MIT Press.
Mithen, S. 1996. *The Prehistory of the Mind*, London: Thames and Hudson.
Nagel, T. 1971. "Brain Bisection and the Unity of Consciousness", in: Nagel, T. *Mortal Questions*. Cambridge: Cambridge U.P. 1979, 147-164.
Nesse, R.M., Williams, G.C. 1994. *Why We Get Sick. The New Science of Darwinian Medicine*. New York: Times Books.
Nordenfelt, L. 1987. *On the Nature of Health. An Action-Theoretic Approach*. Dordrecht: Kluwer.
Northoff, G. (ed.) 1997. *Neuropsychiatrie und Neurophilosophie*. Paderborn: Schöningh.
Phillips Griffiths, A. (ed.) 1994. *Philosophy, Psychology, and Psychiatry*. Royal Institute of Philosophy Supplement 37. Cambridge: Cambridge U.P.
Place, U.T. 1956. "Is Consciousness a Brain Process?" *British Journal of Psychology*, 47: 44-50.
Putnam, H. 1967. "The Nature of Mental States", (orig.: "Psychological Predicates"), in: Capitan, W.H., Merrill, D.D. (eds.) *Art, Mind, and Religion*, University of Pittsburgh Press.
Reznek, L. 1987. *The Nature of Disease*. London: Routledge.
Reznek, L. 1991. *The Philosophical Defence of Psychiatry*. London: Routledge.
Sadler, J.Z., Wiggins, O.P., Schwartz, M.A. (eds.) 1994. *Philosophical Perspectives on Psychiatric Diagnostic Classification*. Baltimore: John Hopkins U.P.
Sadler, J.Z. (ed.) 2002. *Descriptions & Prescriptions. Values, Mental Disorders, and the DSMs*. Baltimore: John Hopkins U.P.
Scadding, J.G. 1988. "Health and Disease: What can Medicine Do for Philosophy?" *Journal of Medical Ethics*, 14: 118-124.
Schramme, T. 2000. *Patienten und Personen. Zum Begriff der psychischen Krankheit*. Frankfurt: Fischer. Reissued as: *Psychische Krankheit aus philosophischer Sicht*. Gießen: Psychosozial Verlag 2003.
Sedgwick, P. 1973. "Illness – Mental and Otherwise", *The Hastings Center Studies*, 1(3), reprinted in Caplan, A. et al. (eds.) *Concepts of Health and Disease. Interdisciplinary Perspectives*. Reading: Addison-Wesley 1981, 119-129.
Smart, J.J.C. 1959. "Sensations and Brain Processes", *The Philosophical Review*, 68 (2): 141-156.

Spitzer, R.L., Endicott, J. 1978. "Medical and Mental Disorder: Proposed Definition and Criteria", in: R.L. Spitzer, D. Klein (eds.) *Current Issues in Psychiatric Diagnosis*. New York: Raven Press, 15-39.
Spitzer, M., Uehlein, F.A., Oepen, G. (eds.) 1988. *Psychopathology and Philosophy*. Berlin: Springer.
Spitzer, M., Maher, B.A. (eds.) 1990. *Philosophy and Psychopathology*. Berlin: Springer.
Stephens, G.L., Graham, G. 2000. *When Self-Consciousness Breaks. Alien Voices and Inserted Thoughts*. Cambridge, Mass.: MIT Press.
Stevens, A., Price, J. 1996. *Evolutionary Psychiatry. A New Beginning. London*: Routledge.
Straus, E.W., Natanson, M., Ey, H. 1969. *Psychiatry and Philosophy*. Berlin: Springer.
Sullivan, M.D. 1990. "Organic or Functional? Why Psychiatry Needs a Philosophy of Mind", *Psychiatric Annals*, 20 (5): 271-277.
Symons, D. 1992. "On the Use and Misuse of Darwinism in the Study of Human Behavior", in: Barkow, J.H., Cosmides, L., Tooby, J. (eds.), *The Adapted Mind. Evolutionary Psychology and the Generation of Culture*. Oxford: Oxford U.P., 137-159.
Szasz, T.S. 1960. "The Myth of Mental Illness", *American Psychologist*, 15: 113-118, reprinted in: R. Edwards (ed.) *Psychiatry and Ethics*. Buffalo: Prometheus 1982, 19-28.
Szasz, T.S. 1987. *Insanity. The Idea and its Consequences*, New York: John Wiley and Sons.
Theunissen, M. 1991. *Negative Theologie der Zeit*. Frankfurt: Suhrkamp.
Thome, J. 1995. *Psychotherapeutische Aspekte in der Philosophie Platons*. Hildesheim: Olms.
Tooby, J., Cosmides, L. 1992. "The Psychological Foundations of Culture", in: Barkow, J.H., Cosmides, L., Tooby, J. (eds.) *The Adapted Mind. Evolutionary Psychology and the Generation of Culture*. Oxford: Oxford U.P., 19-136.
Wakefield, J.C. 1992. "The Concept of Mental Disorder. On the Boundary Between Biological Facts and Social Values", *American Psychologist*, 47 (3): 373-388.
Wakefield, J.C. 1994. "Rejoinder to Professor Kirmayer" in: Kirk, S.A., Einbinder, S.D. (eds.) *Controversial Issues in Mental Health*. Boston: Allyn and Bacon, 9-11.
Wilkes, K. 1988. *Real People. Personal Identity without Thought Experiments*. Oxford: Clarendon Press.

The Relation of Philosophy and Psychiatry

Thus Spake Settembrini: A Meta-Dialogue on Philosophy and Psychiatry[1]

Lou Marinoff

1. What Unites Philosophy and Psychiatry?

> Analysis is good as a tool of enlightenment and civilization – to the extent that it shakes stupid preconceptions, quashes natural biases, and undermines authority. Good, in other words, to the extent that it liberates, refines and humanizes – it makes slaves ripe for freedom. It is bad, very bad, to the extent that it prevents action, damages life at its roots, and is incapable of shaping it. Analysis can be very unappetizing, as unappetizing as death, to which it may very well be linked – a relative of the grave and its foul anatomy. – Thomas Mann, *The Magic Mountain*

Before discussing what unites philosophy and psychiatry, I will attempt to define my terms. This is for the sake of avoiding unnecessary debates that emanate from what philosophers call "equivocations" – ambiguities of language or usage that give rise to disagreements that are semantic but not substantive. As we may find enough substantive matters to dispute, let us at least seek a degree of semantic accord at the outset.

By psychiatry, I understand a branch of medicine concerned with the diagnosis and treatment of so-called "mental" disorders. I say "so-called" because the use of the term "mental" in this context is fraught with philosophical difficulties from the outset, stemming from the unresolved "mind-brain" problem. If mental activity is considered a mere epiphenomenon (i.e. an insubstantive reflection, or ontological chimera) of brain activity, then mental illness is presumably reducible to brain dysfunction. Then again, in so far as thoughts, memories, volitions, intentions, aspirations, dreams, hallucinations and other ostensibly mental phenomena remain unreduced or incompletely reduced to neural, neurochemical, synaptic, engramic or other biological substrates, the dualistic distinction between states of mind and states of brain is bound to bear some weight. By my lights, progress in medical science (including psychiatry) is synonymous with advances in reliable knowledge of the body (including the brain); whereas progress in medical arts is synonymous with advances in reliable knowledge of the integral person, which includes

---

1 I would like to thank Thomas Schramme and Johannes Thome for inviting this contribution, and for making helpful editorial suggestions. I would also like to thank Keith MacLellan for his help with research.

approaches to understanding consciousness and its manifestations for what they are, and not merely for what they are assumed to be. Thus by its very definition, psychiatry entails both implicit philosophical assumptions and explicit philosophical challenges.

As expressed by Venezualen psychiatrist Abraham Genis: "Philosophy has always been a preferential activity of psychiatrists (...) and in many cases, in the course of our psychotherapeutic relations with our patients, we recognize that, inevitably, we are philosophizing." (Genis 2003)

The etymology of "philosophy" is "love of wisdom", but academic philosophers need manifest neither passion nor sagacity in their official capacities as "trade-unionists" of formal thought. Ever since Wittgenstein, analytic philosophers of the Anglo-American tradition gradually divorced themselves from the extra-academic world and its poignantly tangible concerns; while Continental philosophers tended to immerse themselves over-deeply in surreal worlds and their intangible flights of fancy. Either way, and markedly since Wittgenstein, theoretical philosophers have largely succeeded in utilizing their considerable intelligence to make themselves irrelevant to the world at large and inaccessible to ordinary persons seeking practical philosophical guidance. Wittingly or not, they borrowed Poincarré's apocryphal toast "Here's to pure mathematics; may it never be good for anything", and transposed it wholesale to the love of wisdom.

I blame none of this neo-scolasticism on Wittgenstein. He is no more accountable for the cloistering of philosophy than is Darwin for the extrapolations of Social Darwinism, or Einstein and Heisenberg for New-Age sophistry which asserts that everything is either "relative" or "uncertain". Wittgenstein merely provides a convenient (and cult-like) focus for the endless and fruitless debates of the cloister. Since there is little consensus on what Wittgenstein meant by anything he said, his writings afford a richly unclear if ethereal basis for expedient speculation, which serves as both vocational and occupational therapy for cadres of permanently institutionalized philosophers. As such, perhaps the DSM V will identify a new dysfunction: WPD, or "Wittgensteinian Personality Disorder", characterized by aggressively defending the conjunctive proposition that Wittgenstein is the most brilliant philosopher of all time, but that nobody (including himself) knows exactly what he meant by anything he said.

Mercifully, we have other conceptions of philosophy, dating from antiquity, blossoming among the Early Moderns, and flowering during the Enlightenment, that place a greater premium on what Aristotle called "phronesis" – literally, "practical wisdom" – which lends itself to a wide variety of human concerns that unfold far beyond the narrow, stultified and mind-numbingly ecclesiastical groves of academe. It is phronesis that undergirds the re-emergence of worldly philosophy in the latter decades of the 20th century, in both its main branches: applied ethics, and philosophical practice.

All sub-branches of applied ethics – e.g. biomedical ethics, business ethics, computer ethics, engineering ethics, environmental ethics, journalism ethics, and even legal ethics – are concerned with real issues astride the Humean gap between fact and value, and with their appearances and interpretations as conceived in the Cartesian theatre of mind. The brute fact that we possess technologies to do such-and-thus – e.g. harvest and sell transplantable organs, conduct insider stock-trading, engage in data-mining, deforest the planet, manufacture news instead of reporting it, and defend any point of view (no matter how absurd) for money – does not entail any guidelines for effective reasoning on the ineluctable normative questions: *Should* we do such things? If so, why? If not, why not? Applied philosophers contribute to and help foment public debate on these and kindred issues, which in turn inform public policy, regulation and ultimately legislation, thus engendering an ethos that enhances (or at least pays lip service to) effective moral reasoning.

It is but a short step – yet also a "quantum" leap for some – from addressing a generic biomedical ethical issue (e.g. "What are the ethics of physician-assisted suicide?") to counselling a client struggling personally with that issue (e.g. "Should I myself seek physician-assisted suicide?"). This is precisely the step from applied ethics to philosophical counselling. If it is legitimate for philosophers to counsel society as a whole by addressing issues of immediate public concern, then it is surely legitimate for philosophers to counsel individuals by helping them address the same issues in a context of immediate private concern.

Clients nowadays present a host of similar personal issues to philosophers, ranging from duties in marriage to rights in the workplace to moral dilemmas; from decision-theoretic problems concerning relationships or careers or existential crises to generalized searches for meaning, purpose and value in life at any stage. Our typical clients are neither medically ill nor emotionally disturbed. They are rational and functional beings who seek articulation and elucidation of philosophical issues, or of philosophical implications of issues, that hold some sway in their current circumstances. For self-preservative reasons, they are seeking to make sense of their situations, and to find some applicable principles for reframing their adversity, or calibrating their moral compass, or charting their course through whatever external difficulty afflicts them, or understanding the extent to which they may be afflicting themselves with external manifestations of their own internal conflicts.

If we understand practical wisdom in this way, then we can assert a (perhaps the) foundational perspective of mainstream philosophical counselling: that the human being's functionality is empirically operative in at least three interactive domains – the biological, the affective and the noetic. The Greek word "noesis" (from *noein*, to think, and *nous*, the mind) means the exercise of reason, especially in apprehending universal forms. The cognate adjective "noetic" refers to the rational and intellectual faculties of mind.

Medical arts and sciences, including psychiatry, are naturally rooted in the biological domain. Psychological arts, sciences and pseudo-sciences tend to be rooted in the affective domain. Philosophical arts are rooted in the noetic domain. At the same time, there is no strict or impermeable demarcation between and among these domains. Thus one who contemplates the whole person is committed from the outset to interdisciplinary theories as well as to multidisciplinary practices.

For instance, it is clear that problems with affect can themselves be signs of medical illness. Then again, affective disorders can also arise because of inconsistent beliefs (as in cognitive or existential dissonance). By the same token, the kind of medical advice that a patient hypothetically seeks and ultimately follows (e.g. allopathic versus homeopathic) is partly dependent upon that person's web of beliefs about medicine, influenced by reason and experience alike; in other words, is influenced by a patient's informal philosophy and conditioned psychology of medicine itself. Moreover, the availability and quality of medical, psychological and philosophical services themselves, in a given sovereign state or region thereof, depend upon the broader philosophies of politics and economics that undergird, shape and ultimately govern the prevailing ethos.

A person who is medically ill is bound to have reduced functionality in all three domains. Disease in the biological domain almost always entails some distress in the affective domain, which in turn tends to interfere with the higher cognitive functions, such as rational choice. It is the physician's and psychiatrist's tasks to diagnose disease, prescribe treatment, indirectly restore health – and thereby re-instate the patient's overall functionality. At the same time, a person who is philosophically confused or conflicted also has potentially reduced functionality in all three domains. An unresolved moral dilemma, for example, can cause loss of sleep and appetite (in the biological domain), along with anxiety and irritability (in the affective domain). But in such a case, symptomatic treatment by medicine, psychiatry or psychology (e.g. medications or psychotherapies) will not resolve the core problem, which is axiological and subsists in the noetic domain. A philosophical resolution of the moral dilemma is required to re-instate the overall functionality of such a client.[2]

Thus philosophy and psychiatry are united in the first instance by a common mission, albeit grounded in different domains: to restore the functionality

---

2 This is not to assert that philosophical resolutions, where attainable, eschew or obviate affective dimensions of distress. The authoritative sanction that accompanies the invocation and implementation of a given moral principle, e.g. Aristotle's golden mean or Kant's categorical imperative, has indubitable psychological undertones. Yet here the sanctioning authority itself is clearly philosophical; and the medium of deliberation, primarily noetic. E.g., see Marinoff 1995.

of the beneficiaries of their respective services. For most human beings, optimal functionality requires persistent maintenance of an unstable equilibrium of physical health, emotional balance and conceptual order. What divides philosophy and psychiatry, as we shall see more pointedly, is that typical clients of philosophers tend to be affectively well-balanced, whether they are confronting a marital break-up, a career crisis, or even a fatal prognosis. By contrast and almost by definition, typical patients of psychiatry tend to be affectively ill-balanced, for a constellation of possible reasons. As a service provider, the psychiatrist therefore faces a more difficult daily mission than does the philosopher. However, the meta-mission of determining *whose* mission it should be in a given case – i.e. of demarcating more fully between psychiatric and philosophical criteria of functionality – is a collaborative challenge for psychiatrists and philosophers together.

Idiosyncratically, philosophy and psychiatry are united by reciprocal professional relations. Some philosophers do seek (while others should seek) psychiatric help; and some psychiatrists do seek (while others should seek) philosophical help. It is therefore mutually incumbent on philosophers and psychiatrists to participate in meta-dialogues concerning the theory and substance of their reciprocating professional dialogues. I will characterize two such meta-dialogues for you. The first was an indirect exchange, refracted through the distorting medium of a prominent American newspaper. The second was a direct exchange, through an invited course given to European psychiatrists.

Philosophical counselling was introduced to mainstream American culture in the late 1990s, partly through a series of newspaper articles. A formulaic norm by which journalists often feign balanced reporting is to represent (or possibly misrepresent) the position of a story's protagonist, then to provoke precipitous objections (nominally, rebuttals) from the protagonist's competitors or detractors. Thus the Associated Press represented philosophical counselling as help for the "ethically-challenged" in a 1998 article published on the front page of the *Los Angeles Times*.[3] The journalist had elicited her perfunctory precipitous objection from no less a figure than the (then) President of the American Psychiatric Association, Herbert Sacks, who rashly accused philosophical counsellors of "practicing medicine without a license".

This draws two brief retorts from me. First, I assert that any psychiatrist who reflexively equates a moral dilemma with a mental illness might benefit from philosophical counselling himself – in this case an initial consultation on Plato's distinction between appearance and reality, then Hume's distinction between fact and value. This would be followed up by Hume's argument illustrating the

3 *Los Angeles Times*, Sunday, April 5, 1998, A1.

impossibility of deriving "ought" from "is", which applies straightforwardly to most clients facing moral dilemmas. The brute facts of circumstance do not permit the derivation of normative conclusions, unless normative premises are smuggled into the argument. The philosophical counsellor's role in such cases is to conduct a dialogue that helps the client to articulate his or her implicit normative premises, to elucidate their normative prescriptions, and to evaluate moral alternatives and their probable consequences.

Moreover, as I have explained, if moral dis-ease is "diagnosed" and treated as though it were medical or psychiatric disease, the symptoms might be temporarily alleviated, but the moral dilemma would persist until addressed and resolved in its proper domain. That domain is ethical, not medical. This leads to my second retort; namely, that any psychiatrist who diagnoses and treats moral dilemmas (or other philosophical problems) as "mental illnesses" is *practicing non-medicine with a license.*

The power of licensure is such that any physician (or licensed psychologist) can not only mis-diagnose ethical problems as medical ones, but also can legally dispense ethics counselling to patients without necessarily knowing anything at all about ethics. Whereas a philosophical counsellor who so dispenses can attract accusations of practicing medicine (or indeed psychology) without a license. Viewed in one way, such accusations are hubris arising from poor professional formation, from lack of appropriate continuing education, and from perennial corruptions of power itself. In America, an admixture of hubris with profit-motive exacerbates turf-wars between and among professional care-givers, which nonetheless can have the salutary aftereffect of obliging consumers to think more carefully about what might be wrong with them, and therefore also about what kind of help to seek. *Caveat emptor.*

On the whole, Europeans are far better-educated than Americans, whose system is in free-fall, although I gather that one of globalization's unfortunate side-effects is a marked decline in European educational standards as well. Many Americans regard philosophy as a pointless elective study to be avoided at all costs, mostly because it requires intellectual exertions incompatible with hedonism and consumerism, generally because it cannot be done while watching television, playing video games or surfing the world wide web, and specifically because deconstructed "education" in America is no longer predicated on reading, writing or reasoning skills – rather on vacuous pretensions to self-esteem, puerile denigrations of rigor, and sophomoric ideologies celebrating "diversity" as the primary goal and overarching virtue of institutions of erstwhile higher education. Thus even willing students can nowadays barely parse a sentence of any Enlightenment thinker. Unslaked conceptual thirsts, combined with untutored palates, make mainstream Americans so vulnerable to slogans, cults and circuses. Europeans, by contrast, tend respectfully to regard philosophy as a mandatory component of a decent formal education, but not as something especially useful in subsequent personal or professional life. Thus Europeans study philosophy early on, but eschew it as a luxury later. So they too, for manifestly different reasons, miss out on its quotidian benefits.

Pace the peripatetic Golden Mean, it appears that the European extreme of underutilizing philosophy out of misplaced reverence for its antiquity and theoretical complexity is more virtuous than the American extreme of underutilizing philosophy out of received anti-elitism and entrenched mass-marketing of junk food and junk thought alike. This hypothesis would account for the best-selling status of my popular book, *Plato Not Prozac*, throughout Europe but not in America. And perhaps for this reason, I was invited by the Swedish Psychiatric Association to direct an accredited course in philosophical counselling, team-taught along with two outstanding European colleagues (Anders Lindseth and Antti Matilla), at the 2002 EAP conference in Stockholm. Dr. Henrik Nyback, a member of the SPA Board, subsequently commented "Your presentations of various aspects of philosophical counselling were very inspiring to me and to the international audience (...) I'm convinced that in the future the interaction between our disciplines, philosophy and psychiatry, will grow and deepen into further collaboration." Needless to say, this open-minded European view of philosophical counselling is a far cry from the unvarnished buffoonery of the American charge of "practicing medicine without a license."

The nuanced picture, of course, is never so black-and-white. In fact, many rank-and–file American psychiatrists also support the idea of philosophical counselling, and some are even using *Plato Not Prozac* as a philosophical field manual in their own practices. I myself collaborate with a psychiatrist, Dr. Mahin Hassibi, on my *pro bono* philosophical counselling research protocol at City College. Psychiatrist members of the Association for the Advancement of Philosophy and Psychiatry have acknowledged that perhaps 10% of their patients present philosophical, and not exclusively psychiatric, problems. Our potential for collaboration is indeed considerable, and probably universal.

2. What Divides Philosophy and Psychiatry?

> Order and classification are the beginning of mastery, whereas the truly dreadful enemy is the unknown. The human race must be led out of the primitive stage of fear and long-suffering vacuity and into a phase of purposeful activity. Humankind must be informed that certain effects can be diminished only when one first recognizes their causes and negates them, and that almost all sufferings of the individual are illnesses of the social organism. – Thomas Mann, *The Magic Mountain*

Western medicine, of which psychiatry is a special branch, is based on an allopathic (rather than a homeopathic) model whose roots are essentially Newtonian. The body is viewed as a kind of machine, replete with parts and systems. Defective parts can be repaired or replaced; malfunctioning systems can be restored to acceptable levels of functionality. All bodily parts and systems are ultimately subject to biochemical and biophysical laws, greater understanding of which conduces to greater power, in a straightforwardly Baconian sense, over maintenance of health and management of sickness. The role of the mind and its faculties – such as volition, intention, imagination, and the like – are quite marginalized in this materialistic paradigm, which views thought (or ideation) as an epiphenomenal by-product of neural and synaptic activity. Notwithstanding the shortcomings of this view, its successes are undeniable: Life expectancies in the developed world, whose citizens have fair to excellent access to leading-edge medical technologies, have almost doubled in the past century or so.

Psychiatry is in the exciting and also unenviable position of treating the most interesting and least-understood organ in the body: the brain. Notwithstanding Freud's postulated reduction of thought to deterministic cerebral activity, carried on philosophically by eliminative materialists among other physicalists, the issue of substance dualism is far from settled. Even untrammeled idealism of Buddha's, Plato's or Berkeley's kinds, although disparaged by current Western philosophical fashion, is not thereby refuted. Given the organ it treats, psychiatry is *de facto* the most philosophical of the medical arts. However, consistent with the successes of the allopathic model, the received philosophy of current mainstream psychiatry is also inherently mechanistic. In so far as the brain is viewed as a volatile soup of neurochemical transmitters, whose unstable homeostasis is normally auto-regulating but susceptible to uncontrollable perturbations as well as congenital imbalances, the first line of defence against so-called "mental illness" is the restoration of neurochemical balance, effected by the latest generation of serotonin re-uptake inhibitors and other "mood-enhancing" formulations. The default medical treatment is therefore molecular psychiatry, ideally but not necessarily followed by some kind of dialogue.

Given the enormous demands placed upon physicians and psychiatrists, who typically have large case-loads and correspondingly little time to devote to each case, and who are increasingly afflicted (at least in the USA) with mountainous paperwork plus the daily struggle of justifying proposed treatments via telephone to bureaucratic third-party insurers, medical professionals have increasingly little time to talk to their patients. This potentiates a fruitful alliance between psychiatrists, physicians, and philosophical counsellors, provided that the medical profession is willing to admit that faculties of mind also play an active and vital role in maintaining overall well-being. This in turn requires at least two related modifications to the Newtonian model of medicine: first and generally, adopting a more holistic view of the human being; second and particularly, abandoning the notion that psychiatry guarantees an objective perspective from which to study the human being.

The integration of more holistic theories and practices into the extant mechanistic model is ongoing, and its elaboration lies beyond the scope of this essay. It is the second modification that I wish to address: the rejection of the premise that one human being, through the lens of any paradigm, can study another human being with scientific impunity. Just as there are no uniquely "privileged frames" from which one can observe absolute properties of physical objects, there are no uniquely "privileged frames" from which one can make absolute diagnoses of human beings. For example, while "paranoia" entails a set of attitudes and behaviours that are dysfunctional in open and free societies – hence "diagnosable" as a "mental illness" – the same set of attitudes and behaviours might be highly functional – and might therefore become a norm, not an "illness" – in a totalitarian regime. And even if one rebuts such panoramic sociological relativism, one does not thereby avert or remedy the value-ladenness of diagnostic criteria.

In the former Soviet Union, dissidents were routinely confined to psychiatric hospitals instead of political prisons. The rationale was purely dialectical (*qua* Orwellian), and not at all medical. The Soviet Union had been declared, by the Communist Party, to be a "worker's paradise". Anyone who objects to living in paradise is obviously crazy. QED.

Lest we who inhabit less paradisiacal but nonetheless freer polities fall prey to smugness, consider the Rosenhan experiments, in which researchers posed as "mentally ill" patients in order to gain admission to psychiatric wards, where they clandestinely studied the psychiatrists and other staff. Unable to observe ongoing signs of "mental illnesses" in these patients, the staff made pejorative notes on their normal activities – such as, "patient engages in writing behaviour". Surprisingly, only the psychiatric patients were able to penetrate the deception: "You're not crazy. You're checking up on the hospital" said one (Rosenhan 1973).

The Rosenhan experiments raise a serious philosophical problem, which has nothing to do with professional ethics. Let me illustrate the problem with parallel scenarios involving auto mechanics, and surgeons. Some unscrupulous mechanics defraud their clientele, by making unnecessary repairs to cars, or by replacing perfectly functional parts, or by charging for work not done. Similarly, some unscrupulous surgeons malpractice medicine by performing unnecessary surgeries. In both kinds of cases, the dishonest mechanics and the dishonest doctors are obviously aware of their fraudulence. Thus they stand in knowing and wilful violation of their respective professional ethics. In the Rosenhan experiments, by contrast, the psychiatrists and staff did not knowingly or wilfully malpractice medicine. They simply assumed *ab initio* that anyone who came under their care was "mentally ill", and thus they sought observational data that confirmed their hypothesis. Failure to observe such data in specific cases should have suggested disconfirmation, but instead they re-interpreted the data to salvage their unsound hypothesis. Blinded by their pre-conceived notions, they were unable to make objective assessments of their putative "patients".

I do not raise the Rosenhan spectre to attack psychiatry or defend anti-psychiatry; rather, to remind psychiatrists of Plato's salient distinction between appearance and reality.[4] The moral is: Not everyone who appears as a patient is necessarily a patient.

The history of science is riddled with examples of theory-laden obfuscation of observed data – from Penzias's and Wilson's inadvertent discovery of the Big Bang's cosmic echo to Margaret Mead's ironic coming of age in Samoa. These examples among many others, writ large across the entire spectrum of the sciences, are all indicative of the main point: namely, that there is no uniquely privileged paradigm from which to make value-neutral observations. All empirical observations are theory-laden; that is, are made through the lens of imperfect knowledge, and are therefore susceptible to distortion or aberration by received false premises mistakenly held to be true. Moreover, since nothing is more value-laden than states of mind themselves, then states of mind attempting to evaluate other states of mind, and attempting to evaluate responses to those evaluations, are bound to potentiate the drawing of irremediably subjective – and at times ineluctably arbitrary – inferences.

One way to restore a measure of implied objectivity to such an imprecise science, especially in the absence of specifiable causal reductions of many so-called "mental illnesses" to actual brain-states, is via statistical correlation. That is, patients who present with certain symptoms, and who exhibit particular signs, are statistically likely to be suffering from such-and-thus syndrome. On this view, the DSM affords a sensible – perhaps the sole sensible – approach to "diagnosing" dysfunctions of the brain. At the same time, however, such a manual is conspicuously vulnerable to two kinds of defects, which some philosophers and psychiatrists have identified. The two are: reification (an ontological and epistemological problem), and science by democracy (a political and economic problem).

Reification occurs primarily through neglect of the Duhem-Quine thesis, namely the unavoidable underdetermination of theory by data. Simply stated, it means that there are in principle any number of theories that could account for a given observation; and that there is no way, *a priori*, to ascertain which of these theories is in fact the sound one. Consider the empirical proposition "Disorder A produces behavior B". Suppose this is demonstrable, whether causally or correlatively. Now consider the diagnostic inference: "Behavior B evidences disorder A". This is not necessarily true at all on causal grounds, and may or may not be significant on probabilistic ones. For example, the

---

4 See Plato's "Allegory of the Cave" in his *Republic, Book VII.*

empirical proposition that attention deficit disorder (ADD) produces misbehaviours in the schoolroom is statistically if not causally verifiable. However, the diagnostic inference that misbehaviour in the schoolroom evidences ADD is clearly dubious. Any number of factors could induce students to misbehave. But it is precisely on such dubious converse inductions that the so-called "epidemic" of ADD has been "diagnosed" (that is, reified), resulting in the coerced drugging of millions of American schoolchildren with Ritalin. While obstreperous children should certainly be tranquillized on airplanes, the reification of an ADD "epidemic" in the schools is ontologically suspect, commercially motivated and educationally scandalous.

An underlying cause of reification itself, not just of one "disorder", but of many, is indubitably the ballot-box method by which disorders are elected to the DSM. No significant discovery in the history of science, including medicine, has ever been made by such democratic means. On the theoretical side, the Newtons, Darwins and Einsteins all worked alone, had their theories subjected to the most withering scepticism, and their hypotheses rigorously tested, before winning gradual (if not grudging) acceptance by communities of their peers. On the empirical side of medicine, important breakthroughs by the likes of Pasteur, Lister and Semmelweiss met with uniformly vituperative opposition from peers, until finally accepted and adopted. The way of scientific progress is verisimilitudinous but combative; that is, unfolds via asymptotic approaches to truth made by clear-sighted individuals initially opposed by bias-blinded herds.

By contrast, the politicization of science – by any political system – is bound to have the opposite effect, and lead to antiverisimilitudinous scientific regress. Naturally, both fine- and coarse-grained distinctions between various political systems are reflected in their respective politicizations of science, which makes regress a matter of degree, but not of kind. From a copious and lamentable historical catalogue of such cases, one could cite the Roman Church's prohibition of Galilean astronomy, the Anglican censorship of Hobbesian political theory, the Creationist denial of Darwinian evolutionism, the Nazi proscription of "Jewish physics", the Soviet endorsement of Lamarckian agronomy, the Maoist annihilation of its intelligentsia, the African denial of AIDS's aetiology, or the American radical feminist repudiation of science itself. Whether the political interference has been motivated by theocracy, misology, totalitarianism, despotism, or hysterical anti-realism, the result is always the same: retreat from truth, obstruction of progress, increase in suffering, and – in the worst cases – needless death on extravagant scales.

Churchill's stinging aphorism about democracy being the worst form of government – except for all the others – translates into the comparatively benign face of the democratization of science. Nonetheless, one decisive factor in democratic politics is lobbying, and the pharmaceutical industry's ability to lobby the medical profession is undeniable. Thus, when the American

Psychiatric Association elects a "mental illness" like Social Anxiety Disorder to the DSM, and when we witness prime-time television advertisement campaigns for prescription drugs like Paxil, billed as a panacea for life's concerns, we are bound to conclude that the pharmaceutical industry and the medical profession have struck a nefarious albeit democratic bargain to perpetrate fraud on gullible consumers. While this will not result in mass-death, as did the corrupt lobbying of politicians and others by the tobacco industry during many decades, it does represent the undesirable colonization of medicine by *laissez-faire* capitalism.

As long as the DSM remains vulnerable to charges of reification of disease and democratization of science, philosophical aspersions will justifiably be cast on it, and by extension on those who take it and its paradigmatic peculiarities too literally.

So what – if anything – divides philosophy and psychiatry, besides the standard objections raised by medical and professional ethicists, and beyond the paradigmatic critiques that philosophers of science level across the spectrum of such endeavours? Given the plurality of philosophical approaches to psychiatry by psychiatrists themselves, from Karl Jaspers's existentialism to Raymond Prince's transculturalism; from R.D. Laing's unorthodoxy to Thomas Szasz's apostasy – it appears that psychiatrists have recapitulated many of the differences that divide philosophers themselves. The starkly contrasting views of human nature held by Rousseau contra Hobbes, or by Buber contra Foucault, are typical divisions in a discipline defined de facto by diversity of opinion on everything. The operative divide in either profession is between those who view man as a fundamentally sick animal (a position espoused theologically by Augustine, psychoanalytically by Freud, and commercially by the pharmaceutical industry) and those who view man as a circumstantially afflicted but ultimately transcendent being (a position espoused pragmatically by Buddha, idealistically by Emerson, and allegorically by Huxley). So perhaps philosophy and psychiatry are actually united by their respective divisions.

3. What Transcends Philosophy and Psychiatry?

> In general, our pharmacologists would do well not to be too overweening about their knowledge, for they had the same problem with a great many things: they knew this and that about the dynamics and effects of a substance, but any questions as to precise causes all too frequently proved an embarrassment. – Thomas Mann, *The Magic Mountain*

Thomas Mann's *Death in Venice* is not simply an elegant novella, charting the demise of the neo-classical literatus Achenbach; it is an allegory on the demise of classicism itself, which heralds the death of Western civilization. While generally taken to be Mann's last word on the subject, there does remain a plausible alternative view, put forward by Mann himself in his windier classic, *The Magic Mountain.*

Set in the Swiss Alpine village of Davos, whose elegant hotels during the latter 19th and early 20th centuries were sanatoria for the respiratorily-challenged, *The Magic Mountain* hypothesizes that Western civilization is merely ill – perhaps even gravely ill – but has some unascertained prospect of recovery. A central question of the novel is whether that which is yet-to-be-ascertained is in fact ascertainable at all. Interestingly enough, this later became a central question for 20th century epistemology of science.

Much of Mann's characters' colloquy about the diagnosis and treatment of potentially fatal respiratory ailments is straightforwardly transposable from the medical metaphor to the geopolitical, dialectical, eschatological and teleological axes of Mann's (and man's) perspective on the West. In order to explore the intricacies and interstices of this debate more deeply, Mann provides an erudite mouthpiece: a scholar and belletrist by the name of Lodovico Settembrini, who plays metaphysician to our ailing but possibly convalescing civilization.

I have embarked this far on literary interpretation only to introduce to you the character of Settembrini. To those readers already acquainted with him, as well as to those newly-introduced in virtue of the foregoing, I should now like to re-acquaint you, via an unusual missive. Since the letter in question was penned by a psychiatrist, it may prove a more reliable source of re-introduction than the idle speculations of a philosopher. The letter was published in *Psychiatric News*, newsletter of the American Psychiatric Association, and was written in response to an article on philosophical counselling.[5] The article itself had emerged from that seminal piece in the *L.A. Times*, and was penned by the newsletter's editor Richard Karel – not a psychiatrist himself, but an in-house journalist employed by the American Psychiatric Association.

> *Psychiatric News*, Letter to the Editor, May 15, 1998[6]
> Philosopher Therapists
> Richard Karel's piece in the April 17 issue on "philosopher practitioners" (philosophers who claim to practice a form of psychotherapy) brought back memories of Thomas Mann's novel, *The Magic Mountain*. There we meet the humanist scholar, Settembrini, who embodies the enlightened classicism of the Renaissance.
> "There is one power, one principle, which commands my deepest assent", Settembrini says, and this "is the intellect". When spring comes to the Alpine sanitarium, Settembrini is ecstatic: "All the disquieting, provocative elements of spring in the valley were here lacking: here were no seething depths, no steaming air, no oppressive humidity! Only dryness, clarity, a serene and piercing charm."

5 http://www.psych.org/pnews/98-04-17/philos.html
6 http://www.psych.org/pnews/98-05-15/pies.html

> Reading the words of the "philosopher practitioner" Dr. Lou Marinoff, one feels that he and Settembrini are kindred spirits. In a recent article in the *New York Times*, Professor Marinoff holds forth hope to troubled souls, who would "explore and address their dilemma through the long history of thought, rather than through Prozac, for example."
> Let us leave aside Professor Marinoff's admission that "the history of thought" might not suffice for those with "severe personality disorders" – or, presumably, psychotic disorders or suicidal depressions. Let us leave aside the matter of how philosopher practitioners will be trained to recognize when their "clients" are too sick to benefit from Sartre or Nietzsche. Let us defer the critical issue of unrecognized medical and neurological illness in many patients with so-called existential problems. Let us even put aside the huge medicolegal question of whether unvalidated "treatment" by philosophers may delay lifesaving care by mental health professionals.
> We must still return to Settembrini, with his love for dryness and clarity and his distaste for seething depths and steaming air. It is in precisely such a tropical clime that the psychotherapist must often work. The sexually abused individual who experiences traumatic flashbacks, the narcissistic character who bristles with anger at the world's indifference, the substance abuser who explodes after a single drink: these individuals do not live in Settembrini's (or Marinoff's) sunlit world of philosophical humanism. Many are struggling in that darker land of the shattered self, and there – with courage, care, and passion – must be joined by the therapist. This is no place for well-intentioned scholars, armed with the serenity of the Western philosophical canon. Sometimes the text must come close to the flame before its words take wing.
> Ronald Pies, M.D.
> Lexington, Massachusetts

I must offer a well-tempered response to Dr. Pies, whose comments certainly merit one. But before doing so, let me thank him for his flattering – and, as it turns out, prescient – comparison to Settembrini. I will instantiate his prescience in due course; but first, here is my reply to the good Doctor.

First, we need not leave aside my admission, shared by most philosophical practitioners, that great ideas alone will not suffice to remedy severe personality disorders, psychoses, or suicidal depressions. To quote from my IRB-approved research protocol at The City College of New York: "Philosophical counselling is intended for clients who are rational, functional, and not mentally ill, but who can benefit from philosophical assistance in resolving or managing problems associated with normal life experience."[7] The assertion that some people can benefit from philosophical counselling does not entail the assertion that all people can. Thus this objection by Dr. Pies (if it is one) is a straw man.

7 The IRB is the Institutional Review Board, which must approve all research conducted on or with human beings, even if non-iatrogenic. IRBs are governed by Federal Regulatory Law, and NIH guidelines.

Second and more important, let us not leave aside the matter "of how philosopher practitioners will be trained to recognize when their 'clients' are too sick to benefit from Sartre or Nietzsche". My reply is straightforward. Like every other profession, philosophical counselling has a scope of practice. City College's IRB approved this one:

> The most suitable candidates for philosophical counselling are clients whose problems are centered in:
> 1) issues of private morality or professional ethics;
> 2) issues of meaning, value, or purpose;
> 3) issues of personal or professional fulfilment;
> 4) issues of underdetermined or inconsistent belief systems;
> 5) issues requiring any philosophical interpretation of changing circumstances.

Note that the IRB's approval of this scope of practice entails its recognition that all the foregoing issues are intrinsically or primarily philosophical, and that none of them is intrinsically or primarily psychological, medical or psychiatric. The APPA's training and certification of philosophical counsellors is consistent with this scope of practice. We are not trained to diagnose or treat "sicknesses" or other conditions lying outside this scope. We are trained to dialogue with rational and functional clients whose issues lie within it. If during an initial consultation or a subsequent dialogue it emerges that a client's primary problem appears not to lie within this scope, the client is referred for psychological, medical or psychiatric evaluation.

Philosophical counselling is defined by the APPA as an educational activity. It is not radically different than teaching philosophy in a classroom, save that it applies philosophical analysis and insight to issues pre-selected by the client, instead of to texts or topics pre-selected by the professor. One might as well ask "How are university professors trained to know when their students are too 'sick' to study Sartre or Nietzsche"? The answer is that they aren't, and needn't be. Students who lack sufficient rationality or functionality to cope with philosophy courses either drop them or fail them or find other subjects to study, or else seek tutoring to help exercise reason or improve academic performance. Similarly, persons who lack sufficient rationality or functionality to dialogue with philosophical counsellors either don't come to us in the first place, or are referred by us for more appropriate help. In general, clients too "sick" to benefit from Sartre or Nietzsche are usually too "sick" to make and keep appointments with philosophical counsellors, or too "sick" to engage in lucid or coherent dialogue with them – hence merit referrals for psychiatric or psychological evaluation. Thus the good Doctor should be reassured on this score.

Third, let us not defer "the critical issue of unrecognized medical and neurological illness in many patients with so-called existential problems". On the contrary, let us meet it head-on. During the APPA's training of philosophical counsellors, we do indeed make this very point: that a good many illnesses can manifest symptoms that appear as philosophical, psychological or even psychiatric problems, but which in fact require a medical or neurological diagnosis to reveal the underlying disease (Talbot-Stern 2000, Reeves 2000). About 10% of self-referred psychiatric patients have symptoms provoked by medical illness, and that is no small number (Hall et al. 1978).

The most rational conclusion to draw is that, in the best of possible worlds, any person wishing to see a counsellor of any kind – whether psychiatric, psychological, philosophical, pastoral, legal, etc. – should receive a full medical work-up first, to ensure as far as possible that the actual problem is not corporeal. However, in the real world, there are hundreds of thousands of psychiatrists and psychologists seeing millions of patients annually, a substantial proportion of whom apparently have undiagnosed medical problems. In the same world, there are several dozen philosophical counsellors seeing several hundred self-selecting clients annually, many of whom have previously received treatment from psychiatrists or psychotherapy from psychologists, and some of whom are simultaneously under the care of physicians for diagnosed ailments, but still need to make philosophical sense of their lives (and ends-of-lives, when prognoses are fatal). A small fraction of these clients claim to be suffering from *angst*. Where, then, does the crisis of undiagnosed illness manifest most severely? Clearly it does so in the camps of psychiatry and psychology themselves. Thus the medical profession, including psychiatry, ought to be concerned first and foremost with its own epidemic of undiagnosed disease.

As the profession of philosophical practice develops and grows, philosophical counsellors will begin to see enough clients to make statistically-significant studies feasible. Then we'll be able to test this question empirically: What proportion of clients of philosophical counselling have undiagnosed diseases? I predict that this fraction will be significantly smaller than that for patients of both psychiatrists and psychologists. Furthermore, I predict that it will be as small as, or smaller than, that of the general populace. Statistically, this would mean that seeing a philosophical counsellor poses no risk greater than that of going about one's normal business in everyday life – e.g. of crossing the street, or driving to work.

That said, I now shift from a defensive to an offensive posture, to raise a crucial point implied but ignored by Dr. Pies's concern about undiagnosed illness. There are two gross ways in which nosology can err: by failing to diagnose existing disease, or by succeeding to diagnose non-existing disease. Let us re-address the latter possibility. As previously mentioned herein, and as elaborated for lay readers in two popular books (Marinoff 1999, 2003), the DSM IV contains a number of ontologically-suspect "diseases" – either transparently subjective on their face (e.g. "non-compliance with treatment disorder"), commercially contentious in their application (e.g. "attention deficit disorder"), or pretentiously pseudo-scientific in their jargon (e.g. "post-traumatic stress disorder").

The DSM has steadily increased the number of its democratically-elected "mental illnesses"; has encouraged widespread "paint-by-numbers" diagnoses of every conceivable complaint, often as not without any demonstration of causal reductions to putative brain dysfunctions; and has become the definitive instrument of unprecedented and growing pharmaceutical avarice, through which a gargantuan industry of legalized drug-dealing is imposed on consumers by an alliance of big business interests, complicit medical (and pseudo-medical) professionals, and states which license them. They are capitalizing on a myth foisted initially upon gullible and uncritical American consumers, and increasingly propagated throughout the global village, to the effect that every experience of dis-ease (*qua* noetic or emotional discomfort) is a "symptom" of some sickness (*qua* "mental illness" or – as the popular catechism goes – "chemical imbalance in the brain"). It is almost effortless for an intellectually shoddy, technocratically dependent, abjectly ill-educated and consumer oriented populace to ingest this myth wholesale, then to ingest the medications advertised as panaceas for the conspirators' catalogue of reified "diseases". On this issue, Dr. Pies remains regrettably silent.

Fourth, let us not put aside "the huge medicolegal question of whether unvalidated 'treatment' by philosophers may delay lifesaving care by mental health professionals". Rather, let us confront this sublime assertion head-on. How many patients, world-wide, die annually in the so-called "lifesaving care" of so-called "mental health" professionals – whether of suicide, or of undiagnosed diseases, or of related causes? There were 30,575 suicides in the USA alone in 1998.[8] How many thousands of these committed suicide while in the "lifesaving care" of "mental health" professionals? In New York State, such patients have a suicide rate well above the general population – 115.9 per 100,000 versus 9 per 100,000 respectively, in 1985 – and growing.[9] At the same time, to my knowledge *not one single client of any philosophical counsellor has ever committed suicide*, or died of an undiagnosed disease, or died because a philosophical counsellor somehow "delayed" the provision of "lifesaving care". Nor has any philosophical counsellor ever been sued for malpractice. Those who make the most outrageous accusations against our profession cannot present one shred of supporting evidence, while all the evidence extant suggests that they are most vulnerable to the very charges they levy against us! Are critical thinking and scientific reasoning no longer taught to medical students in general, and to psychiatric residents in particular?

And let me re-proportion Dr. Pies's "huge medicolegal question" of so-called "unvalidated 'treatment'". I reiterate that philosophical counselling is defined by the APPA as an educational activity, not a medical one. The APPA

---

8 http://www.menstuff.org/issues/byissue/seniorssuicide.html

9 http://www.cqc.state.ny.us/publications/puboutsu.htm

trains and certifies philosophical counsellors with the explicit authorities of the New York State Department of State, and the New York State Department of Education. Furthermore, philosophical counselling is legislatively unregulated in every state of the union, and thus is not legally proscribed anywhere in the USA. So what becomes of Dr. Pies's "huge medicolegal question"? It is neither medical, nor legal, nor huge, nor even a question at all. As to "unvalidated 'treatment'", philosophical counsellors neither *diagnose* nor *treat* our clients. Rather, we *dialogue* with them, as providers of an educational service. The provision of this service is indeed validated, by a professional association (the APPA) of those best-qualified to validate it. The APPA's Certification Standards and Code of Ethics bind our Certified Practitioners.[10] I trust that the good Doctor is not implying that *all* professional services must be validated by psychiatrists in order to be reputable.

Fifth and finally, "We must still return to Settembrini, with his love for dryness and clarity and his distaste for seething depths and steaming air. It is in precisely such a tropical clime that the psychotherapist must often work (...) Many are struggling in that darker land of the shattered self, and there – with courage, care, and passion – must be joined by the therapist. This is no place for well-intentioned scholars, armed with the serenity of the Western philosophical canon."

I couldn't agree more, save that many of us philosophical practitioners bear two arms; the other being the serendipitous Eastern philosophical canon. Nevertheless, it is clear that psychiatrists must contend daily with the darkest aspects of dysfunctionality, derangement and dementia. So many of the "shattered" selves in their custody suffer metaphorically from "Humpty-Dumpty disorder", in that all the King's horses and all the King's men – not to mention all the King's psychiatrists – cannot put them back together again. By contrast, it is equally clear that philosophers' clients are neither dysfunctional nor deranged nor demented. They inhabit a land not doomed by darkness, though not always flooded with light. They seek, and more often than not find, illumination via bright sparks of philosophical inquiry.

There is a notoriously but understandably permeable demarcation (that is, a "fine line") between cops and criminals. In the small minority of worst cases, only a badge distinguishes one from the other. In all cases, law enforcement officers deal daily with criminals and crimes of every description – not to mention their victims – and so are continuously exposed to the worst of what nominally accountable citizens do to themselves and others. Thus one can understand the cop's conditioned (and probably self-preservative) inclination to view all suspects as guilty until "proven" innocent, even in a criminal

10 http://www.appa.edu

justice system that upholds the presumption of innocence and lays the burden of proof of guilt upon the prosecution.

A similar demarcation obtains between psychiatrists and their patients. In the small minority of worst cases, only a license distinguishes one from the other. In all cases, psychiatrists deal daily with human dysfunctions and dysfunctional deeds of every description, and so are continuously exposed to the worst of what citizens nominally unaccountable (by reason of diminished autonomy) to do themselves and others. Thus one can understand the shrink's conditioned (and probably self-preservative) inclination to view all patients as dysfunctional until proven functional, in other words as "mentally ill" until proven mentally well, even in a Republic whose civil and criminal justice systems jointly if implicitly uphold the presumption of sanity, and lay the burden of proof of insanity upon the State.

Even so, the vast majority of human beings are neither criminally inclined nor mentally ill, and yet require care or guidance from myriad helpers at different stages of their lives – whether from parents, teachers, friends, spouses, lawyers, doctors, coaches – and sometimes even from philosophers. The very best of these helpers, like the very best law enforcement officers and the very best psychiatrists, all join courage, care and passion to their helpful services. Here endeth my reply to the good Doctor, a reflective and conscientious professional, who perhaps sustains understandable regret that so little light from the blazing suns of human mentation at its best can ever penetrate the murky depths of human dysfunction at its worst. At the same time, I am sure he would encourage (rather than obstruct) the delivery of philosophical services, properly construed, to those who can benefit from them.

4. Thus Spake Settembrini

> Letting oneself go, in fact, was doubtless a definition of madness in many cases, inasmuch as it was a way of fleeing from great affliction and served weak natures as a defence against the overpowering blows of fate, which such people felt they could not withstand in their right mind. But then anyone could use that excuse, so to speak; and he, Settembrini, had brought many a madman back to reality, at least temporarily, by confronting his fiddle-faddle with a pose of unrelenting reason. – Thomas Mann, *The Magic Mountain*

Dr. Pies may not realize that he is also somewhat prophetic. Unbeknownst to us both, his flattering but fanciful comparison of me to Settembrini would, within three years of its publication, become more actual than either of us could have imagined.

Since the early 1970s, the sleepy ski resort of Davos has become home to the Annual Meeting of the World Economic Forum. Each year in late January, the world's business, political and cultural leaders gather to deliberate and shape the planetary agenda for the evolution of the global village and the amelioration of the human estate. Owing to my pioneering labours in philosophical practice, and its positive reception in many countries and cultures around the world – and notwithstanding assorted critiques by psychiatrists, psychologists and philosophers as well – I was invited to participate in the 2001 and subsequent WEF Programmes. Thus, in January 2001, I found myself in Davos. More to the point, the closing luncheon traditionally takes place on the parapets of the majestic Schatzalp, in the very hotel in which Thomas Mann wrote *The Magic Mountain* and invented the character of Lodovico Settembrini.

There on the Schatzalp, surveying the vista Mann surveyed when he deliberated the fate of Western civilization in the mouths of Settembrini and his interlocutors, I have been implicated in a sequel to that scene, in a latter act of our long-running play. What could we say about the West and its undeniable decline, that had not already been said more eloquently by Mann, more dramatically by Nietzsche, more apocalyptically by Wagner, more historiographically by Spengler?

Lodovico Settembrini had been involved in a multidisciplinary project to catalogue the world's sufferings, with the positivistic aspiration that an accurate taxonomy would abet their alleviation. In retrospect, the myriad historical sufferings that Settembrini contemplated classifying pale in comparison to the unprecedented horrors of the 20th century, during which the very scale of human conflict and its needlessly imposed miseries was recalibrated several times over, to accommodate the escalating excesses, before being consigned to that special obsolescence reserved for instruments that measure too much too well. Just as the obese have little use for bathroom scales and mirrors, so moralists have little use for Sivard indices and daily newspapers.

It is Job's comfort to tens of millions of victims – butchered in but one of many wings of the 20th century's sprawling slaughterhouse – that Erich Fromm "diagnosed" Joseph Stalin posthumously as "a clinical case of non-sexual sadism" (Fromm 1973). Shall we consult a political DSM, to discover what "disorders" motivated not only Stalin, but also Hitler, Hirohito, Mao, Pol Pot, Amin and Milosevic, among other noteworthies in the pantheon of mass-murderers of that agonized century? Shall we consult the fatalist Tolstoy, who believed that kings are History's slaves? Shall we consult Henri Bergson, Aldous Huxley, and Karl Popper, who understood all too well the aetiology and pathology of 20th-century mass-slaughter, but whose ideas were powerless to prevent it?

And in the wake of September 11, 2001, shall we consult Thomas Carlyle, who claimed that no false man could found a religion? The great proselytizing faiths, Christianity and Islam, also have their hallowed places in the fulsome annals of wanton carnage. The havoc wrought by men in the names of their Gods rivals that wrought by Gods in the names of their men. If the monumental arrogance and rabid intolerance of fanatical Christianity at its worst attracted diagnoses of infantilism from Freud and epithets of enslavement from Nietzsche, while Christianity at its best helped sustain the high culture that nurtured them both (two stars twinkling in a veritable galaxy of luminaries), what dare we say about Islam, whose worst is possibly yet to come – on both the giving and receiving ends? I travel across America and around the world these days, heightening the philosophical awareness of individuals, groups and organizations, and everywhere I am asked searching questions about Islamic terrorism. People in America and the world over remain profoundly perturbed by the events of 9/11 and what they portend, and are dissatisfied with pseudo-explanations they have received – from expedient half-truths told by politicians, to half-baked analyses by television's talking heads, to half-witted pronouncements by celebrity ignoramuses. And what can pharmacology and psychotherapy offer to survivors and relatives of victims of 9/11, save temporary symptomatic diminution of their grief and "validation" of their emotions? What can pharmacology and psychotherapy offer to millions who live in fear of terrorism, or who cannot possibly begin to make sense of it in our prevailing ethos of the slogan and the sound-byte, and in the absence of coherent historical exegesis, realistic political analysis, and cogent philosophical insight?

And what does psychiatry say about the perpetrators themselves? Will the APA elect "Islamic terrorist disorder" to the DSM V? Probably not, and with good reason. In America, the "temporary insanity" defence has deservedly lost popularity and currency, along with other juridical vestiges of radical liberalism's illiberal campaign to eradicate individual responsibility for thought, speech and deed. Since the domestic terrorist-bomber Timothy McVeigh was tried and convicted of multiple premeditated murders, one can hardly expect suspected foreign terrorists to find a safe psychiatric haven in the USA, except perhaps among those extreme liberals whose militancy has immunized them against reason, suggesting that they themselves need psychiatric care. For example, the American Civil Liberties Union recently defended the alleged "right" of a fundamentalist Muslim woman to remain completely veiled for her driver's license photo. Prudently, the Court ruled that official identification photos really ought to identify someone's face, as opposed to their costume. Only on the campuses of America's politically correct universities, which have for thirty years engendered toxic hatred for Western civilization and fatuous contempt for its hard-defended liberties, do Islamic terrorists continue to be accorded the heroic status of "freedom fighters" – but soberingly sane ones withal.

At the same time, no enlightened political philosophy hitherto conceived, nor any psychopathology yet elected, can begin to circumscribe the farrago of convoluted fatalism, revisionist historicism, exquisite anti-realism, venomous hatred, enduring enmity, fulminating prevarication, hyperbolic Schadenfreude, tortuous casuistry, and disregard for chivalry that characterizes Islamic among other fanaticisms, excludes its adherents *en masse* from the realm of eudaimonic possibility, and represents a greater threat to Western civilization than even Western civilization itself.

Viewed from the Schatzalp, the world-at-large is neither a charnel house, nor a prison yard, nor a psychiatric ward, nor a café-philo. From the dry, clear, serene and piercing charm of the Schatzalp's perspective, civilization is but a thin, transparent and fragile veneer over humanity's perennial barbarism and congenital savagery, applied and maintained by the few for the many, by dint of profound vision, prodigious effort, unstinting optimism, courageous leadership and consummate civility. The masses – now billions – of civilization's beneficiaries are fed, clothed, sheltered, networked, acculturated, employed, amused and retired by processes they barely understand, but upon which their very lives, limbs and longevities, along with their scant knowledge of the past and abundant hope for the future, are utterly reliant. They do not know where their food comes from, nor their clothing, nor their shelter, nor their electricity, nor their fuel, nor their entertainment, nor their scant knowledge, nor their abundant hope.

Those who view the world from the Schatzalp do know these things, and more, for they are charged with providing them. For the most part, they tirelessly sustain, defend, implement and improve the blueprint for our global civilization. Those who err on the side of avarice, and indulge in excess for its own sake, are justly sent to prison like common criminals. But the majority of the business and political leaders whom I have met safeguard the manual of best practices for a decent life, a commodious society, and a prosperous humanity. Without them, anarchy would prevail, evil triumph, and suffering proliferate even more than it does despite their best efforts. Yet the masses are given to protest this civilized state of affairs, egged on by radical agitators or naïve reformers; preyed on by murderous revolutionaries or maniacal gangsters; harried by hustlers, swindlers, parasites and bureaucrats – the endless baggage-train of camp-followers that civilization is condemned to pull.

Viewed from the Schatzalp in these early years of the 21st century, the world today is a more ample study in contradiction than a sanatorium brimming with cloned Settembrinis could fathom. It is at once a more hopeful place than Lodovico could have imagined, and yet a place of greater despair than he could have feared. Human progress remains both credible and measurable, yet has developed even greater resistance to metaphysical analyses. Human regress too remains, incredible at times yet no less irreversible, compassed partly by the scope of meta-dialogue between philosophers and psychiatrists, but lying well beyond their joint and several capacities to redress. Here even Bacon may have erred – not all knowledge is power, if by power we mean more than understanding – while Ecclesiastes hit nearer the mark: "For in much wisdom is much vexation; and he that increaseth knowledge increaseth sorrow." And Lord Acton too was quite mistaken: Not all power corrupts. In actuality, power can even purify, as long as its wielder judiciously tempers a Nietzschean Weltanschauung with a Kantian good will, and exercises contemplation in quintessential quietude, avoiding Promethean flames and eschewing Daedalian wings alike.

"Human reason needs only to *will* more strongly than fate, and it *is* fate."
– Thomas Mann, *The Magic Mountain*

References

Fromm, E. 1973. *The Anatomy of Human Destructiveness*, New York: Holt, Rinehart & Winston.
Genis, A. 2003. "Maieutics and Philosophy", 4th Virtual Congress of Psychiatry, 10/02/03, http://www.psiquiatria.com/interpsiquis2003/9661.
Hall, R.C.W., Popkin, M.K., Devaul, R., et al. 1978. "Physical illness presenting as psychiatric disease", *Arch Gen Psychiatry*, 35: 1315-1320.
Marinoff, L. 1995. "On the Emergence of Ethical Counseling: Considerations and Two Case Studies", in: Lahav, R. and Tillmanns, M. (eds.) *Essays on Philosophical Counseling*. Lanham, MD: University Press of America, 171-191.
Marinoff, L. 1999. *Plato Not Prozac*, New York: HarperCollins.
Marinoff, L. 2003. *The Big Questions*, New York and London: Bloomsbury.
Reeves, R.R. 2000. "Unrecognized medical emergencies admitted to psychiatric units", *Am J Emerg Med*, 18(4): 390-393.
Rosenhan, D. L. 1973. "On being sane in insane places", *Science*, 179: 250-257.
Talbot-Stern, J.K. 2000. "Psychiatric manifestations of systemic illness", *Emerg Med Clin North Am*, 18(2): 199-209, vii-viii.

Ten Principles of Values-Based Medicine (VBM)[1]

K.W.M. (Bill) Fulford

Values-Based Medicine (VBM) is the theory and practice of effective health-care decision-making for situations in which legitimately different (and hence potentially conflicting) value perspectives are in play.

As a theory, VBM is the values-counterpart of Evidence-Based Medicine, or EBM. VBM and EBM are both responses to the growing complexity of decision-making in healthcare: EBM is a response to the growing complexity of the relevant *facts*; VBM is a response to the growing complexity of the relevant *values* (see Principles 1-5, Table 1, and Table 2 below). As a practice, VBM is a skills-based counterpart of the currently dominant quasi-legal form of clinical bioethics. Quasi-legal ethics prescribes good *outcomes* in the form of increasingly complex ethical rules and regulations. VBM emphasizes the importance of good *process* in the form particularly of improved clinical practice skills (see Principles 6-10, Table 1, and Table 3 below).

The Theory

1st Principle of VBM
All decisions stand on two feet, on values as well as on facts, including decisions about diagnosis (the "two feet" principle)

2nd Principle of VBM
We tend to notice values only when they are diverse or conflicting and hence are likely to be problematic (the "squeaky wheel" principle)

3rd Principle of VBM
Scientific progress, in opening up choices, is increasingly bringing the full diversity of human values into play in all areas of healthcare (the "science driven" principle)

4th Principle of VBM
VBM's "first call" for information is the perspective of the patient or patient group concerned in a given decision (the "patient-perspective" principle)

5th Principle of VBM
In VBM, conflicts of values are resolved primarily, not by reference to a rule prescribing a "right" outcome, but by processes designed to support a balance of legitimately different perspectives (the "multi-perspective" principle)

1 First published in: Radden, J. (Ed) The Philosophy of Psychiatry: A Companion. New York: Oxford University Press 2004. Reprinted with kind permission.

The Practice

6th Principle of VBM
Careful attention to language use in a given context is one of a range of powerful methods for raising awareness of values (the "values-blindness" principle)

7th Principle of VBM
A rich resource of both empirical and philosophical methods is available for improving our knowledge of other people's values (the "values-myopia" principle)

8th Principle of VBM
Ethical Reasoning is employed in VBM primarily to explore differences of values, not, as in quasi-legal bioethics, to determine "what is right" (the "space of values" principle)

9th Principle of VBM
In VBM, communication skills have a substantive rather than (as in quasi-legal ethics) a merely executive role in clinical decision-making (the "how it's done" principle)

10th Principle of VBM
VBM, although involving a partnership with ethicists and lawyers (equivalent to the partnership with scientists and statisticians in EBM), puts decision-making back where it belongs, with users and providers at the clinical coal-face (the "who decides" principle)

Table 1: 10 Principles of Values-Based Medicine (VBM)[2]

Philosophy and Values-Based Medicine

VBM is derived primarily from philosophical value theory, i.e. that part of ethics (and of aesthetics) that is concerned with the logic, with the meanings and implications, of value terms (paradigmatically, good, bad, right, etc; and, in aesthetics, beauty). VBM draws on philosophical value theory particularly as developed through careful attention to language use.[3]

---

2 Adapted from Fulford, K.W.M. (forthcoming) *Values-Based Medicine: Effective Healthcare Decision-Making in the Context of Value Diversity.* Cambridge: Cambridge University Press.

3 This approach, associated particularly with Oxford analytic philosophy, is sometimes called the "Oxford school". Exemplars include Philippa Foot (1959), R.M. Hare (1952; 1963), J.O. Urmson (1950) and G.J. Warnock (1971). Although focusing particularly on moral values, philosophical value theory seeks to characterize the logical properties of value terms of all kinds. Von Wright defined several hundred kinds of values in his compendious, The Varieties of Goodness (von Wright 1963). In the current pandemic of ethical issues in medicine, we tend to forget that many other kinds of value bear on decision-making at all levels in healthcare, policy, managerial, clinical, and indeed in research (see Sadler, 1996; also Principle 1 below.)

Being an analytic rather than substantive branch of philosophy[4], philosophical value theory has in recent years been largely neglected in favour of ethical theories seeking to establish what for want of a better word might be called moral "facts" (see, e.g., MacIntyre 1985 and Dancy 1993). The charge against philosophical value theory has been that, if not actually incoherent, it has little relevance to practical issues (Williams 1985).[5] Bioethics, similarly, while drawing extensively on substantive ethical theories such as deontology (in rights-based codes connecting ethics with law), consequentialism (as in health economics (Williams 1995), and virtue theory (in professional education, e.g. May 1994), has made little use of philosophical value theory. Yet it is precisely in being an *analytic* discipline that philosophical value theory is a potentially rich resource for an *empirical* discipline like healthcare.[6] In my *Moral Theory and Medical Practice* (1989) I showed how ideas derived from philosophical value theory help to transform the traditional fact-centred "medical" model of the conceptual structure of healthcare into a more balanced fact+value model. VBM is the practitioner's "cut" of this fact+value model of healthcare.[7]

VBM: The Theory (Principles 1-5)

As noted above, VBM stands to the values bearing on clinical decision-making much as Evidence-Based Medicine (EBM) stands to the facts (see Table 2). There is of course considerable debate, not least among those concerned with the development of EBM (Eddy 1991, Hudson Jones 1999, Straus et al. 1999), as to whether, in its current form, EBM is a sufficient response to the "fact" side of healthcare decision-making. A fact+value model, nonetheless, suggests that in the increasingly complex environment of modern healthcare, to the extent that we need EBM (albeit an enlightened EBM), so, too, do we need VBM.

Principles 1-5 of VBM thus define the theory of VBM as a values-counterpart of EBM. For Principles 1-3, as we will see, VBM and EBM run closely parallel. For Principles 4 and 5, VBM and EBM are anti-parallel, though still complementary (see Table 2).

---

4 E.g. a branch of philosophy that is concerned to clarify meanings rather than (directly) to produce "answers".

5 I return to the practical importance of analytic ethical theory below, see especially footnote 16.

6 Cf. the contribution of mathematics to the physical sciences.

7 The ten principles of VBM outlined in this chapter are based on Fulford KWM, Values-Based Medicine (forthcoming) Cambridge: Cambridge University Press.

	VBM (Values-Based Medicine)	EBM (Evidence-Based Medicine)
Principles of VBM	**Similarities**	
1. The "two feet" principle	Key role in clinical decision-making (the values input)	Key role in clinical decision-making (the fact input)
2. The "squeaky wheel" principle	VBM a response to growing complexity of values	EBM a response to growing complexity of facts
3. The "science driven" principle	Complexity (of values) generated primarily by scientific progress	Complexity (of facts) generated primarily by scientific progress
	Differences	
4. The "patient-perspective" principle	At the top of the "values hierarchy" are the value perspectives of individual patients or patient groups	At the top of the "evidence hierarchy" are facts which are as perspective-free as possible
5. The "multi-perspective" principle	Disagreements over values are resolved primarily by processes which seek to balance legitimately different value perspectives	Disagreements over facts are resolved primarily by research methods aimed at establishing perspective-free facts

Table 2: VBM and EBM

- Values and Clinical Decision-Making

1st Principle of VBM: All decisions stand on two feet, on values as well as on facts, including decisions about diagnosis. (The "two feet" principle)

The origins of VBM, then, are in the growing complexity of the values involved in all areas of healthcare decision-making. The most obvious evidence of this growing complexity is the recent explosion of ethical issues. But values come in many varieties, epistemic, aesthetic and prudential, for example, as well as moral and ethical; they also take different logical forms (e.g. needs, wishes, desires); they have many origins (e.g. personal, professional, cultural); and they have a rich grammar (encompassing nouns, verbs, adverbs, etc). Matters are further complicated by the fact that the very word "value", besides its central use of judgements of good and bad, has a number of other meanings.[8]

8 As when mathematicians speak of evaluating an equation, for example.

VBM is concerned with values in healthcare in the central sense of the term, as covering any judgement of good and bad. A unifying feature of such judgements, as a former White's Professor of Moral Philosophy in Oxford, Richard M. Hare, pointed out, is that they are prescriptive or *action-guiding* (Hare 1952).

It is this action-guiding property of values which explains why values are one of the two feet on which all decisions in healthcare (and indeed in any other context) stand. All our decisions, conscious or unconscious, deliberative or reflective, are guided in part by matters of fact. EBM, as I noted a moment ago, is a response to the growing complexity of the facts guiding clinical decision-making. But values, too, are essential. We need facts to guide our decisions; but we also need values. This is illustrated by the relatively straight-forward decision about prescribing lithium given in Box 1.

Box 1 –
Diane Abbot's (overtly evidence-based) decision to start on lithium

Diane Abbot, a 64-year old artist and art historian, was referred by her GP (family doctor) to a psychiatrist, Dr Kirk.[9] She had a history of occasional but increasingly disruptive episodes of hypomania. One of her academic colleagues had been successfully treated for a similar condition with lithium. She wanted to discuss the latest evidence on efficacy, on possible adverse side effects, etc., before deciding whether to start on lithium herself. The resources of EBM were essential to this process. Combined with Dr Kirk's individual expertise, and Diane Abbot's understanding of her colleagues' experience, the resources of EBM allowed everyone concerned to be satisfied that her eventual decision to start on lithium was securely evidence-based. But values, too, although not explicitly part of the decision-making process, were also essential. For without values those concerned would have had no basis on which to take a decision "on the evidence". In any decision about treatment, then, EBM is an increasingly essential resource. But it is the *values*, implicit or explicit, attaching respectively to clinical *effectiveness*, to *cost*, to *adverse* side-effects, and so forth, which have to be balanced in coming to a decision in a given case.

The importance of values in treatment decisions is relatively self-evident. The fact+value model of VBM, though, suggests that values are important also in

9 Diane Abbot's story is described in Fulford, forthcoming (Evidence-Based Medicine: Thomas Szasz' Legacy to Twenty-First Century Psychiatry).

areas of healthcare decision-making that, in the traditional fact-centred medical model, have been assumed to be exclusively matters for science, notably diagnosis. Principle 2 of VBM explains why this is so.

- Values Visible and Invisible

2nd Principle of VBM: We tend to notice values only when they are diverse or conflicting and hence are likely to be problematic. (The "squeaky wheel" principle)

Values are sometimes more and sometimes less visible in relation to healthcare decision-making. For example, values are highly visible in the current furore over whether cheap anti-AIDS drugs should be made available for developing countries. By contrast, values are more or less invisible in a "crash team's" decision over what drugs to use in a cardiac emergency.

The fact that values fall on a scale, from implicit to explicit, from invisible to visible, has led many to think of decisions in medicine as being divided into two distinct types, scientific and ethical. On this view, the anti-AIDS drug manufacturer's decision is a matter for ethics while the crash team's decision is a matter for science. It is on this view, too, that as noted at the end of the last section, treatment in general is considered a matter *inter alia* for ethics while diagnosis is considered a matter exclusively for science.

A different way of interpreting the visible/invisible scale of values, which again we owe to Hare and others in the "Oxford school", is that it is a function of *diversity*. Hare pointed out that where values are uniform, where they are largely shared, they tend to be implicit. It is only where values are *not* shared, where *different* values are operative in a given context, that they tend to become visible (Hare 1952, 1963). Thus, the crash team's decisions are driven by the shared value of saving the life of their patient. The furore over anti-AIDS drugs, by contrast, directly reflects a clash of clinical and commercial values. This is a case of what is sometimes said to be "the squeaky wheel getting the grease!" As Box 2 illustrates, it is only where values cause trouble, it is only when there is conflict or disagreement over them, that we notice they are there.

Box 2 –
Diane Abbot's (overtly values-based) decision to stop lithium

A few months after starting on lithium, Diane Abbot returned to Dr Kirk with a letter from her GP explaining that she had decided to stop taking lithium. He, the GP, was concerned about this because her mood had been well stabilized and she had had no significant side effects "medically speaking". The implication was, could Dr Kirk make her see sense? Diane Abbot explained that although she had had no "real" problem with the lithium, and that although her mood had indeed been more stable, she could no longer "see colours". No, she did not mean colour blind! But colours had lost their emotional intensity, which, for her as an artist, was a disaster. She recognized her GP's concerns, which were indeed shared by her colleagues – that in her hypomanic episodes she risked embarrassing and potentially costly consequences of her disinhibited behaviour. But from her point of view, what mattered above all was her work as an artist. This was why she had decided to stop taking lithium.[10]

Whereas, therefore, Diane Abbot's decision to start lithium (described in Box 1) was overtly evidence-based, her decision to stop lithium was overtly values-based. Both decisions, of course, on closer inspection, are seen to be based on facts (evidence) as well as values. In the present case, the relevant fact was that lithium was blunting Diane Abbot's appreciation of colour. There is evidence, from personal narratives (Jamison 1996 as well as from wider field trials (Keller et al. 1992)), that a degree of blunting of normal mood is a common side effect of lithium. It is a side effect to which little attention has been paid because, to most people, it is relatively unimportant. Hence it did not figure in the evidence-based discussions which led to Diane Abbot's decision to start on lithium. Had Diane Abbot appreciated the extent to which lithium might impair her ability to "really see" colours, her values as an artist might have surfaced more explicitly at that stage. In the event it was only when her values led to her decision to stop treatment, it was only when her values thus became discrepant with those of her GP and colleagues, that they became fully visible. The same principle, of values tending to become visible only when they are discrepant, explains the overtly value-laden nature of psychiatric diagnosis compared with diagnosis in most areas of physical medicine (see text).

Hare's interpretation of the visible/invisible scale of values can now be applied to the relative visibility of values in relation to treatment decisions compared with decisions about diagnosis. In the traditional fact-centred model of medicine, as noted above, diagnosis is assumed to be essentially a matter for medical science. This is because in most of medicine diagnosis does indeed appear to be value free. But this in turn, according to Hare's interpretation, is because

10 She was reluctant to experiment with lower doses of lithium (she had started at the bottom of the normal "therapeutic" range). Instead she worked out with Dr Kirk and her GP an advance directive for early intervention with further hypomanic episodes (see below, Box 3).

in the acute, life-threatening and often painful conditions with which medicine has traditionally been concerned, the operative values are largely shared. A "heart attack" (myocardial infarction), for example, involving as it does severe physical pain and imminent death, is, in and of itself, a bad condition by anyone's standards. Over such conditions, that is to say, our values are largely shared; hence they tend not to be problematic; hence, consistently with Hare's interpretation of the visible/invisible scale, the values involved in taking a heart attack to be a *bad* condition (and, hence, to this extent a disease[11]), go largely unnoticed. Yet the values are there, nonetheless.

The values involved in diagnosis come close to being fully visible in psychiatry.[12] Indeed, psychiatric diagnostic classification is more overtly value-laden than its counterparts in other areas of medicine in no less than four respects: 1) the language of psychiatry's official classifications such as the American *Diagnostic and Statistical Manual,* is value-laden, 2) some of the specific categories are defined in part by value judgements (e.g. personality disorders and the paraphilias), 3) the differential diagnosis of many psychiatric disorders includes moral categories (e.g. alcoholism v. drunkenness, psychopathy v. delinquency, hysteria v. malingering), and 4) Criterion B (social/occupational dysfunction) for schizophrenia, and corresponding criteria for other functional psychoses, are overtly evaluative in form.

The diagnosis of functional psychotic disorders makes fully explicit the need for a fact+value conceptual framework for diagnosis. What is required for a diagnosis of schizophrenia, say, is *both* the presence of certain specific experiences and/or behaviours (defined descriptively and listed under Criterion A) *and* a change in social and/or occupational functioning which is a change

---

11 The value judgements involved in taking a condition to be a disease/illness, etc., express not just negative value but a particular *kind* of negative value, i.e. disease is different from ugliness (negative aesthetic value), delinquency (negative moral value), foolishness (negative prudential value), etc. The characterization of the particular kind of negative value expressed by disease, illness, etc., is an important task for philosophy particularly in relation to psychiatry: see my *Moral Theory and Medical Practice*, chapters 6-10, and work by the Swedish philosopher, Lennart Nordenfelt (1987), for one approach to this via agency. VBM, however, as presented here, is not dependent on this further characterization. A negative value judgement, according to this approach, is at least a necessary, albeit not sufficient, prerequisite for a condition to be a disease/illness; and VBM is based on the generic properties shared by all value terms rather than the properties that mark out "medical" value judgements from value judgements of other kinds.

12 See, Fulford 1989, chapters 8 and 9; also 1994a. For an account of Criterion B for schizophrenia and the dependence of the differential diagnosis between psychosis and religious experience on value judgements, see Jackson and Fulford 1997. Values in the diagnosis of manic-depressive disorder are discussed in Moore, Hope and Fulford 1994. For recent work on values in psychiatric diagnosis, see the edited collection by John Sadler (2002), *Descriptions & Prescriptions: Values, Mental Disorders, and the DSMs*; and his forthcoming monograph, *Values and Psychiatric Diagnosis*.

for the worse (defined by one or more of the negative value judgements specified by Criterion B). The same fact+value framework is implicit in all areas of medicine. In other areas, though, the evaluative element remains implicit because the operative values are largely shared. There is no 'Criterion B' for a heart attack, not because the diagnosis of a heart attack is *more* scientific than that of schizophrenia, but because a heart attach is *less* complex evaluatively. A heart attack, as described above, is a bad condition by anyone's standards. Hence the evaluative part of the diagnosis is unproblematic. Hence it can be (and properly is) ignored in practice.

In the traditional fact-centred medical model, the more value-laden nature of psychiatric diagnosis is taken to be a mark of the (supposedly) primitive state of psychiatric science (Boorse 1976, Phillips 2000). In the fact+value model supporting VBM, it is a mark of the evaluatively (as well as scientifically) more complex nature of psychiatry. Psychiatry, that is to say, and consistently with Hare's interpretation of the visible/invisible scale of values, is concerned with areas of human experience and behaviour, such as emotion, desire, volition and belief, over which human values vary widely and legitimately. This is why we need a Criterion B for the diagnosis of schizophrenia but not for a heart attack. Schizophrenia is evaluatively (as well as descriptively) complex. A heart attack is not.

- More Science equals More Values not Less

3rd Principle of VBM: Scientific progress, in opening up choices, is increasingly bringing the full diversity of human values into play in all areas of healthcare. (The "science driven" principle)

The "squeaky-wheel" principle, however, raises a question: human values, we must assume, have always been diverse. So why should it be only now, in the first years of the twenty-first century, that values have become so visible in medicine? From the perspective of the traditional fact-centred medical model, this is counter-intuitive. According to the traditional model, as science progresses so the importance of values in healthcare will become less not more. The fact+value model of VBM, by contrast, as we will see in this section, anticipates that as science progresses, so the importance of values in healthcare should become, as thus far they have become, more not less.

The increasing visibility of values in healthcare at this time is capable of different interpretations. Some ethicists and lawyers see it as a case of medicine finally waking up, or finally being woken up, to ethical issues: and about time too, is the implication! Hare's interpretation of the visible/invisible scale of values, however, that the degree to which values are visible is a function of diversity, suggests rather that medicine has been moving from a time when the operative values were shared to a time in which they are increasingly divergent. The growing visibility of values in medicine, Hare's interpretation suggests, reflects a growing diversity of the values guiding decision-making in healthcare.

So where has this growing diversity come from? We do not have to look far for possible candidates. First, there is the diversity of values themselves, noted above. Needs, wishes, interests, etc., may all be relevant to, and yet all pull in different directions in medicine. Then again, there is the variety of origins of values: individual, cultural, professional. Again, these may pull in different directions. A third source of diversity, less well recognized but no less important, is the diversity of our values as individual human beings. For human values differ widely and legitimately, from person to person, for the same person in different contexts or at different times, from culture to culture, and at different historical periods (Fulford, Dickenson and Murray 2002a).

These sources of diversity of values, however, are all largely static. Hence there must have been some other factor or factors involved in opening the stopcock, as it were, in letting the diversity of human values through into medicine at the present time. Again, we do not have to look far for likely candidates, some external and others internal to medicine. Externally, there is our increasing individualism (we are less inclined to take our values from each other), and our rejection of authority (of handed-down values). There is also global travel and communication (exposing us to a wider range of values) and our increasingly cosmopolitan society (bringing different cultural values into direct contact).

In addition to these external factors, however, significant as they have been, there is a factor of even greater importance which is internal to medicine, namely *scientific progress.* On the traditional fact-centred medical model noted above, this may sound a bit far-fetched, viz. that scientific progress, instead of increasingly eliminating values from medicine, is actually letting them in. But the link between scientific progress and the growing visibility of values in medicine is in fact entirely straightforward. It is that scientific progress increasingly *opens up choices,* and with choices go *values.* So long as I have no choice in a given situation, my values are irrelevant. It is only where I *have* a choice that my values become relevant to guiding the choice I make. This is illustrated for psychiatry by the story of Diane Abbot, in Box 3. But in all areas of healthcare, technological and scientific advances are increasingly giving us an ever wider range of choices over an ever wider range of aspects of our lives.[13]

---

13 Reproductive medicine is a case in point. Even a few years ago, reproductive medicine was concerned mainly with major pathology, like "impacted foetus" or infertility, over which people's values are largely shared (like a 'heart attack', these are *bad* conditions, in themselves, for anyone). But now a series of remarkable advances in "assisted reproduction" are giving

Box 3 – Science gives Diane Abbot choices

Diane Abbot's decisions were made possible by advances in the medical sciences underpinning psychiatry. Without the Australian psychiatrist John Cade's original observation of the mood stabilising properties of lithium, and subsequent studies clarifying its effects and side effects, Diane Abbot would not have been in a position to start on lithium. Equally importantly, though, without the availability of other options for managing her hypomanic mood swings, she might not have been in a position to stop taking lithium. Had her options been either to take lithium and to continue working albeit with less emotional intensity, or to stop lithium and risk potentially damaging periods of hypomania, she might well have opted for lithium. As it was, she worked out with Dr Kirk, her psychiatrist, an 'advance directive', which she agreed with her GP and colleagues, on the basis of which they could insist on early treatment with neuroleptics, if necessary as an involuntary in-patient, when she showed warning signs of a relapse. This was a feasible strategy in Diane Abbot's case because her warning signs were clear-cut, notably that she stopped sleeping and that she consistently misinterpreted these signs, at the time, as "entering a productive phase". But Diane Abbot's decision to stop lithium, nonetheless, was made possible, ultimately, by science. It was science which made lithium available and it was science which made the alternatives to lithium available. The sciences, particularly the "brain" sciences, have had a bad press recently. For many in the user movement, indeed, there has been something of a moral imperative to refuse treatments, such as ECT, even where an individual has found such treatments helpful (Perkins 2001). But as Peter Campbell, a user advocate who writes about his own experience of manic-depressive illness, has pointed out, what matters, is not that a particular treatment is or is not used. What matters is that the use or otherwise of a given treatment is guided primarily by the values of the person receiving it (Campbell 1996). In psychiatry, as described in the text, the values guiding treatment decisions are necessarily diverse (i.e., because human values are inherently diverse in the areas of experience and behaviour with which psychiatry is concerned). But scientific progress, in opening up an ever wider range of choices, is increasingly allowing the full diversity of human values through into clinical decision-making in all areas of medicine.[14]

---

us choices in areas that until recently were the stuff of science fiction: we can reverse the menopause, we can select foetuses, we are close to "designer" babies. Small wonder, then, that the full diversity of human values has been brought into play in this area of medicine!

14 The effect of scientific progress in opening up choices and hence bringing the full diversity of

- Patient Centred Practice

4th Principle of VBM: VBM's "first call" for information is the perspective of the patient or patient group concerned in a given decision. (The "patient-perspective" principle)

Thus far we have seen that values guide all decisions (Principle 1), that values become visible where they are diverse rather than shared (Principle 2), and that they are becoming increasingly visible in medicine because scientific progress, through opening up choices, is allowing the full diversity of human values into play in healthcare decision-making (Principle 3). In these three respects, as anticipated above, VBM runs parallel with EBM (see Table 2). We now come to two respects in which EBM and VBM, although still complementary, run anti-parallel.

The first anti-parallel between VBM and EBM is in their respective "first calls" for information. In EBM, our first call is objective information, i.e. information which is as free as possible from the particular subjective perspective of this or that individual or group. The aim of science, classically conceived, is what the American philosopher, Thomas Nagel, has called the "view from nowhere" (Nagel, 1986). This is why, in EBM, the information derived from meta-analyses of high quality research is at the top of the "evidence hierarchy" (Sackett et al. 1997). Such information is as perspective-free as it is possible to get.

Box 4 –
Diane Abbot's values as the "first call" in her decision to start on lithium

Given the prominence afforded autonomy of patient choice in medicine, at least in industrialized countries (Okasha 2000), it may seem self-evident that when it came to stopping lithium, Diane Abbot's values should have taken precedence over those of her colleagues and GP. Importantly, though, her values were also the "first call" in her original decision to start treatment. Yet that decision, with hindsight, turned out to have been wrong, "wrong", that is, as judged by her values as an artist. Had her need to be able to "really see" colours been more apparent at the time, then the evidence of lithium's "emotional blunting" effects would probably have been discussed at that stage. Diane Abbot might still have decided to start

human values into other areas of medicine, is illustrated by a number of articles in Fulford, Dickenson and Murray 2002b: see e.g., J. Raphael-Leff on gamete donation and Paul Cain on cardio-pulmonary resuscitation.

on lithium; but with her eyes open to the possibility of this side effect; and with her GP, also, aware that this was a concern.
The skills which would have allowed Diane Abbot's values to have been more accurately weighed in the decision to start on lithium are discussed below (under Principles 6-9). It is worth noting, though, that Diane Abbot herself was guided to a significant extent by the positive experiences of her colleague on lithium. So this is not a case of being misled by a naïve use of EBM. Narrative, as well as meta-analytic, sources of evidence were in play. Yet still the wrong decision was made.[15] Things worked out well. But this was because of the way in which the subsequent decision to stop lithium was handled (see Box 5, below).

In VBM, by contrast, as Box 4 illustrates, our "first call" is the perspective of the particular patient (or group of patients) concerned in a given decision. This follows from the diversity of human values noted above. The point is that human values are not, merely, different but *legitimately* different.[16] Hence, in a given clinical situation, while we may have a great deal of general information about the values that are likely to be operative, and while such information is indeed an important part of the knowledge base of VBM (see Principle 7), it can never be a substitute for the *actual* values of the *particular* individuals concerned.

---

15 Or, more accurately, the right decision (to have a *trial* of lithium) on the wrong or incomplete grounds (because the possibility of emotional blunting had not been discussed).

16 The central importance of individual perspectives as our "first call" in VBM is sufficiently grounded on the given diversity of human values in healthcare (illustrated by the edited collection, Fulford, Dickenson and Murray 2002a). That our values are not only different but *legitimately* different also follows analytically from the logical separation of fact and value (or, more exactly, of description and evaluation) insisted on by "non-descriptivism" in philosophical value theory. The 18th century British empirist philosopher, David Hume, is generally credited with the first explicit account of the claim that no description of a state of affairs in the world can ever, in itself, add up to a value judgement of that state of affairs: "no ought from an is" is how Hume's "law" is often summarized. Hare is perhaps the clearest exponent of this position among twentieth century philosophers (Hare 1952). The opposing school, descriptivism, points to situations in which we feel compelled to make a given value judgement on the basis of a given description (e.g. Warnock 1971). Exponents of the Hume-Hare version of *non*-descriptivism argue that in such cases the "compulsion" to make a given value judgement is only a psychological not a logical compulsion. The compulsion, that is to say, arises from the fact that in response of the situation in question, most or even all people would in fact, human values being what they are, make the same value judgement. But this leaves the analytic separation (the separation of *meaning*) intact. In *Moral Theory and Medical Practice* (1989), and in two subsequent papers, Fulford 1999 and 2000a, I have argued that the Hume-Hare separation of fact and value applied to concepts of disease and illness has a rich crop of implications for practice in psychiatry and medicine. The phenomenology specifically of delusion, furthermore, has interesting implications for the

- Resolving Differences

5th Principle of VBM: In VBM, conflicts of values are resolved primarily, not by reference to a rule prescribing a "right" outcome, but by processes designed to support a balance of legitimately different perspectives. (The "multi-perspective" principle)

Principle 4, in centring VBM firmly on the values of the person (or group) concerned in a particular decision, is, in this rather precise sense, "patient-centred" (Fulford 1995). The diversity of human values, however, has a second and in a sense opposite corollary, namely that disagreements are *inevitable*. The given diversity of human values makes it inevitable that the values of a particular patient may well be different from those of their doctor; and both may be different from those of a nurse or social worker, or from those of the informal carers concerned, and so forth.

How, then, to resolve such differences? This brings us to the second anti-parallel between VBM and EBM. In EBM differences of view about the facts are resolved, in principle, by consensus: more facts (more data) are accumulated, crucial experiments are carried out, or a wider evidence-base is accessed, all with the aim of deciding which view is right. But when it comes to values, there may be no uniquely right view. And if Principles 2 and 3 of VBM are

---

debate about fact and value in philosophical value theory. (The traditional debate has been in "horizontal" terms, i.e. directly between fact and value: the phenomenology of delusion, however, in particular that delusions may take the form of value judgements as well as of factual beliefs, points to a "vertical" connection between fact and value, i.e. that both depend on and hence are (logically) related through, a background structure of practical reasoning; see Fulford 1989, ch. 10). Many of the practical implications of philosophical value theory, however, can be derived equally from descriptivist theory, to the extent that healthcare is concerned with areas in which human values are largely *shared* (Fulford 1991). The practical dangers of descriptivism arise from the temptation to extrapolate the claimed derivation of "values" from "facts" to areas in which human values are legitimately *different*. In such areas, i.e. in areas in which people's values are *not* shared, descriptivism is at risk of abusive consequences though imposing the values of one group or individual on those whose values are different. This risk is greatly increased through our tendency to underestimate the extent of the differences of values between us (see below, Principle 7). And it is a risk to which psychiatry, as an area of particular diversity of human values (Principle 3 above), has been peculiarly vulnerable in practice (Fulford 1998). In psychiatry, through much of the twentieth century, abusive practices arose, not primarily from malicious intent but through one person or group's beliefs about "best" practice being allowed to exclude all other views (Fulford 2000a and 2000b). In psychiatry, then, a non-descriptivist rather than descriptivist basis for VBM is required. VBM's Principle 3, furthermore, suggests that scientific progress is driving all areas of medicine increasingly into areas of value diversity. A non-descriptivist rather than descriptivist basis for VBM is thus likely to be increasingly important in all areas of medicine if we are to avoid the abusive imposition of one person's or group's values on others. See also Principle 10, below.

right, value diversity rather than uniquely right values, will become increasingly the norm in healthcare. Values-Based Medicine, then, aims to resolve differences, not by consensus but by what I have called elsewhere "dissensus" (Fulford 1998), i.e., by *processes which support effective action through a balance of legitimately different value perspectives.*

It will be worth looking at this notion of dissensus in a little more detail since it is at the heart of the practice of VBM. Thus, in the quasi-legal model of bioethics differences of values are resolved, in principle, by reference to a rule (embodied in a code or guideline and often supported by law), which has been settled in advance by consensus. Differences of interpretation may arise, of course. But these are settled, again in principle, by reference to a regulatory body with executive decision-making powers.[17] Quasi-legal bioethics is thus outcome-focused. It seeks to determine the outcome of decisions by reference to rules expressing particular values. In this respect quasi-legal bioethics is like EBM. Both are outcome-focused. Both, that is to say, aim to provide rules (or guidelines) on what to do in a given situation. These rules are based on consensus respectively on the facts (EBM) and the values (quasi-legal bioethics) guiding clinical decision-making.

Box 5 –
Diane Abbot's values and the "dissensual" basis of her decision to stop lithium

As noted in Box 2, and described in the text (under Principle 2), Diane Abbot's decision to stop lithium was overtly values-based because the operative values were contested. When she started on lithium her values were concordant with those of her GP and colleagues. But when it came to stopping lithium, what mattered to Diane Abbot was her ability to "really see" colours, while what mattered to her GP and colleagues was the potentially damaging effects of a further episode of hypomania. And her GP and colleagues had a point! Diane Abbot, when hypomanic, was a considerable liability to herself and to everyone else. Moreover, whatever her subjective impression, objectively her output as an artist had been enhanced rather than restricted while on lithium. Stabilising her mood may have taken some of the excitement out of her work; but this, in the view of her colleagues, was more than compensated for by her greater consistency. Even in her own terms, then, it seemed (to everyone else) imprudent, to say the least, that she should come off lithium.

17 In the UK, for example, the Human Fertilisation and Embryology Authority has such powers.

Quasi-legal ethics and VBM, in these circumstances, lead to the same outcome, that Diane Abbot should stop taking lithium. But whereas in quasi-legal ethics stopping lithium is an outcome prescribed by a rule expressing a "right" value (patient autonomy), in VBM stopping lithium is the product of a process aimed at achieving a balance of different, and legitimately different, values. As described in the text, the quasi-legal rule is justified by a (supposed) consensus (on the value of autonomy); whereas the VBM process, of balancing legitimately different value perspectives, starts from the premiss that there is often no one right perspective – hence the neologistic "dissensus". The shift in VBM from outcome to process, from *what* is done to *how* it is done, depends critically on the skills summarized under Principles 6-9 below.

VBM, as Box 5 illustrates for the case of Diane Abbot, shifts the emphasis from outcome to process. In VBM there is a clear place for rules and regulation in providing a framework for practice. Such a framework, as we will see at the start of the next section, is essential. In VBM, though, the framework of rules and regulation is limited to those values which for a given community are largely shared, and hence over which consensus (agreement on a particular value) is appropriate. A key insight of VBM, however, summarized in Principle 3 above, is that, as scientific advances open up choices, so diversity rather than shared values will increasingly become the norm in healthcare decision-making. Increasingly, then, dissensual, as well as consensual, approaches to clinical decision-making will be needed. Increasingly, that is to say, instead of relying solely or even primarily on rules and regulation to prescribe outcomes, we will need to develop processes which allow effective decision-making through a balance of legitimately different value perspectives.

This 'multi-perspective' approach, in the context of healthcare decision-making, depends critically on a number of key clinical skills. This is one specific sense in which VBM is process rather than outcome focused. In VBM, good clinical decision-making, in the increasingly values-diverse context of modern healthcare depends, in the well-worn phrase, not just on *what* is done but on *how* it is done. It is to the skills base of VBM that we turn in the next section.

VBM: The Practice (Principles 6-10)

As a strategy for resolving differences, dissensus, in VBM, is anti-parallel not only with EBM but also with bioethics. As a theoretical discipline, bioethics is a rich and varied discipline fully cognizant of the diversity of human values.

In its connections with practice, however, it has taken a predominantly quasi-legal form premised on the (generally unacknowledged) assumption of "right values". The growing mountain of ever-more complex rules and regulations governing all areas of healthcare aim to give effect to these right values: the rules tell us what the values are; regulatory bodies have executive authority to interpret the rules in equivocal cases.[18]

Principles of VBM	VBM (Values-Based Medicine)	Quasi-Legal Ethics
6. The "values-blindness" principle	Values important in all areas of healthcare	Values concerned with ethical issues
7. The "values-myopia" principle	Full range of empirical methods used for increasing knowledge of values	Empirical methods subject to prior values
8. The "space of values" principle	Ethical reasoning used to explore differences (the space of values)	Ethical reasoning used to decide "what is right"
9. The "how it's done" principle	Communication skills have substantive role	Communication skills have a merely executive role
10. The "who decides" principle	Primarily patients and practitioners	Primarily ethicists and lawyers

Table 3: VBM and Quasi-Legal Ethics

It is no part of VBM to suggest that we can do without rules and regulation altogether (Fulford and Bloch 2000). To the contrary, as already noted, VBM incorporates rules and regulation but as a framework for practice defined by the values shared within a given community.[19] Such values, then, set bench-

18 It is no coincidence that the form of ethical regulatory codes is similar to that of practice guidelines derived from EBM. Both assume a unique 'right' answer (in principle) for every situation; both assume that we approximate to the right answer by consensus. Quasi-legal bioethics, I have argued elsewhere, has indeed adopted this model (unwittingly) from scientific medicine (Fulford 2000b). In this respect, then, although developed originally as a guardian against the misuse of medical technology, bioethics has taken on the colours of its enemy!

19 VBM, in emphasising value diversity, might be thought to risk ethical relativism and, hence, ethical chaos! There are several reasons why this is not so: 1) Human values, if more diverse than has generally been recognized, at least in healthcare, are not chaotic (if they were, law, which is self-evidently values-based, would be chaotic!); 2) The shared values which, in VBM, are the proper remit of the rules and regulation of quasi-legal ethics, provide, for a given group, a framework for decision-making; 3) Where values are not shared, VBM starts not

mark outcomes against which decisions taken within the relevant community can be measured. By the same token, though, quasi-legal ethics is *in*appropriate in situations in which legitimately *different* values are in play.[20] In such situations, we should rely not on "good outcomes" but on "good process", not on *what* is done but on *how* it is done. The next four principles outline some of the key skills supporting the "how" of VBM.

- Skills Area 1 – Awareness of Values

6th Principle of VBM: Careful attention to language use in a given context is one of a range of powerful methods for raising awareness of values. (The "values blindness" principle)

At the heart of many of the problems with values in healthcare is what might be called "values blindness". Problems arise in practice, that is to say, not so much from direct conflicts of values as from a failure to recognize values for what they are. In multi-disciplinary teamwork, for example, a recent empirical study has shown that deep but largely unrecognized differences of values between psychiatrists, social workers, community nurses, patients and informal carers, may be a key factor behind failures of collaborative decision-making (Colombo et al. forthcoming, Fulford 2001).

This "values blindness" has many sources: the tendency of values to become invisible when shared (see principle 2, above); the development of professional identity (which includes a shared value system, Fulford 1994); and the success of science (tending to eclipse values and other humanities-related aspects of medicine, e.g. in medical education, Hope and Fulford 1993).

A key skill underpinning VBM, then, is greater awareness of where, what and how values come into healthcare. Improved knowledge of values, and the reasoning and communication skills described later in this chapter, all contribute to this. A distinct skill, however, is greater alertness to language

---

from the post modern "anything goes", but from a principle of *mutual* respect with a range of clear and definite implications for policy and practice (mutual respect, for example, precludes racism because racism is incompatible with respect for differences). Far from being a recipe for ethical chaos, then, VBM is more like the values-equivalent of a political democracy. Like a political democracy, VBM might be thought to be weaker than an authoritarian autocracy, such as a monarchy or a totalitarian regime. And in situations of extreme danger (e.g. war or famine) an autocracy may be more effective (indeed we declare "marshal law" when a single shared value of survival is at stake). But the lesson of the twentieth century is that totalitarian solutions, in our civilization, however well intentioned, collapse into abusive ideology; and that democracy, is, in practice, the stronger system (see also Principle 10, below).

20 I.e. because the "right" values expressed in the rules and regulations governing the decision in question will necessarily be in conflict with the necessarily different values of many of those to whom the rules and regulations are intended to apply. See also below, Principle 10.

use, to the words and phrases actually used in a given context. This approach is based on the work of the Oxford philosopher, J.L. Austin (Austin 1956/7). Austin argued for what he called "philosophical field work", i.e. rather than just thinking about meanings in the abstract, Austin said that we should examine the language people actually use as a guide to understanding. This approach has been applied as a method of enquiry across a range of issues in the philosophy of psychiatry (Fulford 1990), and, combined with empirical social science methods, in research (Fulford 2001). It is illustrated for the case of Diane Abbot in Box 6.

Box 6 – Awareness of the values operative in Diane Abbot's case

As described in the text, a first, and essential, skill for VBM is raised awareness of values. The effectiveness of linguistic analysis, of careful attention to language use, as a method for raising awareness of values is illustrated by the account of the opening stage in Diane Abbot's story in Box 1. In the first part of this Box, Diane Abbot's overtly evidence-based decision to start on lithium was described in the language of a clinical case history. Here we were concentrating on the message, viz., the importance of EBM, combined with Dr Kirk's clinical experience and Diane Abbot's legal colleague's positive personal experience, as the basis of her decision. In the second part of the Box, by contrast, we were made aware of the significance of values, alongside evidence, in her decision. This was done by standing back for a moment from the message (the importance of EBM) and looking at the actual words in which the message (as a standard clinical case history) was delivered. The key words, italicized in Box 1, were *value* words – "effectiveness", "cost" and "adverse". The values awareness workshop and other new training initiatives, described in the text, are based on this linguistic-analytic approach.

Recently this language-based approach has been developed as part of a new training programme in values-based practice for healthcare professionals (nurses, social workers, psychologists, etc.) working in such areas as assertive outreach, community care and acute in-patient care. In this context, in particular, Austin's methodology has turned out to be a particularly powerful method for raising awareness of the often very wide differences of values between different team members, and between providers and users of services (Fulford, Woodbridge and Williamson 2002).

Having raised awareness of the extent to which values permeate healthcare, however, what is the next step? Where do we go from there?

- Skills Area 2 – Knowledge of Values

7th Principle of VBM: A rich resource of both empirical and philosophical methods is available for improving our knowledge of other people's values. (The "values-myopia" principle)

Where Principle 6 is concerned with values blindness, Principle 7 is concerned with "values myopia", i.e. with our tendency, even when aware of values, to assume that other people's values are the same as our own. Within health-care this tendency is evident, for example, both in clinical interactions and, on a larger scale, in needs assessment (Marshall 1994) and service planning (Campbell 1996). But values myopia, as Box 7 illustrates, may have subtle and complex interactions with the evidence-base of practice.

Box 7 – Knowledge of the values operative in Diane Abbot's case

Knowledge of values in VBM includes knowledge both of the extent of the *differences* between people in their values and of the extent to which people *underestimate* these differences: we all tend to assume that other people's values are similar to our own. In Diane Abbot's case this "values myopia" (see text) led to one of the fault lines in her original decision to start lithium. The evidence-base for this decision, in so far as it was derived from EBM, was the effects and side-effects of lithium as characterized by the results of meta-analyses of high-quality research. But the effects and side-effects described in such studies are picked out by reference to values which are widely shared – an "effect" of a drug is one which is positively valued by most people in most contexts, a side-effect is one which is negatively valued by most people in most contexts.

There is nothing wrong with this as such. To the contrary, such values, positive and negative, are essential: they pick out, severally, variables (the effects and side-effects) relevant to a given research paradigm; and taken together, they determine whether the research is "worth" doing in the first place. But a failure to recognize the (inevitable and appropriate) skewing of research towards values that are largely shared, can lead to decisions which fail to reflect the sometimes very different values of a given individual in a particular context. The emotional blunting side-effect of lithium was known. But being a side effect of relative unimportance to most people, it had not figured prominently in EBM analyses of lithium, nor indeed in Dr Kirk's clinical experience. Hence, although emotional blunting turned out to be a key side effect from Diane Abbot's perspective as an artist, it was not on Dr Kirk's agenda in his initial discussion with her. Again, this is not a fault with EBM as such. Diane Abbot was equally misled by the narrative information from her colleague. The fault line runs rather from a "values-myopic" use of evidence, whether meta-analytic, clinical or experiential, in clinical decision-making.

A second skill underpinning VBM is thus, straightforwardly, knowledge of the values bearing, or likely to bear, on a given decision in a given context. Our resources in this respect are partly empirical, partly philosophical. Empirical methods for gaining better understanding of other people's values include first hand narratives (the growing "user literature", for example), the use of poetry and other literary sources, anthropological methods (such as ethnography), psychological techniques (cognitive-behavioural; psychoanalysis), and surveys. Among philosophical methods, Continental philosophy, which is more text-base than Anglo-American Analytic philosophy, is a rich resource. This includes phenomenology (concerned with the structure and content of experience) and hermeneutics (concerned with revealing meanings).[21]

There is no shortage of methods, then, empirical, literary, philosophical, and so forth, for building up our knowledge of the values likely to be operative in a given case. In some instances this may be enough to resolve difficulties; greater knowledge of the values in play in a given clinical context may help to remove misunderstandings, to increase mutual respect, and so forth. To understand all is to forgive all! Sometimes, though, conflicts and difficulties will remain. It is here that reasoning skills may be helpful.

- Skills Area 3 – Reasoning about Values

8th Principle of VBM: Ethical reasoning is employed in VBM primarily to explore ***differences*** *of values, rather than, as in quasi-legal bioethics, to determine "what is right". (The "space of values" principle)*

Methods for reasoning about values can be derived from any area of ethics (Dickenson and Fulford 2000, chapter 2). Methods commonly used in healthcare include consequentialism (e.g. the utilitarian basis of much health economics) and deontology (e.g. rights-based documents; and standards). In the clinical context, two methods have gained wide currency,

21 Illustrations of each of these resources, empirical and philosophical, with practical relevance for healthcare, and drawing on a rich international literature, are given in an anthology combining first-hand narratives from patients and carers with academic articles, poetry and other literary sources (Fulford, Dickenson and Murray 2002b). The aim of this anthology is two-fold: first, to illustrate the remarkable diversity of human values relevant to every aspect of healthcare decision-making (from first contact, through diagnosis to treatment and outcome); and second, to build up a picture of the extent of the arsenal of methods available for improving our knowledge of values in relation to health-care decision-making.

- principles – "top down" reasoning from general principles
- casuistry – "bottom up" reasoning, direct from cases.

All of these methods may be helpful in VBM. The aim of ethical reasoning in VBM, however, is radically different from its aim in the quasi-legal form of bioethics (Fulford, Dickenson and Murray 2002a). In quasi-legal ethics, as in legal reasoning itself, the aim is to decide "what is right". As noted above, this is appropriate where values are more or less shared. In VBM, by contrast, in the context of value *diversity*, the aim is rather to explore the nature and extent of *differences* of values. There are limits, of course, and these are reflected in the framework for practice provided by quasi-legal ethics and law (limited to situations where values are shared). But in situations of value diversity the first aim of ethical reasoning is to explore the "space of values" (Fulford and Bloch 2000).

Box 8 – Reasoning about the values operative in Diane Abbot's case

The fault line in Diane Abbot's original decision noted in Box 7, viz. a values-myopic use of evidence, illustrates the key difference between quasi-legal ethics and VBM in their approaches to reasoning about values. The quasi-legal aim of coming to an agreement on the "right" outcome (consensus), inevitably leads to a focus on shared values. This is especially true of casuistry, or case-based reasoning, the very justification of which is that agreement on actual cases reflects shared values (Fulford and Bloch 2000). Diane Abbot was, in a sense, guided in her decision to start lithium by casuistic reasoning, i.e. by the case of her colleague on lithium and his positive experience of that treatment.
The aim of ethical reasoning in VBM, by contrast, is to explore *differences* of values. In Diane Abbot's case, such reasoning might have alerted her, and Dr Kirk, to a key difference between herself and her colleague, viz. that whereas she was a creative artist, he was a lawyer. Both were successful academics whose work required high levels of sustained attention. For both, therefore, the attention disrupting effects of hypomania were highly negatively evaluated. But whereas for the lawyer emotional blunting was *de minimis* (it was not indeed a side effect of which he had even been aware), for the artist it was of the essence. Casuistic reasoning, it is important to add, is not the only way in which this difference of values might have been anticipated. Principles reasoning, although much criticized in bioethics, offers a powerful tool for exploring differences of values.[22]

---

22 Tom Beauchamp and James Childress, in their original description of the role of principles reasoning in medicine (Beauchamp and Childress 1989), are much closer to VBM than to

The radically different aim of ethical reasoning in VBM, i.e. to explore differences of values, has important implications for practice. These are illustrated by the case of Diane Abbot in Box 8. But it also carries with it a radically different way of thinking about differences of values themselves in healthcare. In quasi-legal ethics, the assumption of uniquely "right" values carries with it the implication that differences of values are a problem to be "solved" (by consensus, by *dictat*, or whatever means). The assumption in quasi-legal ethics is that differences of values are a barrier to effective clinical decision-making. In VBM, by contrast, differences of values, while indeed sometimes requiring resolution, may also be a *resource* for clinical decision-making. For as management theorists rather than ethicists have recognized (Heifetz 1994[23]), we are all better at understanding other people's values when they are similar to our own. In VBM, then, different value perspectives, as represented by different members of a multi-disciplinary team for example (see below), operate as a series of lenses or filters for highlighting the often very different value perspectives of individual clients or patients. Different value perspectives within the clinical team, on this VBM model, far from being an impediment to effective clinical decision-making, offer a positive resource for matching decisions as closely as possible to the values of those concerned.

There will be situations, though, in which, despite being fully aware of the origin of a problem in differences of values (Principle 6), and despite having fully explored the values concerned (Principles 7 and 8), conflicts still remain. This is inevitable (and indeed to be welcomed!) if, as VBM suggests, *legitimately* different value perspectives are the norm in healthcare. In healthcare, moreover, matters can never be left in the air (Fulford 1994). Practical situations demand practical action, even if this means leaving well alone. It is here that communication skills become important in VBM.

- Skills Area 4 – Communication Skills

9th Principle of VBM: In VBM, communication skills have a substantive rather than (as in quasi-legal ethics) a merely executive role in clinical decision-making. (The "how it's done" principle)

In VBM, awareness, knowledge and ethical reasoning are combined with communication skills to effect action. Educationally, this is an extension of a

---

quasi-legal ethics. Their "prima facie" principles are, in effect, dimensions along which the values operative in a given case can be analysed (Fulford, Dickenson and Murray 2002).

23 Heifetz was a psychiatrist before moving into management and leadership studies. His book, *Leadership Without Easy Answers*, develops a theory of "adaptive work" supported by a series of clear practical strategies for effective decision-making in contexts of conflicting values.

model of "ethics training" for medical students developed in Oxford, in which traditional ethics and law are fully integrated with communication skills in a clinical problem-solving approach to ethical reasoning (Hope, Fulford and Yates 1996).

A wide range of communication skills are important in VBM. Two particular kinds of skill stand out, though, as being essential.

- *Patient-perspective skills:* i.e., the skills of listening to and exploring the values of a client or patient. These are the basis of the patient-centred principle of VBM (Principle 4). Raised awareness (Principle 6), improved knowledge (Principle 7) and ethical reasoning (Principle 8) may all be helpful in this respect, particularly where there are difficulties of communication. But as Principle 4 emphasizes, the values of the particular individual concerned are irreducible.
- *Multi-perspective skills:* i.e., the skills involved in coming to a balance of values in situations of conflict and disagreement. These are the basis of the multi-perspective principle of VBM (Principle 5), the principle that replaces consensus with dissensus, i.e., with effective action in the context of legitimately different value perspectives. Relevant perspectives in healthcare include those of other colleagues (medical and non-medical), of informal carers, of managers, and so forth. Mutual understanding and respect are fundamental in this respect. But specific skills, such as negotiation and conflict resolution, are also essential.

Box 9 –
Communication skills and the values operative in Diane Abbot's case

Both patient-perspective and multi-perspective communication skills, as described in the text, were important to securing the good outcome achieved in Diane Abbott's case. These skills were especially important at the apparently unproblematic initial stage, i.e. when everyone agreed with Diane Abbot's decision to start on lithium. A quasi-legal approach would have endorsed Diane Abbot's choice on grounds of the "right" value of autonomy. As such, there would have been a risk of alienating her colleagues and GP when her decision to stop lithium ran counter to their concerns for her welfare: such concerns, expressed in terms of beneficence in Beauchamp and Childress' *Four Principles*, tend to be relabelled pejoratively in quasi-legal bioethics as "paternalistic".

In VBM, by contrast, the dissensual nature of decision-making starts from (the meta-value of) respect for differences of values. A pre-condition of such respect is that the voices of those concerned, of *all* those concerned, are listened to. This is not as easy as it sounds! First, it is time consuming – although the time spent in coming to an understanding of the relevant perspectives tends to pay off in the longer term through those concerned, as in Diane Abbot's case, feeling understood and fully engaged (see Principle 10, below). Second, it is not always easy to understand other people's values where they are different from one's own. As noted in the text, this is one reason (among many others) why the different value perspectives represented by a well functioning multi-disciplinary team may be crucial to good clinical care. These perspectives operate as a series of "lenses" sensitive to the different values operative in a given case. A further and increasingly important series of such lenses is provided by support groups and networks of those with first-hand experience of the situation in question. Talking with people who have "been through it" provides invaluable experiential information. Diane Abbot's lawyer colleague was helpful to her not just in starting lithium but also in her decision to stop it. Given the differences in their values, though, it might have been helpful, too, if Diane Abbot had been able to talk to someone from the creative arts with personal experience of lithium therapy. A key role of advocacy groups in VBM is to support decision-making by helping to put service users with similar backgrounds and experience in touch with each other.

Communication skills, although of course important also in quasi-legal ethics, have a deeper importance in VBM. In quasi-legal ethics communication skills are *executive*, their role being primarily to help in implementing the rules (which in turn are taken to express "right" values, see above). In VBM, by contrast, as Box 9 illustrates for the case of Diane Abbot, communication skills have a *substantive* role. In VBM, communication skills are central, 1) to establishing the different value perspectives bearing on a given situation (complementing, at an inter-personal level, the philosophical and empirical methods outlined above under Principles 6 – 8), and 2) to resolving a course of action where the operative value perspectives are genuinely in conflict. This is why, as noted under Principle 5 above, in VBM good practice depends not just on *what* is done but on *how* it is done.[24]

24 Exploring values may sound like a tall order (a luxury perhaps?) in the contingencies of day-to-day practice. But the practical importance of values in modern healthcare has been recognized in the UK by the priority afforded values in the work of the National Institute for Mental Health (England). The NIMHE is a department of the Modernization Agency in the UK's National Health Service (NHS) with responsibility for implementing the UK government's key strategy for mental health, the National Service Framework for Mental Health. The first action of the NIMHE was to establish a Values Project Group to develop a framework of values and, importantly, a "process for implementation" (Ministerial Announcement, 2001), for all stakeholders, both users and providers, in mental health. The Values Project Group is working in partnership with each of the other NIMHE programmes, including such key areas as recovery practice, equality, inclusion and "users as experts". Its work is also connected

- Taking back the territory

10th Principle of VBM: VBM, although involving a partnership with ethicists and lawyers (equivalent to the partnership with scientists and statisticians in EBM), puts decision-making back where it belongs, with users and providers at the clinical coal-face. (The "who decides?" principle)

Where Principles 6-9 of VBM are concerned with the skills base of decision-making in the context of value diversity, Principle 10 is concerned with "who decides?"

In quasi-legal ethics, the assumption of "right" values, and its consequent proliferation of rules and regulatory authorities, inevitably leads to a model of the ethicist as an expert. And ethicists, like scientists, may indeed bring a range of relevant expertise to policy, practice, education and research in healthcare. As we saw earlier, however, where legitimately different values are in play, the particular value prescribed by a quasi-legal ethical rule, however enlightened, will necessarily conflict with the very different values of many of those to whom the rule is intended to apply.

The complaint of ethicists against doctors has been "doctor knows best". Bioethics has thus rightly emphasized the importance of patient autonomy in healthcare decision-making. Quasi-legal ethics, however, if extended from areas of value uniformity to areas of value diversity, risks a new culture of "ethicist knows best" (Fulford, Dickenson and Murray 2002, Introduction). VBM, in starting from the legitimately different value perspectives increasingly in play in all areas of healthcare, puts ethical decision-making back where it belongs, with those concerned, as users and providers, as patients, professionals and as managers, at the clinical coal face.

Box 10 – 'Who decides?' and the outcome in Diane Abbot's case

The shift in the locus of decision-making in VBM from ethicists and lawyers to patients and professionals, carries with it a shift from rights to responsibilities. The "right values" of quasi-legal ethics creates a culture of legal rights. The meta-value of respect for differences in VBM creates a culture of mutual responsibility. In Diane Abbot's case, Dr Kirk's failure

---

with other NHS modernization initiatives, such as the Black and Ethnic Minority strategy. NIMHE thus recognizes that understanding patients' values and the values of colleagues is an *investment* in time. It is an up-front cost which could pay huge dividends in terms of the quality of the patient's experience, the job satisfaction of providers, compliance, responsiveness to change, and so forth.

to mention emotional blunting as a potential side-effect of lithium, might have led a rights-minded lawyer to consider an action for breach of duty of care. The action would probably not be pursued because the damages, in this case, were negligible. But an increasingly defensive approach to practice is the result of an over-reliance on such rights-based approaches. In Diane Abbot's case, the defensive strategy would have been to give her a checklist of potential side-effects of lithium and to ask her to "sign" a consent form, or such like. Instead, a positive relationship of trust was built up, between all those concerned, such that Diane Abbot, her colleagues and GP, all felt engaged in and hence a sense of ownership of, the decisions made.

This had a number of positive therapeutic effects. First, the experience of emotional blunting helped Diane Abbot to appreciate that her mood swings were not, as such, pathological, but (within limits) a positive aspect for her work as an artist. Second, it allowed her to take responsibility (with help from others) for managing future over-swings. As noted in the text, her positive decision to stop lithium was combined with an advance directive for early intervention in a future hypomanic episode. This was felt to be important (by Diane Abbot as well as her GP and colleagues) because of her lack of insight in the past into the warning signs of a relapse. In the event, when these signs eventually recurred it was Diane Abbot herself who initiated contact with her GP. Somehow, her engagement in the process of managing her condition had given her improved insight at this crucial early stage. We can only speculate on the mechanisms involved here; some combination, perhaps, of her improved understanding of her condition, of her new trust in her GP, Dr Kirk and her colleagues, and of her confidence that she would be treated with due regard to her values. This improved insight may not prove to be a permanent change, of course. But her recognition of the positive as well as negative aspects of her mood swings, and her ability to take responsibility as well as to receive help, are consistent with the improved prognosis associated with recovery approaches to the functional psychoses (Mueser et al. 2002).

As the outcome of Diane Abbot's story (described in Box 10) illustrates, this re-engagement of those concerned with the decisions they make, is the basis of a close connection between VBM and the emphasis on agency which is at the heart of the recovery model of mental health practice (Mueser et al. 2002).

Conclusions – Psychiatry First

Although this chapter has been about Values-Based *Medicine*, the main driver for the development of the ten principles outlined here has been psychiatry. In one sense, this is how it should be. Psychiatry, as noted under Principle 2 above, is more value-laden than any other branch of medicine essentially because it is concerned with areas of human experience and behaviour in which human values are particularly diverse. Hence, it would seem, it is natural that it is here, in psychiatry, that VBM should be developed first.

In the traditional fact-centred model of medicine, however, the development of VBM in psychiatry would be interpreted very differently, viz. as an apology or as a substitute for its (supposed) lack of a mature underpinning scientific theory. According to this model, as we also noted under Principle 2, psychiatry's more overtly value-laden nature is a mark of scientific deficiency. Correspondingly, therefore, according to the fact-centred traditional medical model, psychiatry needs VBM because it lacks science. Philosophical value theory, by contrast, suggested that the more value-laden nature of psychiatry is a mark, not of scientific inadequacy but of values complexity. Psychiatry is more value-laden than other areas of medicine because it is concerned with areas of human experience and behaviour, such as emotion, desire, volition and belief, in which human values are highly (and legitimately) diverse (Fulford 1989, ch. 5).

It is as a response to value complexity, then, not as a substitute for scientific sophistication, that VBM has developed first in psychiatry. Principle 3 of VBM, furthermore, the "science driven" principle, showed that with future progress in medical science and technology, similar value complexity will increasingly become the norm in *all* areas of medicine. Far from lagging behind medical science, therefore, psychiatry, in developing the theory and practice of VBM, is providing a lead that other areas of medicine, under the pressure of scientific progress, will eventually be obliged to follow. VBM, then, is indeed a first for psychiatry. And given its origins in philosophical value theory, the extent of the penetration of VBM already into policy and practice in mental health makes it also a first for the *philosophy* of psychiatry.

Acknowledgements

I am grateful to the many colleagues who have contributed with suggestions, examples and case studies, to the development of the ideas set out in this chapter. My particular thanks go to Gillian Bendelow, Jeremy Dale, Melissa and Paul Falzer, John Geddes, Christa Kruger, Eric Matthews, Sarah Matthews, John Sadler, Werdie van Staden, and the members of the Values Project Group of the National Institutes of Mental Health in England (NIMHE), Piers Allott

(Chair), Simon Allard, Catherine Laurence, Liz Mayne, David Morris, Albert Persaud and Kim Woodbridge.

References

Austin, J.L. 1956-7. "A plea for excuses", *Proceedings of the Aristotelian Society* 57:1-30. Reprinted in White, A.R., (ed.) (1968) *The Philosophy of Action*. Oxford: Oxford University Press.

Beauchamp, T.L., Childress, J.F. 1989; 4th Edition 1994. *Principles of biomedical ethics*. Oxford: Oxford University Press.

Boorse, C. 1975. "On the distinction between disease and illness", *Philosophy and Public Affairs*, 5: 49-68.

Campbell, P. 1996. "What We Want From Crisis Services", in: Read, J., Reynolds, J. (eds.) *Speaking Our Minds: An Anthology*. Basingstoke, England: The Macmillan Press Ltd for The Open University, 180-183.

Colombo, A., Bendelow, G., Fulford K.W.M., Williams, S. forthcoming. "Evaluating the Influence of Implicit Models of Mental Disorder on Processes of Shared Decision-making within Community-based Multi-disciplinary teams", *The International Journal of Social Science and Medicine*.

Dancy, J. 1993. *Moral Reasons*. Oxford: Blackwell Publishers.

Dickenson, D., Fulford, K.W.M. 2000. *In Two Minds: A Casebook of Psychiatric Ethics*. Oxford: Oxford University Press.

Eddy, D.M. 1991. "Clinical decision-making: from theory to practice. Rationing by patient choice", *JAMA*, 265: 105-108.

Foot, Ph. 1959. "Moral Beliefs", *Proceedings of the Aristotelian Society*, 59: 83-104.

Fulford, K.W.M. 1989, reprinted 1995 and 1999; 2nd ed. forthcoming. *Moral Theory and Medical Practice*. Cambridge: Cambridge University Press

Fulford, K.W.M. 1991. "The concept of disease", in: Bloch, S., Chodoff, P. (eds.) *Psychiatric Ethics* (second edition). Oxford: Oxford University Press, 77-99.

Fulford, K.W.M. 1994a. "Closet logics: hidden conceptual elements in the DSM and ICD classifications of mental disorders". ch. 9, in: Sadler, J.Z., Wiggins, O.P., Schwartz, M.A., (eds.) *Philosophical Perspectives on Psychiatric Diagnostic Classification*. Baltimore: Johns Hopkins University Press.

Fulford, K.W.M. 1994b. Not more medical ethics. ch. 15, in: Fulford, K.W.M., Gillett, G.R., Soskice, J.M. (eds.) *Medicine and moral reasoning*. Cambridge: Cambridge University Press.

Fulford, K.W.M. 1994c. "Medical Education: Knowledge and Know-how", ch. 2, in: Chadwick, R. (ed.) *Ethics and the Professions*. Aldershot, England: The Avebury Press.

Fulford, K.W.M. 1995. "The Concept of Patient-Centred Care", ch. 1, in: Fulford, K. W. M., Ersser, S., Hope, T. (eds.) *Essential Practice in Patient-Centred Care*. Oxford: Blackwell Science.

Fulford, K.W.M. 1998. "Dissent and dissensus: the limits of consensus formation in psychiatry", in ten Have, H.A.M.J., Saas, H-M. (eds.) *Consensus Formation in Health Care Ethics*. Kluwer: Philosophy and Medicine Series, 175-192.

Fulford, K.W.M. 1990. "Philosophy and Medicine: The Oxford Connection", *British Journal of Psychiatry*, 157: 111-115.

Fulford, K.W.M. 1999. "Nine Variations and a Coda on the Theme of an Evolutionary Definition of Dysfunction", *Journal of Abnormal Psychology*, 108: 412-420.

Fulford, K.W.M. 2000. "The Paradoxes of Confidentiality: a Philosophical Introduction", ch. 1, in: Cordess, C. *Confidentiality: Philosophy and Practice*. London: Jessica Kingsley Publishers.

Fulford, K.W.M. 2000a. "Teleology without Tears: Naturalism, Neo-Naturalism and Evaluationism in the Analysis of Function Statements in Biology (and a Bet on the Twenty-first Century)", *Philosophy, Psychiatry, & Psychology* 7/1: 77-94.

Fulford, K.W.M. 2000b. "Philosophy Meets Psychiatry in the Twentieth Century – Four Looks Back and a Brief Look Forward", in: Louhiala, P., Stenman, S. (eds.) *Philosophy Meets Medicine*. Helsinki: Helsinki University Press, 114-31.

Fulford, K.W.M. 2001. "Philosophy into Practice: The Case for Ordinary Language Philosophy", ch. 2, in: Nordenfelt, L. *Health, Science and Ordinary Language*. Amsterdam: Rodopi.

Fulford, K.W.M., Bloch, S. 2000. "Psychiatric Ethics: Codes, Concepts, and Clinical Practice Skills", in: Gelder, M., Lopez-Ibor, J. J., Andreasen, N. (eds.) *New Oxford Textbook of Psychiatry*. Oxford: Oxford University Press. ch. 1.5, 27-32.

Fulford, K.W.M., Dickenson, D., Murray, T.H. 2002a. "Introduction: Many Voices: Human Values in Healthcare Ethics", in: Fulford, K.W.M., Dickenson, D. and Murray, T.H. (eds.) *Healthcare Ethics and Human Values: An Introductory Text with Readings and Case Studies*. Malden, USA, and Oxford, UK: Blackwell.

Fulford, K.W.M., Dickenson, D., and Murray, T.H. (eds.) 2002b. *Healthcare Ethics and Human Values: an Introductory Text with Readings and Case Studies*. Oxford: Blackwell Publishers.

Fulford, K.W.M., Williamson, T., Woodbridge, K. 2002. "Revealing Values in Mental Health Practice: A Values Awareness Training Workshop. Published as Values-Added Practice", *Mental Health Today*, October, 25-27.

Hare, R.M. 1952. *The language of morals*. Oxford University Press.

Hare, R.M. 1963. "Descriptivism", *Proceedings of the British Academy* 49: 115-134. Reprinted in: Hare, R.M. 1972. *Essays on the moral concepts*. London: The Macmillan Press Ltd.

Heifetz, R. 1994. *Leadership Without Easy Answers*. USA: Harvard University Press

Hope, R. A., Fulford, K.W.M. 1993. "Medical Education: Patients, Principles and Practice Skills", ch. 59, in: Gillon, R. (ed.) *Principles of Health Care Ethics*. Chichester, England: John Wiley and Sons.

Hope, T., Fulford, K. W. M. and Yates, A. 1996. *The Oxford Practice Skills Course: Ethics, Law and Communication Skills in Health Care Education*. Oxford: The Oxford University Press.

Hudson Jones, A. 1999. "Narrative in Medical Ethics", *BMJ*, 318: 253-256.

Jackson, M., Fulford, K.W.M. 1997. "Spiritual Experience and Psychopathology", *Philosophy, Psychiatry, & Psychology*, 4/1: 41-66. Commentaries by Littlewood, R., Lu, F.G. et al., Sims, A., Storr, A. and response by authors, 67-90.

Jamison, K.R. 1996. *Touched With Fire: Manic Depressive Illness and the Artistic Temperament*. California, USA: Touchstone Books.

Keller, M.B., Lavori, P.W., Kane, J.M. Gelenberg, A.J., Rosenbaum, J.F., Walzer, E.A., Baker, L.A. 1992. "Subsyndromal symptoms in bipolar disorder. A comparison of standard and low serum levels of lithium", *Archives of General Psychiatry*, 49(5): 371-376.

MacIntyre, A. 1985. *After virtue: a study in moral theory*. London: Duckworth.

Marshall, M., 1994. "How Should We Measure Need? Concept and Practice in the Development of a Standardized Assessment Schedule", *Philosophy, Psychiatry, & Psychology*, 1/1: 27-36.

May, W.F. 1994. "The virtues in a professional setting", ch. 6, in: Fulford, K.W.M., Gillett, G.R., Soskice, J.M. (eds.) *Medicine and moral reasoning*. Cambridge: Cambridge University Press.

Ministerial Announcement at launch of the National Institutes for Mental Health in England (NIMHE), 2001

Moore, A., Hope, T., Fulford, K.W.M. 1994. "Mild Mania and Well-Being", *Philosophy, Psychiatry, & Psychology*, 1/3: 165-178.

Mueser, K.T., Corrigan, P.W., Hilton, D.W., Tanzman, B., Schaub, A., Gingerich, S., Essock, S.M., Tarrier, N., Morey, B., Vogel-Scibilia, S., Herz, M.I. 2002. "Illness Management and Recovery: A Review of the Research", *Psychiatric Services*, Vol 53, No 10: 1272-1284.

Nagel, T. 1986. *The View from Nowhere*. Oxford: Oxford University Press.

Nordenfelt, L. 1987 *On the nature of health: an action-theoretic approach*. Dordrecht, Holland: D. Reidel Publishing Company.

Okasha, A. 2000. "Ethics of Psychiatric Practice: Consent, Compulsion and Confidentiality", *Current Opinion in Psychiatry*. 13: 693-698.

Perkins, R. 2001. "What constitutes success? The relative priority of service users' and clinicians' views of mental health services", *British Journal of Psychiatry*, 179: 9-10.

Phillips, J. 2000. "Conceptual Models for Psychiatry", *Current Opinion in Psychiatry*, 13: 683-688.

Sacket et al. 1997. *Evidence-Based Medicine: How to Practice and Teach EBM*. London: Churchill Livingstone.

Sadler J.Z. 1996. "Epistemic Value Commitments in the Debate over Categorical vs. Dimensional Personality Diagnosis", *Philosophy, Psychiatry, & Psychology*, 3/3: 203-222.

Sadler, J.Z. (ed.) 2002. *Descriptions & Prescriptions: Values, Mental Disorders, and the DSMs*. Baltimore: The Johns Hopkins University Press.

Sadler, J.Z. (forthcoming). *Values and Psychiatric Diagnosis*. Oxford: Oxford University Press.

Straus, S.E., McQuay, H.J., Moore, R.A., Sackett, D.L. 1999. "A proposed patient-centred method of delivering information about the risks and benefits of therapy: the likelihood of being helped versus harmed", *Int. Clin Psychopharmacology Journal* (Full) ID: 2966.

Straus, S.E. 2002. "Individualizing Treatment Decisions: The Likelihood of Being Helped or Harmed", *Evaluation & The Health Professions*, Vol. 25, No. 2: 210-224. Sage Publications.

Urmson, J.O. 1950. "On grading", *Mind*, 59: 145-169.

von Wright, H.G. 1963. *The Varieties of Goodness*. London: Routledge and Kegan Paul. New York: The Humatics Press.

Warnock, G.J. 1971. *The Object of Morality*. London: Methuen & Co Ltd.

Williams, B. 1985. *Ethics and the limits of philosophy*. London: Fontana

Williams, A. 1995. "Economics, QALYs and Medical Ethics – a Health Economists Perspective", *Health Care Analysis* 3 (3): 221-226.

Classification and Conceptual Considerations

The Concept of Psychiatric Nosology

Pierre Pichot

Nosology, a term created in the 18th century, is, according to the dictionaries, the division of medicine designated to determine the specific characteristics of the diseases, whereas nosography refers to their systematic classification. Nosology is a variation of taxonomy, initially the classification of plants, later of all species of living beings and now understood as the general science of classification. Classification constitutes a fundamental place in all empirical sciences based on the assumptions of the orderliness of natural phenomena and of the rational apprehension of this order by man. The classificatory grouping of phenomena and the signification of the rationale for classification are in fact codifications of the existing state of knowledge in a scientific discipline. Classification has two functions. It creates order out of the potential chaos of discrete, discontinuous or heterogenous observations, in other words, it is a technique to condense information. But it has also a predictive value in that it permits the observer to predict the relationships between phenomena not obviously connected. Thus in medicine, diagnosis, that is the attribution of a patient to a specific class, allows prognosis – the prediction of the evolution of a disorder– and the choice of optimal therapy.

Nosology rests, according to its definition, on the concept of disease, the birth of which is attributed to Sydenham. "Nature", wrote the English physician in 1682, "in the production of diseases is uniform and consistent: so much so, that for the same disease in different persons the symptoms are for the most part the same; and the self-same phenomena you could observe in the sickness of a Socrates, you would observe in the sickness of a simpleton. Just so the universal characters of a plant are extending to every individual of the species; and whoever (I speak in the way of illustration) should accurately describe the colour, the taste, the smell, the figure, etc. of the single violet find that his description held good, there and thereabout, for all the violets of that particular species upon the face of earth".

The 18th century was the initial golden age of classifications. The "Systema Naturae" and the "Genera Plantarum" became model principles for medicine, published in 1735 by Carl von Linné, who claimed to have been the first to introduce the concept of "natural classification", i.e. the only classification based on the rational order followed by Nature in the creation of species. Sydenham had already spotted the comparison of a disease with a botanical species and the original extensive nosological system covering the whole of medicine, the "Nosologia Methodica" (1768), was subtitled "Sistens Morborum Classes, Genera et Species Juxta Sydenham Mentem et Botanicorum Ordinem" (Consisting of the Classes, Genders and Species of Diseases Based on the Principles of Sydenham and the System of the Botanists). The author, Boissier de Sauvages, a physician of Montpellier where he taught botany at the medical school, enumerated and described briefly more than 2,400 diseases in his book. It was in fact mostly a compilation of the works of his predecessors and the main influence of Linnaeus lies in the adoption of a binary nomenclature. In the genre Melancholia 14 species are described, often with picturesque names such as Melancholia vulgaris, amatoria, religiosa, anglica or enthusiastica. But Boissier had clearly recognized the nature of his nosography by affirming that "a disease consists of a cluster of several independent symptoms, named syndrome by the Greeks", probably the first use of the term in a modern medical text.

The second important nosological system of the same period, presented by the Scottish physician Cullen in "Apparatus ad Nosologicam Methodicam" (1769), and in "First Lines in the Practice of Physics", is of a radically different orientation. Inspired by his predecessor in Edinburgh, Whitt, a follower of Sydenham and Willis, he abandoned the old humoral theory in favour of the concept of "nervous disease". Cullen proposed in this domain a classification based on a combination of the aetio-pathogenic mechanisms involved and the body functions impaired. Opposing the "local diseases" produced by a known local lesion to the "general diseases", he described among the latter, the "neuroses", general non-lesional dysfunctions of the nervous system. They are divided according to the types of manifestations, in comas, adynamies, spasms and vesanies, the latter ones including mostly the different forms of insanity. Cullen's influence is associated with the introduction of the concept of neurosis, the content of which has varied considerably, but which still today plays a significant role in the nosological literature.

The classifications of Boissier and Cullen were rejected as "artificial" by their direct successor, Pinel, the founder of modern psychiatry, in his epoch-making "Treatise of mental alienation" (1801). For Pinel mental alienation is a single disease: he uses the term in the singular in the title of his treatise. It has different modes of expression: mania, melancholia, dementia and idiotism recognized by the "deep study of the symptoms". They are not categories of ontological quality, rather they provide a convenient instrument only for the management of the patients. The same view was defended by his pupils and followers for half a century. On the basis of clinical observations they eventually modified the boundaries of Pinel's four forms of insanity, included new ones yet still remained convinced of its unity. When the most influential of his pupils, Esquirol, wrote in 1838 a book on "mental diseases" he used the term in its plural form only to conform to the general usage: his isolation of "lypemania" and the various "monomanias" rested on conceptual foundations radically different from those which had inspired the "nosographs" of the previous century. The conviction that mental alienation constituted a single disease, which had remained implicit in the French psychiatric school, was, however, systematically elaborated in Germany in the doctrine of the "Einheitspsychose", first developed by Zeller. It acquired a temporary reputation through the adoption by Griesinger (Vliegen 1980).

Around 1850, a new period began in the history of psychiatric nosology. Jean-Pierre Falret, a pupil of Esquirol, was convinced in mental pathology that one could isolate "natural forms" of diseases, as had been done in other branches of medicine through the anatomo-clinical approach. In 1822, Bayle described general paralysis in this way, associating a succession of pathological manifestations of alienation (mania, monomania, dementia) and lesions of the arachnoid discovered at autopsy. But the importance of this discovery was not recognized and, moreover, further anatomo-pathological studies of the brain of the insane turned out to be disappointing. Falret believed that each disease held a corresponding specific symptomatology and therefore, even if for the time being little could be expected from anatomo-pathology, it was possible to isolate mental diseases by the "clinical method" alone. But only on two conditions: Firstly, one must not rely on a single, arbitrarily chosen, superficial symptom, as Esquirol had done in his definitions of the various monomanias, but on a cluster of relevant "basic symptoms". Furthermore, one must be aware of the major significance of the evolution of the disease, formed by the succession of different syndromes. In 1851, Falret described "circular madness" – our present bipolar disorder – defined by the succession of manic and depressive episodes separated by free intervals. Circular madness and general paralysis for him were the only "true" mental diseases, isolated so far from the chaos of mental alienation. By mentioning the name of a naturalist, who was then considered the greatest taxonomist, he concluded that psychiatry was "awaiting its Jussieu".

His expectation was to be fulfilled by Emil Kraepelin. He had been preceded by Kahlbaum, whose pupil Hecker had isolated hebephrenia, and who, in his reputable description of catatonia, had explicitly used Falret's approach as his model. In the foreword to the fifth edition of his Treatise (1896), Kraepelin announced that, from this time on, he would adopt exclusively a clinical perspective based on his concept of disease (Hoff 1985). According to Kraepelin, finite categories exist in psychiatry. They could be determined if we had all scientific facts at our disposal, either by symptomatic, pathogenic or aetiological criteria. The three nosologies would be identical, he claimed, thereby postulating a perfect correspondence between the three levels. Accordingly, if we do not yet possess sufficient knowledge of the causes and of the mechanisms, the study of the symptoms, their conditions of appearance, their nature and their evolution will result in the "natural" nosology. The emphasis on evolution, originating from Falret, resulted in the creation of the major categories of the psychoses, Dementia praecox and Manic-depressive Insanity.

Kraepelin was far from being dogmatic about aetiology, in that he accepted the existence of both biological and psychological factors, and recognized that they were generally unknown. But his main contentions were the strictly categorical structure of nosology and the unequivocal relation between symptoms, mechanisms and causes. Kraepelin's nosology rapidly gained recognition worldwide, despite the existence of divergent conceptions in Germany, such as those of Wernicke (1900) and Hoche (1912), and of the resistance of national schools, such as the French one, who firmly adhered to their own traditions. The categories delineated by Kraepelin were eventually modified: Examples are the introduction of the concept of schizophrenia by Bleuler (1911), which emphasized the existence of a specific psychopathological mechanism in all cases of Dementia praecox, or the sub-division by Angst and Perris (1966), of the manic-depressive psychosis in uni- and bipolar forms. Around 1950, the nosologies in official use, such as the ICD or the DSM-I were still basically Kraepelinian in their structure, and deeply implicated in the principles on which they were based.

Doubts about the values of those nosologies originated from psychoanalysis. It is true that Freud himself, in his early description of Anxiety neurosis, had followed Kraepelin's principles: the new disease was specified by its symptomatology, aetiology and pathogeny. It is also true that Freud later used Kraepelin's nosological terminology. But his main interests lay elsewhere. He concentrated on the elucidation of the psychological mechanisms, which in relation to the maturation of the drives and their disturbances through early life situations were, according to him, responsible for the symptoms observed. Since around 1940, particularly in the United States, his ideas have been adopted and expanded by his followers and the so-called psychodynamic school, which dominated psychiatric thoughts for several decades. In this country, the anti-Kraepelinian and the more widespread antinosological trends led to a disregard of diagnostic practices. For example, the diagnosis of schizophrenia was applied indiscriminately in such a way that, in 1961, it was shown that in the admission statistics of mental hospitals the rate of schizophrenia was in the U.S. five times higher than in England. Even the legitimacy of a psychiatric nosology raised an element of doubt: Masserman (1951) condemns "the tendency to 'define' and classify 'mental disorders' into categories comparable to those used in general medicine, despite the fact that in the case of most mental disorders, little justification for such a classification exists on aetiologic, clinical and even heuristic grounds".

Similarities exist between the two periods during which nosology contributed to one of the major areas of research and controversy in psychiatry. The first period, at the end of the 19th century, saw the emergence of Kraepelin's concept of disease and of his classification, the second period was symbolized by the publication of the third edition of the Diagnostic and Statistical Manual of Mental Disorders (DSM-III) in 1980 by the American Psychiatric

Association. Both had forerunners, the first with Falret and Kahlbaum, the second in the works of the Saint Louis School and of the Biometric Laboratory of Columbia University. Both were efforts to "remedicalize" psychiatry, the first by replacing the old implicit idea of the unity of mental alienation with the description of independent diseases, like in the rest of medicine, the second by opposing the psychodynamic anti-classificatory attitudes. Despite initial controversies, the DSM-III saw the principles on which it was based and its structure and elements rapidly adopted internationally, as in the ICD-10 (1992). Numerous researches aimed at improving the new system, which was completed by the DSM-III-R (1987) and DSM-IV (1994). Hailed by one of his promoters as a "return to Kraepelin", one of the main features of the DSM-III demonstrated a congruence with Kraepelin's nosology in its strictly categorical nature. Because of its claim to be based only on "scientifically demonstrated" facts, it is primarily descriptive, and its categories syndromic. The refusal of hypothetical aetio-pathogenesis has led to the rejection – still strongly criticized by many- of such time-honoured concepts and terms as Neurosis, Hysteria, or endogenous depression. Among its technical innovations, beside the multi-axial structure, the introduction of the diagnostic criteria is of importance. It reflects, similar to the extended use of rating scales in another domain, the growing trend towards quantification in descriptive psychiatry. As one of the leading authors of the DSM-III humorously noted, if the validity of its categories is subjected to the object of discussions, at least their reliability cannot be contested thanks to the use of diagnostic criteria.

From the Nosologia Methodica of Boissier de Sauvages to the DSM-III, psychiatric classifications have been established as typologies. The concept of type, defined by the mathematician and philosopher Cournot (1861) as "a cluster of characteristics, constituting an organic whole, whose clustering cannot be explained by chance", takes into account the fact that in many of the natural sciences, a perfect homogenity of each class is an abstract ideal. Contrary to Sydenham's assertion, the violets of a given species do not have exactly the same colour, taste, smell, or form. In a typological classification, the characteristics of a member of a class may differ to a limited and defined extent from those of the "typical" or "focal" member. The typological nature of psychiatric symptomatic nosologies is illustrated by the DSMs. Nine symptomatic criteria are enumerated in the definition of the "Major depressive episode". A patient is subsumed under a diagnostic label if five or more criteria are fulfilled (an additional condition is the presence of at least one of the first two criteria on the list). The "typical" subject exhibits all nine symptoms. The patients whose symptomatology is made up of one of numerous possible combinations of eight down to five symptoms are given the same diagnosis, but those with four symptoms are excluded from the category. Typologies are usually hierarchical, additional criteria allowing the individualisation of sub-types. Thus the Major depressive episode admits several sub-types, defined by the presence of "specifiers" such as "melancholic", "catatonic" or "atypical" additional features. According to Cournot, typologies are "natural, rational abstractions" as opposed to "artificial" ones. Since Linné, the concept of natural classification has been extensively defined. The pragmatic modern definition is based on the principle of effectiveness: it is the classification that allows the greatest number of predictions. Therefore, in each domain there exists only one natural classification. Artificial ones, based not on a cluster of characteristics – the "organic whole" of Cournot – but on a single one, arbitrarily chosen, may also be fruitful, but in a limited way. In the Middle Ages, plants were classified according to their height and this is still of significance today for the gardener. In the same way, the classification of mental disorders according to their acute and chronic evolution determined in the time before Pinel – and even after him – to which medical institution the patient was to be admitted.

Historians have pointed out that the first classifications have been generally of a descriptive nature, based on easily observable characteristics. With the progress of knowledge, they have relied increasingly on more theoretical criteria. But, if the original descriptive classification was indeed natural, it has not been greatly modified by the use of the new criteria. The botanic taxonomy of the 18th century, based mainly on the morphology of the reproductive organs, was largely confirmed by the study of the chromosomes much later. Mendeleiev's classification of the elements, derived from their atomic weights and chemical properties, was validated by the discovery of the structure of the atom. In medicine, from this perspective, the syndromic nosology would correspond to the descriptive level and the aetiological classification to the more theoretical, scientific one. In many branches of medicine, such as infectious diseases, the discovery of the causes has often confirmed the natural character of the syndromic classification. The supposition of the nosologists has been that it would also hold true for mental disorders, when Falret spoke of "natural forms", Kraepelin postulated the correlation between symptomatology, pathogeny and aetiology, or the DSM-III affirmed that "undoubtly, with time, some of the Disorders of unknown aetiology will be found to have (...) specific aetiologies".

Our present psychiatric nosologies consist of two classifications, one syndromic, concerning all the disorders, and one aetiological, restricted to those whose cause has been proven. Each classification has to be considered separately. Some of the formal elements of the syndromic classification, such as its reliability, have been improved. It is, however, doubtful that the efforts made to increase the homogeneity of each class, leading to a progressive increase of their number, have presented a more natural character to this classification. We are compelled to disregard the requirement of exclusivity, already formulated by Aristotle, according to which each element of a population can be attributed to one, but only one class. In the DSM-IV it is not unusual for a patient to receive several diagnoses, indeed it is even the rule within the Personality Disorders. Co-morbidity depends on factors well known in the other fields of medicine but, in psychiatry, as evidenced by epidemiological surveys, the rate is so high that it may be relegated to the inadequacies of the nosology. Its predictive value being the test for the natural character of a classification, the existence of a treatment specific to each diagnostic class would be a decisive argument in its favour. But the action of our psychopharmacologic agents is clearly not causal, rather it is directed at the neurophysiological intermediaries between the – generally unknown – cause and the symptoms. Many of the existing drugs are put into active use in a large number of differing classes: neuroleptics in schizophrenia and mania; serotonin recapture inhibitors in depressive and obsessive-compulsive disorders. The only possible conclusion is that complex relations exist, at the pathogenic level, between the allegedly homogenous symptomatic classes.

The classification of psychiatric disorders whose cause is proven demonstrates that the correlation between syndrome and aetiology is low in present nosology. When, as in the majority of cases, the identified cause is "organic", i.e. a lesional or functional impairment of the central nervous system, a striking contrast exists between the number and the heterogenity of the known causes, and the few syndromic expressions observed: cognitive global deficit (mental retardation and dementia), delirium, amnestic disorders. Moreover, many syndromes identified within the mental disorders of yet unknown aetiology appear also in the "organic" cases: they belong, among others, to the mood disorders (depressive, manic, bipolar), the psychotic disorders (delusional, hallucinatory, catatonic) or to the anxiety disorders (generalized anxiety, panic attacks, obsessive-compulsive) and there exists no clear relation between those syndromes and the causes.

Over the last decades, this situation has led to the conviction, now frequently expressed, that the nosological categorical system is inadequate for psychiatry. It has proved useful in most medical domains but, according to its critics, its application to the mental disorders should be rejected. One of the main claims of the DSM-III was that it should be of a strictly categorical nature. Seventeen years later the authors of the DSM-IV felt compelled to devote a chapter in their introduction to "the limitations of the categorical approach". The alternative model proposed at the descriptive level is the dimensional one. Its origins lie in psychology, which has traditionally favoured the concept of trait. Both the categorical and the dimensional models condensate the information provided by observation of the characteristics of the individual subjects, the first model by dividing the population in sub-populations whose members possess the same characteristics, the second model by substituting the multitude of characteristics by a few linear dimensions. A statistical method, factor analysis, has been developed to determine empirically from the matrix of correlations between the characteristics, the latent dimensions (factors) accounting for this matrix, and the contribution of each characteristic to each factor (its saturation in regard to the factor). An individual case is no longer described by the enumeration of its many characteristics but by its factorial profile, i.e. by its position in relation to the factors identified, the number of which is much smaller. The description of the personality in terms of factors by the psychologists has been followed by the psychiatrists since about 1950. It has been mainly used to identify the psychopathological dimensions measured by the various rating scales and for the construction of homogenous instruments. However, the influence of the results of those studies on the descriptive nosologies remains limited so far. The only exception concerns schizophrenia. In the last decades, the factorial dimensions underlying its symptomatology have been studied and the DSM-IV offers the possibility of drawing a factorial profile of a schizophrenic patient instead of attributing him to one of the five subtypes: paranoid, disorganized, catatonic, undifferentiated, or residual. The profile includes three dimensions: psychotic, disorganized, and negative, while the position of the subject is determined by the presence and intensity of the symptoms previously related to this dimension by factor-analysis. The introduction of this approach was evoked by the authors of the DSM-IV who, although rejecting it for the time being, expressed their hope that "increasing research on, and familiarity with the dimensional system may eventually result in its greater acceptance as a method of conveying information and as a research tool".

Have we reached a turning point in the history of psychiatric classification? The medical categorical model stemming from Sydenham's concept of disease encounters obvious difficulties in its application to psychiatry. At the descriptive level, the categories are not independent and notions such as comorbidity or disease-spectrum merely recognize the existence of interrelations without actually explaining them. Today's research generally uses diagnostically homogenous groups of patients when aiming to discover the impairment of brain function by studying the anomalies of neuro-transmitters, the location of the disturbance by cerebral imagery, or when trying to identify genetic causal factors. Researchers thereby implicitly assume that the symptomatic homogeneity is based on a corresponding homogeneity of the pathogenic mechanisms and the causes. The results, however, have been, on the whole, disappointing. On the one hand, they tend to show that in a given syndromic category even when appearing homogenous, several biochemical anomalies can be detected whose interrelations are still vague and further, that the genetic mechanisms cannot be analysed with precision even when their causal role is obvious. On the other hand, however, they have also shown the relative lack of specificity of the observed anomalies. Identical disturbances of the neuro-transmitters are involved in several syndromes, dysfunctions of similar zones of the brain are detected by cerebral imagery, and their eventual genetic background does not appear to be strictly specific. The syndromes only observed in the disorders of a known "organic" cause, are much more related to the severity, duration and reversibility of the impact of multiple possible aetiological factors than to the nature of the factor. The syndromes isolated in the "non-organic" disorders are frequently observed in the "organic" ones, so that altogether syndromes and causes present no clear correlation.

In no other domain of medicine has so much time and effort been devoted to the classification of the observed manifestations. The fact that the organisation WHO felt bound to include a detailed glossary defining each of the diagnostic categories in the chapter on Mental Disorders of the ICD (the only chapter in which such a glossary exists), and a supplement of the research devoted to the improvement of the DSM, as published in the "DSM-IV Source Book", demonstrate just two illustrations as to the extent of these efforts. Their relative failure is attributed by some to a certain specificity of psychiatry. The number of significant types – following Cournot's definition – of abnormal psychological and behavioural manifestations is relatively small, much smaller than the present diagnostic categories. They are reactions of the organism to the multiple psychological, social and biological factors mediated by the brain, by far the most complex organ of the human body in its structure and its function. This contrast would explain the difficulties in assessing the relations that supposedly exist between symptomatology, pathogeny and aetiology.

David Goldberg has recently endorsed the proposal to abandon the categorical nosological model in favour of the dimensional one on the grounds that the first is basically inspired by Plato in its postulating the existence of non-observable "essences", i.e. the diseases, whereas, the second, based only on observable facts, conforms to the basic rule of the Aristotelian philosophy of science. From a pragmatic point of view, the dimensional model is more economical at the descriptive level. It could be extended by further research transnosologically, instead of being restricted to a group of mental disorders such as the schizophrenic forms. The existence of widely used transnosological rating scales, such as the Brief Psychiatric Rating Scale (Overall and Gorham 1962), or the Symptom Check List (Derogatis 1977), suggests it is possible for the dimensional system to cover large segments or even the whole of symptomatology. The technical difficulties in the determination of relevant dimensions and in the choice of their optimal number – eventually in a hierarchical structure – could be solved by further research. However, it remains to be proved that the superiority of the dimensional model extends beyond the descriptive level and has a better predictive value than the categorical model. Hypotheses have been made about existing correlations between behavioural traits and the action of some neuro-transmitters, but it must be pointed out that the specific dimensional profile of a patient would allow a better choice of an adequate therapy than a diagnosis in the present nosological system.

No predictions can be made about the future directions psychiatric nosology might take. The categorical approach of today is essentially descriptive, i.e. refuses to rely on "unproven" hypotheses. The more recent dimensional model, not yet applied to the whole field, has by its nature the same character. All previous nosologies, Cullen's classes of neuroses, the "Einheitspsychose", Kraepelin's concept of disease and the various psychopathological, psychodynamic and biological constructs, were based on theories. Despite the fact that those theories have been later partially or totally disproved, they have nevertheless contributed to the progress of our conceptions. In the process of incorporating the results of empirical research in a classification which is, as already stressed, a codification of the existing state of knowledge, one must dispose of a theoretical framework. The present "a-theoretical" attitude corresponds to a probably necessary, but transitory stage in the long and varied history of psychiatric nosology which, as Falret wrote one and half a centuries ago, still "awaits its Jussieu".

References

American Psychiatric Association. 1980. *Diagnostic and Statistical Manual of Mental Disorders* (Third Edition) DSM-III. APA. Washington.

American Psychiatric Association. 1987. *Diagnostic and Statistical Manual of Mental Disorders* (Third Edition-Revised) DSM-III-R. APA. Washington.

American Psychiatric Association. 1994. *Diagnostic and Statistical Manual of Mental Disorders* (Fourth Edition) DSM-IV. APA. Washington.

Angst, J. 1966. *Zur Ätiologie und Nosologie endogener depressiver Psychosen*. Berlin: Springer.

Bayle, A.L.J. 1822. "Recherches sur les maladies mentales (Thèse de Medecine, Paris)", in: Centenaire de la thèse de Bayle (1922). Masson, Paris.

Bleuler, E. 1911. *Dementia praecox oder Gruppe der Schizophrenien*. Leipzig-Wien: Deuticke.

Boissier de Sauvages, F. 1768. *Nosologia Methodica, Sistens Morborum Classes, Genera et Species Juxta Mentem et Botanicorum Ordinem*. Amsterdam: de Tournes.

Cournot, A.A. 1861. *Traité de l'enchainement des idées fondamentales dans les sciences et dans l'histoire*. New edition (1911). Paris: Hachette.

Cullen, W. 1775. *Apparatus ad Nosologiam Methodicam seu Synopsis Nosologicae Methodicae in Usum Studiorum*. Amsterdam: de Tournes.

Cullen, W. 1777-1784. *First Lines of the Practice of Physics*. Edinburgh: Elliot.

Derogatis, L.R. 1977. *SCL-90 R (revised) Version Manual. Clinical Psychometrics Research Unit*. Johns Hopkins University Medical School, Baltimore.

Esquirol, E. 1838. *Des maladies mentales considérées sous les rapports médical, hygiénique et médico-légal*. Paris: Baillière.

Falret, J.P. 1854. "Memoire sur la folie circulaire, forme de maladie mentale caractérisée par la reproduction successive et régulière de l'état maniaque, de l'état mélancolique et d'un intervalle libre plus ou moins prolongé", *Bull Acad Imp Méd*, 19: 382-400.

Falret, J.P. 1864. *Des maladies mentales et des asiles d'aliénés. Leçons cliniques et considérations générales*. Paris: Baillière.

Hoche, A.K. 1912. "Die Bedeutung der Symptomenkomplexe in der Psychiatrie", *Ztschr f d ges Neurol u Psych*, 12: 540-551.

Hoff, P. 1985. "Zum Krankheitsbegriff bei Emil Kraepelin", *Nervenarzt*, 56: 510-513.
Kraepelin, E. 1896. *Psychiatrie. Ein Lehrbuch für Studierende und Ärzte*. Leipzig: Barth.
von Linné, C. 1735. *Systema Naturae Sive Regna Tri a Naturae Systematica Propoista per Clases, Ordines, Genera et Species*. Leyden: Haak.
von Linné, C. 1735b. *Genera Plantarum Eorumque Caracteres Naturales, Secundum Numerum, Figurem, Sitium et Proportiones Omnium Fructificationis Bartum*. Leyden: Wishoff.
Masserman, J.E. 1953. *Principles of Dynamic Psychiatry*. Philadelphia: Saunders.
Overall, J.E., Gorham, D.R. 1962. "The Brief Psychiatric Rating Scale", *Psychol Rep*, 10: 799-812.
Perris, C. 1966. "A study of bipolar (manic-depressive) and unipolar recurrent depressive psychoses", *Acta Psychiatr Scand*, 42 (Suppl 194): 15-152.
Pinel, P. 1801. *Traité médico-philosophique sur l'aliénation mentale et la manie*. Paris: Richard, Caille et Ranvier.
Sydenham. 1682. *Dissertatio Epistolaris ad C. Cole de Observationis Nuperis circa Curationem Variolarum Confluentium, necnamde Affectionis Hystericis*. London: Kettelby.
Vliegen, J. 1980. *Die Einheitspsychose. Geschichte und Probleme*. Stuttgart: Enke.
Wernicke, C. 1900. *Grundriss der Psychiatrie*. Leipzig: Thieme.
World Health Organization. 1992. *The ICD-10 Classification of Mental and Behavioural Disorders: Clinical Descriptions and Diagnostic Guidelines*. WHO, Geneva.

The Legacy of Antipsychiatry

Thomas Schramme

Antipsychiatry is famous – and infamous – for its claim that there is no such affliction as mental illness.[1] If this proved to be true, the status of psychiatry would change radically. The field of psychiatry would no longer be accepted by many as an integral part of medicine because the primary task of medicine is to cure the ill. The statement that there is no such thing as mental illness appears so highly radical that many hold doubts as to its plausibility. Indeed, it could well be viewed as a totally absurd assumption, because in some cases we can even "see" the illness with persons who are hearing voices or hallucinate. Nevertheless, the claim appears absurd in the first instance only due to the fact that the existence of the phenomena is not denied, rather reference to the meaningful use of the concept of illness is denied. This would indicate that critics of the concept of mental illness do not contest that there are many people with serious mental problems, but maintain that we should not refer to them as being *ill*. The first cross-purposes in the debate on the concept of mental illness start at this point. For example, antipsychiatrists are sometimes accused of taking a cynical attitude against those human beings who are seriously afflicted and deny the "factum brutum psychopathologicum" and, consequentially, question social assistance by their statements (Moore 1975, p. 110, Kisker 1979, p. 820, Häfner 1981, p. 19).

In this article, I shall examine different variants of the objection to the concept of mental illness. The authors who have raised these objections are usually united under the label "antipsychiatry". I am not in favour of using this term, mainly because it was coined in a polemic intention by adherents of the "classical" psychiatry to suggest that the "antipsychiatrists" would indeed like to abolish psychiatry and to leave the mentally ill to their fate. This is, as indicated above, wrong. Many critics of the concept of mental illness opted mainly for another kind of psychiatry, primarily focused not on the disease to be treated, but one that includes as its starting point a human being with his particular mental problems.[2] Therefore, the label "antipsychiatry" was

1 This essay is based on a chapter of my book *Patienten und Personen. Zum Begriff der psychischen Krankheit*, Frankfurt: Fischer 2000, which was recently reissued (Schramme 2003). I should like to thank Psychosozialverlag for giving permission to translate it for this occasion.

2 Although there are important differences between the concepts of illness, disease, disorder etc., I will use them interchangeably, since they are not significant for my purposes.

rejected (cf. Bopp 1980, Kick 1990). Whenever I refer generally to theories, which reject the concept of mental illness as insignificant, I will use the term "sceptical psychiatry" and "sceptics" in the case of the corresponding authors. I hope that I have selected a name which has no negative connotations – especially to philosophers.[3]

Sceptical psychiatry is not a homogenous movement. The best known authors include Thomas Szasz, Michel Foucault, Ronald Laing, Erving Goffman, Franco Basaglia, Thomas Scheff, and David Cooper, all of whom differ considerably in their reasoning. But the one common goal of all was to challenge the traditional conceptualization of mental illness. Hence the leading question of this chapter will be: Can we in a meaningful way use the concept of illness regarding the mental sphere? This question is supplemented by a similarly related question, based on the fact that not all sceptics rejected the concept of mental illness as such, but imparted a radically new meaning to it. The notion stands firm in some approaches, but since it differs extremely from the ideas of "classical" psychiatry, it will no longer be necessary to talk of 'illness'. It seems to me as if these sceptics were reluctant or just neglected to take the last conclusive step, i.e. to abandon outrightly the concept of illness. So the second question of this essay is as follows: Are we to define the concept of illness for mental problems in a more radically different way than ever before?

At the beginning of the 1960's, four books were published which together formed the basis of sceptical psychiatry and contained a large extent of the common sceptical arguments: Thomas Szasz's *The Myth of Mental Illness*, Michel Foucault's *Madness and Civilisation*, Ronald Laing's *The Divided Self* und Erving Goffman's *Asylums*. These books attacked the identity of psychiatry in numerous ways.

Goffman, a sociologist, examined the status and role of psychiatric inpatients and unmasked mechanisms which led him to the conclusion that psychiatry shares attributes of a "total institution", i.e. works by means of comprehensive use of power. This examination, which is more or less focused on psychiatric practice, was supplemented by the thesis that "mental illness" is produced by institutional psychiatry itself, namely, by means of reconstructing cases of patients, already sent to a clinic, in such a way so as to correspond to a certain picture of illness.

Laing had worked as a psychologist in a clinic before practicing alternative methods of therapy that should ideally be performed outside institutional psychiatry. In his work, his primary intention was to bring about a better understanding of the situation of psychiatric patients, to interpret their behav-

3 Wakefield (1992) also refers to "sceptical" arguments.

iour as a reasonable reaction to an unbearable situation, and to divert the focus from a supposed disease to a person living his own particular life. He referred strongly to Existentialism, especially to Sartre's approach.

Foucault, in his writings concerning psychiatry, showed its historical involvement in the interests and constellations of power. He regarded the alleged scientific progress in psychiatry as a chimera. The focus on "madness", in his opinion, has been penetrated by social norms ever since, especially the ideal of reason.

Szasz is a psychiatrist and psychoanalyst. He attacked the psychiatric concept of illness in a direct manner like no one else before him. He used various strategies which will be introduced in detail in the following. Without doubt, his critique is the most radical of all the sceptics named above. His works and the literature dealing with his approach alone are numerous and would fill a multitude of shelves. Not only because of his importance, but also because Szasz put forward his arguments with comparatively more clarity, I shall base my discussion of sceptical psychiatry mainly with his theses.

I shall not deal with every author individually, but distinguish between various types of argumentation and scrutinize their validity. Some sceptics advocate more than one variant so will warrant a mention in several parts. Of course, the categorization is often difficult because a particular critique concerning the concept of mental illness is rarely formulated explicitly and therefore must be reconstructed from the texts. But for my purpose the categorization for the different types of argumentation has the advantage of placing the focus not on an overall estimation of sceptical psychiatry and its representatives, but only on the question, whether or not their proposals reduce the concept of mental illness *ad absurdum*. So a detailed reconstruction of particular texts and persons will be abandoned in favour of ideal-types. Admittedly, taking sceptical psychiatry as an object of classification may seem a little awkward since their representatives often rejected the very inclination to categorize. But maybe this can be used to anticipate a first objection to the sceptics: the fact that constant classification and organization help to gain clarity.

In the following, I shall introduce five types of argumentation. The first form I shall refer to as *functional* objections. They do not really bring forth reasons but rather recommendations like: when referring to mental problems, one should not talk of illness or X, whereby X refers to a negative consequence of the use of the term. The second type of objection is *historical*. It does not reject the concept of mental illness in principle, but calls attention to its history, which – according to the argumentation – contradicts its common use in psychiatry. The next three types are based on an implicit engagement with questions like: what, if anything, is meant by 'mental illness'; what do we refer to by using this concept; what is the characteristic attribute of the phenomena we call 'disease' etc. The third type of argumentation, which I call *interpretative*, puts forth a particular approach of the concept of mental illness, but only to show on this basis that it does not refer to many phenomena that are allegedly cases of mental illness. The fourth type attends to a new interpretation, developed from a societal perspective. It should lead to a better explanation of the phenomena than does the "official" theory by means of its medical conceptualization. I refer to this argument as *sociological.* The fifth category of objections is *conceptual.* These objections claim significant differences between the usage of the concept of illness when we refer to bodily or mental events, hence deny the analogy of somatic and mental illness. Because this type of argumentation generally challenges the concept of mental illness it represents the most serious of objections to psychiatry.

1. Functional Arguments

Functional arguments are supposedly the most unsatisfactory ones for philosophers (but probably not for them alone), because they do not bring about general reasons, but refer to alleged negative consequences of the concept of illness. It might be true – so claims a supporter of the functional strategy – that we may in fact regard particular mental problems as illnesses but we should nevertheless treat this concept with suspicion, since illness causes a therapeutical impulse in doctors who will certainly find ways and means to persuade the patient of the need for treatment. The common interpretation of disease as an enemy of human beings, together with the interest of the medical complex in treating as many "ill" people as possible, will inevitably lead to a medicalization of human life. Individual needs and the specific suffering of patients will be objectified and subjected to the "medical gaze".

This type of argumentation was introduced in the works of Michel Foucault, Klaus Dörner and Ivan Illich (Foucault 1976, pp. 83ff., Dörner 1975, Illich 1976). It is supported by the obvious and undeniable medicalization of many human problems in modern societies. The rising costs for medical supplies and the extension of "technical medicine" actually result in a depersonalization of medical practice. But the question follows: Is the most effective form of "therapy" for overcoming this situation the radical change or even abandonment of the concept of mental illness? To my mind, it does not seem so. To be sure, the abuses of medical practice are related to the expansion of the concept of illness – but this needs to deblamed rather more on the fact that it is fairly demanding to define exactly what illness is. If there were a more specific agreement to this question, then the medicalization of new "diseases" would not be possible without certain qualifications. It is unlikely that a change in medical practice would result just from terminating our common use of medical terminology.

A second variant of the functional argument can be found in Franco Basaglia's, Erving Goffman's and Thomas Szasz's contributions (Basaglia

1971, pp. 114ff., Goffman 1961, Szasz 1977). They refer, in particular, to the sometimes intolerable practice of clinical psychiatry. According to this approach, the concept of mental illness provides psychiatry with a medical façade, hence conceals its punishing, pedagogical character and the extreme social consequences of the stigma of mental illness.

We can rebuke this argument in a similar fashion as mentioned above. Even if the concept of mental illness were to be abandoned (e.g., in the DSM the notion 'illness' has indeed been replaced by 'disorder') this would not necessarily lead to a change of clinical practice and its social consequences. On the contrary, as one learns from experience, reforms are possible even if we still use the term 'mental illness'. There is no necessary relation whatsoever between the attribution of a mental illness and "incarceration".

In summary, functional arguments generally lack plausibility insofar that they need to show a valid connection between the usage of the concept of illness and the negatively valued practice of medicine. In my opinion this has not deemed successful.

2. Historical Arguments

Most historical arguments operate by means of a radically new version of the history of psychiatry which differs considerably from the "official" histography. The latter is based mainly on the grounds that there have always been mental illnesses, even if the phenomena were conceptualized in a different way. The sceptics using historical arguments suggest on the contrary, that particular periods and cultures interpreted the phenomena in an entirely different fashion. In their opinion this establishes the relativity of the concept of mental illness, hence undermines its alleged solid basis. If the concept of mental illness depends on cultural constellations alone, there will be no good reasons not to abandon it for the mental sphere.

Foucault, for example, suggests in *Madness and Civilisation* that the concept of mental illness was not introduced purely on scientific grounds, e.g. by the discovery of clear causes of "mad" behaviour, but because of specific social problems and interests concerning the practice of internment. Foucault asserts that especially moral norms influenced society's relationship to "madmen". Szasz believes that Charcot and Freud invented the concept of mental illness at the turn of the century when they had passed over from the merely metaphorical use – "Mental illness is like somatic illness, but..." – to a literal use of the concept. Szasz asserts that there was absolutely no reason for doing this (Szasz 1974, pp. 17ff.).

It is not quite clear how a historical argument could in any way undermine the foundation of the concept of mental illness. Every concept has a history and changes of meaning are often connected to particular interests, as one can see in the more recent debate on the concept of death. But the fact that these variations exist is not in itself sufficient evidence for the futility or ineffectivity of a particular concept, just as it does not prevent any progress in conceptualization, i.e. a better or more reasonable definition. There may have been good reasons for Charcot and Freud (disregarding the question whether or not it is historically correct to attribute to them the introduction of medical terminology in psychiatry) for expanding the concept of illness to include mental problems as well.

To show the futility of the concept of mental illness as such by means of historical arguments, one needs more than just the example of crude and interest-laden conceptualizations e.g. of the French classical age, which is Foucault's example. One would have to prove further that the concept, which has been running through culture- and interest-laden definitions, can never be rid of this flaw. This is not provided by the historical argumentations I am familiar with. General arguments against the concept of mental illness do not seem to work merely on a historical foundation.

To recapitulate: the historical and cultural relativity of the concept of mental illness does not prove its insignificance or that mental illness cannot exist. There may indeed be more significant or reasonable conceptualizations of the term 'mental illness'.

3. Interpretative Arguments

Interpretative arguments claim that, although the concept of mental illness may possibly be used in a reasonable way, it does not apply to several of the phenomena which are allegedly covered by the concept. This is an approach that does not reject the concept of mental illness in principle, but narrows its scope considerably or re-interprets it in a way that it could be abandoned altogether.

This argument has been put forth by Laing in *The Divided Self*. His intention was to supplement the objectifying gaze of a doctor on the supposed mentally ill with the subjective standpoint of the patient himself. Instead of regarding the human being as an object, as an organism, one has to see and understand him as a person in his own particular living conditions to gain sufficient comprehension of his mental problems. The "abnormal" behaviour, which is regarded as a symptom of mental illness in the common psychiatric interpretation, should instead be decoded as an expression of his way of existence. If this had been done, the behaviour of so-called mentally ill people would often lose its unintelligibility, and therefore question the dichotomy of mental health and illness.

Laing is not very clear about what he regards as criteria of mental illness. For example he writes: "I suggest, therefore, that *sanity or psychosis is tested by the degree of conjunction or disjunction* (in the judgement concerning one's own and the other's identity, T.S.) *between two persons where the one is sane by common consent*" (Laing 1960, p. 37). In the first instance, this appears like an operational definition of the concept of mental illness because it entails a test for determining its extension. But on scrutinizing this definition more carefully, it turns out to be unclear – e.g. what is meant exactly by "general consensus"? We would need to know in advance who is mentally healthy in order to determine who is not. But Laing seems to accept, at least implicitly, an interpretation of mental illness as unintelligible mental states (wishes, beliefs, emotions etc.) or behaviour. This interpretation is common and by no means absurd. It is sometimes claimed even by representatives of "classical" psychiatry.[4]

Laing's thesis is that unintelligible mental states and the resulting behaviour become intelligible as soon as one tries to understand them from the inner perspective of the concerned person, since the "pathological" behaviour is often a completely reasonable reaction to threats of the self. These threats can, for example, follow from particular constellations in the family which prevent an united identity. The reaction of the person to the "insecurity of the self" could then be interpreted as an "attempt to achieve secondary security from the primary dangers facing him in his original ontological insecurity" (ibid., p. 95).

This strategy of building a "false-self system" is full of threats, e.g. the problem of the need to both affirm one's own existence and to be a visible object for others who could question this existence. Attempts of the "ill" to be incognito, anonymous, nobody, someone else etc. in order not to risk the "self-created" identity occasionally follow from this impasse. The step towards psychosis is not undertaken, in Laing's opinion, unless the original reaction of protection piles up to a wall which holds the self captured. Since her own identity becomes "real" only in relation to other persons, this confinement leads to a kind of death of the self. "It (i.e. psychosis, T.S.) can be stated in its most general form as: *the denial of being, as a means of preserving being*" (ibid., p. 161).

To summarize: It is Laing's intention to show that many alleged pathological kinds of behaviour can be understood as completely normal and possibly healthy reactions (because they protect the threatened self), if one would only abandon or supplement the restrained, objectifying focus of psychiatry. Laing's claim exemplifies an interpretative argument in the suggested categorization, because he accepts a particular conceptualization of illness in psychiatry – mental illness as unintelligible mental states and behaviour – just in order to show that the phenomena which are often regarded as mental illness are not covered by the concept. Consequently, in Laing's interpretation, many of

4 For example theorists, who refer to irrationality as a criterion of mental illness, like Moore (1975), Edwards (1981), Gert (1990).

the alleged ill people are people in existentially threatening living-conditions who are reacting in a completely normal manner. Despite this, one can speak of illness (psychosis) in some extreme situations. Thus, if we accept Laing's radical reinterpretation, the concept of mental illness would be considerably narrowed in its scope.

But Laing's argumentation is still not convincing: Firstly, he does not show clearly why the mere fact that we can attribute reasonable motives to the behaviour of a supposedly mentally ill person (e.g. a threat to his self) should suffice to qualify or even prevent a psychiatric diagnosis. Admittedly, it may be possible to explain his "pathological" behaviour by means of a "double-bind"-situation in the family, but this explanation would not be crucial for judging whether or not the person is ill. To take a different example, psychosomatic illness is also often explained as an understandable reaction to an unbearable or threatening situation in life. But it is nevertheless usually regarded as illness for good reasons. Mere intelligibility of beliefs, wishes, emotions, behaviour etc. does not rule out the possibility to explain them as basically disordered and therefore to regard the person as mentally ill.

It is wrong to argue that only because mental problems are influenced or caused by social constellations, they cannot be termed as cases of mental illness. It is of course true that society provides generating and sustaining factors, but this does not speak against the conceptualization of severe mental disturbances as illness. Whether or not we are able to understand the behaviour of someone else cannot be a decisive criterion of mental health and illness.[5]

---

5 In passing, I would like to mention briefly Laing's conception of "madness" as a "radical trip", as a journey into inner-life. This interpretation was introduced in the book *The Politics of Experience* in 1967. Thereafter, he was often accused of "romanticizing" mental illness (Laing almost always deals with Schizophrenia), but he rejected that objection vehemently (Mullan 1995, pp. 2, 357).

Laing presupposes that there is no known aetiology or pathology which could back the concept of illness for mental phenomena. Hence Laing believes that he is justified to replace the medical with an "existential" approach. For him, "madness" is a "transcendent", a quasi-religious experience. Since, in his view, modern men are alienated from the "inner world", inner absorption is judged as dangerous or ill. But because inner occupation is essential to human life, madness needs to be accepted as a possible way to recover from a condition of alienation. To refer to other human beings as mentally ill loses its significance if we judge this aspect from an already alienated perspective. "From the alienated starting point of our pseudo-sanity, everything is equivocal. Our sanity is not 'true' sanity. Their madness is not 'true' madness. The madness of our patients is an artefact of the destruction wreaked on them by us, and by them to themselves. Let no one suppose that we meet 'true' madness any more than that we are truly sane" (Laing 1967, p. 118). But even if Laing's normative assertion were true, i.e. that mankind is alienated from the inner realm, this would not explain how the attribution of alleged madness works, since surely not all "inner-absorbed" people can be regarded as mentally ill. In exactly what way the alleged alienation is connected to the relativity of attributions of "madness" still remains unclear.

Some sceptics, e.g. David Cooper, the Sozialistisches Patientenkollektiv and, in some statements, Foucault suggest an even stronger thesis than Laing (Cooper 1978, Roth 1972, Foucault 1976, cf. Bopp 1980, Jervis 1979). They begin with a similar conceptualization of mental illness, identifying *deviant* behaviour as a decisive feature of mental illness (not just unintelligibility). This criterion too is not unfounded. But in this variety of the interpretative argumentation deviant behaviour is evaluated positively, e.g. because it is revolutionary or because it breaks social norms and eventually questions their significance. Hence, according to the named sceptics, mentally ill people become the avant-garde of a political and cultural transformation that is essential. Since illness is usually regarded as a negatively valued condition, the concept of mental illness seems to be led *ad absurdum* by this argumentation. An approval of a particular conceptualization, together with a reversal of the evaluation, supposedly proves the social determination of the concept and therefore the relativity of judgments of mental illness. If the argumentation proves true, it will no longer be significant to talk of mental *illness* because the phenomena in question would pose political and not medical problems.

But this argumentation is also not convincing. Firstly, it is not quite clear what is meant by 'deviance'. The ambiguity of this concept is exploited by the sceptics in order to identify illness in the case of social nonconformity and acquire a positive evaluation of the behaviour. Obviously, there is no mention that one may understand deviation in a different way, e.g. as a violation of psychological norms. For example, compulsive behaviour would then be interpreted as deviant behaviour in the sense that a usually available ability to prevent an action by means of an act of will is disturbed. This claim, of course, is in need of further clarification, nevertheless it suffices in order to criticize the presented sceptical argumentation. In the same way, this ambiguity demonstrates why deviant behaviour does not present a reasonable criterion for the ascription of mental illness, however it may be assessed.

In general, interpretative arguments first need to justify the conceptualization of mental illness on which they base their approach. This step is often skipped tacitly. The exemplary argumentations introduced here postulate a certain interpretation of the concept of mental illness which is not sufficiently vindicated. Hence they fail to secure a foundation for rejecting the concept of mental illness altogether as well as for indicating the need to interpret it in a radically new way. Nevertheless, the interpretative argumentation demonstrates that it is worth to engage in more detail the concept of mental illness since many existing definitions are not apt in their description. And this is a conclusion which is often neglected by "classical" psychiatry.

4. Sociological Arguments

The sociological argumentation attempts to provide better explanations of the phenomena than is the case in classical psychiatry. Alternatives are presented to the "usual" concept of mental illness, either as a supplement or as a substitute. Explanatory arguments differ from interpretative arguments in their outright abandonment of the medical terminology in order to make way for new explanations. In this alternative explanation, mental problems are not explained as psychiatric illnesses but as social phenomena.

The most famous version of this argumentation is dedicated to Thomas Scheff. He advocated this argumentation for the first time in 1966, in his book *Being Mentally Ill.* In 1984, he published an extended and slightly revised edition. Scheff, like Laing, tried to divert the focus from the person as bearer of a disease to the social context in which mental problems appear. Scheff regards medical definitions as implausible, mainly because they are unable to identify an essential characteristic or a common basis of the phenomena. Although at this time neurotransmitters and their probable relation to particular symptoms of illness were discovered, he does not see this as leading to any greater persuasive power of psychiatric conceptualizations (Scheff 1984, p. X). As long as explanations of medical science are not sufficiently validated he sees himself justified in providing rival explanations. According to him, the decision as to which theory proves to be more useful is an empirical matter (Scheff 1984, p. 91). Although Scheff explicitly states that it was not his intention to reject psychiatric interpretations altogether (Scheff 1984, pp. 179, 190), his book does indeed entail propositions which do not stand in accordance with common convictions in psychiatry.

Scheff proposes an explanation of mental problems as forms of "residual rule-breaking". Crime, perversion, drunkenness and bad manners are also violations of norms but these are denoted as such officially on the grounds of particular types of norms. Scheff refers to them as "deviance" in order to distinguish them from violations of residual rules. Mental disorders fall into a category that does not carry an explicit cultural label, contrary to deviant behaviour. They violate the norms which are so fundamental that they are even shared in society without any questioning. Examples of residual rules are rules of conversation, like looking at an interlocutor's face or keeping an adequate distance to her. In our culture, according to Scheff, particular forms of violations of residual rules are condensed in a specific category, or labelled 'mental illness'.

Scheff tries to show that a violation of a residual rule as such does not necessarily lead to labelling. On the contrary, a violation is often "denied" by others because it is transitory. (Scheff changed this notion into "normalized" in the second edition of his book). So the social reaction to a violation of norms determines whether someone is labelled as 'mentally ill'.

The label 'mental illness' itself is generated by social stereotypes, i.e. clichés which are transferred in mass media and eventually form traditions. An essential difference of the alleged mentally ill is suggested ("outgrouping"). According to Scheff, stereotypes explain why the labelling of alleged mental illness is homogenous in society.

The question arises as to why violators of residual rules accept the social label. Scheff believes that this is due to a social and psychiatric system of reward and punish, which – in addition to the vulnerability of a person going through a crisis – leads to an acquiescence to the role of the "mentally ill". Scheff made a point of declaring his controversial thesis: "Among residual rule-breakers, labelling is among the most important causes of careers of residual deviance." (Scheff 1984, p. 69).

It should be emphasized that Scheff does not assert that labelling is one of the most important causes of individual mental problems. This is an attribution which has often been made (e.g. Reznek 1991, pp. 105, 108, Roth and Kroll 1986, p. 15) and which suggests that he would explain the phenomena of mental disturbances by labelling – which, in my opinion, is clearly absurd. But Scheff only asserts that labelling is one of the most important causes of *taking the role* of someone who is mentally ill.

We can draw several conclusions from Scheff's approach: Firstly, attributions of mental illness depend decisively on accidental factors, i.e. whether a rule-violation happens in public or in a tolerant environment, whether the person in question is prepared to accept the label and to submit to the social sick-role and what the stereotypes look like and whether they succeed. Secondly, labelling decisively determines the future social judgement of the offender. By being labelled, a possibly passing transgression may take on a chronic character. Thirdly, mental illness is first and foremost not something a person has, but something which is attributed. Fourthly, the concept of mental illness is a cultural construction, a label, which arises from particular violations of residual rules. Its criteria are determined by stereotypes. To be sure, there are indeed proposals in psychiatric medicine to define the concept of mental illness without these stereotypes, but they are neither plausible nor able to prevail in public opinion.

Nevertheless, Scheff's explanation seems to me lacking in several points. To begin with, it is striking that he is also (like some interpretative accounts) concerned with behaviour. This probably follows from his rejection of "somaticist" or physiological theories of mental illness, i.e. explanations of mental illness by means of physiological disorders. But Scheff does not mention that one might refer to other causes of behaviour than merely the physiological ones and that therefore an essential characteristic of mental illness might exist. Somaticist theories of mental illness are not the only alternatives to Scheff's labelling-theory.

Scheff's problem in explaining why particular violations of residual rules and not others evoke the label 'mental illness' follow directly from the restriction to behaviour. His explanation works on the basis of existent social reactions which are primarily coined by stereotypes and therefore evoked rather incidentally. But there are several examples of labelled mental illness, where social judgement is entirely indifferent or diverse, hence Scheff's thesis does not hold firm.

Scheff's explanation also remains vague in cases of labelled illness, which is not characterized by any violation of residual rules, e.g. eating disorders like anorexia nervosa or certain phobias. If Scheff nevertheless wished to regard these mental problems as violations of residual rules, he would have had trouble in explaining why only these types and not the "normal" manifestations of the same behaviour, e.g. denial to eat, are labelled as mental illness. For that purpose, he would have had to refer to the foundation of behaviour, to its causes, i.e. mental phenomena like desires, beliefs etc. Again, adequate explanations of mental illness cannot merely refer to behaviour and social reactions.

It has been established that Scheff wishes to avoid any reference to causes of behaviour since he regards them as unknown (Scheff 1984, p. 189). Instead he wishes to explain how social reactions create a "chronic" violation of residual rules, i.e. the role of the mentally ill. So his question is not: What is mental illness as compared to other cases which may go along with violations of rules? But: How does the label "mental illness" come into existence? As I have already tried to point out, Scheff was unable to come up with an appropriate answer to this question. But even if he had done so, the first question would still be left unanswered and therefore unproven that the label 'mental illness' is based on accidental and culturally determined components alone. The practice of labelling is preceded by a particular conceptualization of what mental illness is. Since such an analysis does not have to be founded on stereotypes only, but could be supported by convincing reasons – depending on the theory of mental illness maintained – the label 'mental illness' does not have to be accidentally or socially determined. Hence, I do not feel that Scheff's theory presents a better explanation of the phenomena than does the approach of psychiatric medicine, which assumes mental illness as the cause of "deviant" behaviour and therefore of the label.

The strength of Scheff's theory surely lies in his demonstration of accidental contributions to the labelling-practice, which do not fit in accordance to the official viewpoints of medical professionals (Scheff 1984, p. 183). But I believe that we should observe these as serious shortcomings, and so it seems obvious to look for a definition of mental illness beyond labelling. Diagnoses of mental illness must not rely on social reactions to certain behaviour but on a convincing theory of mental illness.

5. Conceptual Arguments

Conceptual arguments express a general scepticism against the concept of mental illness, i.e. they are – contrary to some of the other approaches listed so far – not consistent with the survival of the concept of mental illness. Hence they are particularly provocative. The sceptical conclusion of this argumentation follows from certain dissimilarities between bodily and (supposed) mental illness or between bodily and mental states. So this approach makes use of the dualism between mind and body, which seems to be the basis of the concept of mental illness. Szasz, the main proponent of the conceptual argumentation, states different kinds of divergence.

Firstly, Szasz points at the difference between the generation of somatic and psychiatric disease-kinds. There is, he claims, a basic discrepancy between the establishment of diagnostic units like 'Cancer', 'Tuberculosis', 'AIDS' etc. and classificatory kinds like 'Schizophrenia', 'Hysteria', 'Anorexia Nervosa' etc. The difference consists in the *discovery* of somatic disease-kinds by detecting the nature of it, contrary to the *invention* of mental disease-kinds by attributing an alleged common nature of the phenomena.

Secondly, Szasz sees a dissimilarity between diagnoses on the grounds of signs of disease. These can be identified by *objective* methods in the case of somatic illness but only *subjective* complaints in the case of alleged mental illness.

Thirdly, he shows a discrepancy by first suggesting an answer to the question what *illness* is in general and then proving that the concept of illness cannot refer to mental phenomena. According to this view, mental illness is merely a *metaphorical illness.*

Fourthly, he stresses a general difference between *bodily* and *mental* processes or states. According to this objection, 'body' and 'mind' are two entirely different categories to which notions like 'illness' do not apply in the same way.

Fifthly, Szasz identifies a dissimilarity between the norms underlying different attributions of illness. He believes that in the case of somatic illness the norms are *value-neutral*, whereas in the case of mental illness they are *value-laden*, i.e. the concept of mental illness contains value-judgments contrary to the concept of somatic illness.

a) Discovery – Invention

The difference between the creation of somatic disease-kinds and psychiatric classification cannot be denied. Two examples may suffice to illustrate: In 1882, Robert Koch discovered the so-called Tuberculosis Bacillus which was identified as the cause of a form of disease referred to as 'Consumption' and later – after the discovery of affected tissue – as 'Tuberculosis'. With the discovery of the bacillus it was proved that particular phenomena, previously referred to as 'Tuberculosis', were not caused by the same germ and therefore did not belong to the same category. Koch discovered, one could argue, the nature of the disease Tuberculosis.

In contrast, the abolition of the alleged mental illness Homosexuality from the DSM was mainly owed to the pressure exerted by the gay-rights-movement. This obviously indicates the political structure of psychiatric diagnostic units. Since the installation of new illnesses works along the same principle, i.e. by voting, one may claim that mental illnesses like 'Hyperkinetic Syndrome' or 'Post-traumatic Stress-Disorder' have been invented. So this difference seems to prevent us from justly speaking of mental illness in the same way we speak of somatic illness.

But we can object to this argumentation as follows: All diseases are in some form or other inventions or constructs. It may be true that Koch discovered a bacillus but certainly he did not discover the disease Tuberculosis. It is just a name for particular phenomena collected under a specific disease-concept, i.e. a disease-kind (Blankenburg 1989, Häfner 1989). Tuberculosis, just like Schizophrenia, cannot be discovered because the unification in the disease-kind could have happened in another way. The fact that particular phenomena were no longer regarded as Tuberculosis after the discovery of the Tuberculosis Bacillus does not indicate that they were not cases of "true" Tuberculosis or the like, but only proves an alteration of our knowledge about the nature of particular phenomena. There is no mistake in principle in referring to some illnesses as Tuberculosis even if they are not caused by the same germ. But since disease-kinds are usually best classified by their causes – for the supposedly best therapy – a reclassification is generally implemented when the aetiology is known. In the history of medicine, one may find many examples of these conceptual alterations which are owed to findings on the nature of illness phenomena.[6] Here we can also see the variety of criteria underlying classifications (and, in fact, they vary in existing nosologies like DSM or ICD). Either particular symptoms or a syndrome, i.e. the unification of several symptoms, or pathological anatomy, dysfunction, or causes can be used as criteria. This variety shows why there can be no discovery of disease-kinds.

Disease-kinds are categories guided by human interests and not entities found in nature (Margolis 1980, Sadler et al. 1994). It may be said that somatic or mental phenomena, which we collect under a specific concept of disease, exist independent of human interests. But the disease itself does not appear

6 By referring to a nature of disease-kinds it is suggested only that there can be regularities of the phenomena. It is not intended to claim that diseases are natural kinds (cf. Reznek 1987).

without an organism, which is diseased, and hence in individual forms.[7] The unification of all these similar – but nevertheless non-identical – phenomena into one category cannot be regarded as a discovery. In some formulations our common language veils the ontological status of disease-kinds.[8] For example we sometimes say: "I have caught a cold" or "Ronald has Alzheimer's disease", as if a disease would be an entity whizzing about in the environment, e.g. entering into the body through the ear. Because this is not so, one cannot discover a disease-kind like measles as one discovers an unknown virus. The Mycobacterium Tuberculosis *is* not the disease Tuberculosis, but its cause. Hence, its discovery cannot be regarded as *discovery* of a disease.

But this defence against the discovery-invention-objection does not appear to be the last word, because, so far, it has only been shown that one cannot discover disease-*kinds*. This follows from the fact that the unification under a specific disease concept is always a human intervention. But Szasz's argument can be interpreted at a deeper level, namely, to the general concept of illness. We have – so the argument could run – a rough idea – even if we do not have a clear definition – what an illness is in general. If we feel pain or are no longer able to do particular things, then we are *presumed* to have a disease. Here we are still placing a judgement on the level of symptoms. This presumption will usually be confirmed if a lesion, a disorder or the like is found as the basis of these symptoms. We could then claim that we have discovered a disease if we find the underlying pathology. If we cannot find a lesion or the like, we are unable to explain the condition of the patient. We then either have to accept that our diagnostic abilities are not yet up to standard and that we will someday discover an underlying pathology or come up with another explanation, e.g. that the patient is malingering. But the discovery of the disease follows from the discovery of the underlying pathology. If a new form of pathology is discovered, e.g. as in the example of AIDS, a new form of disease is discovered, even if it cannot be said, as suggested above, that *AIDS* was discovered.

---

7 That does not include the thesis that there are no diseases but only diseased persons, which was proposed by so-called individual pathology (e.g. Karl Menninger). Cf. Häfner 1981, Sadegh-Zadeh 1977. A related question is, whether a disease state can exist beyond the death of the diseased person. For example, Szasz claims – in my opinion against common intuitions: "Every 'ordinary' illness that persons have, cadavers also have" (*The Second Sin*, p. 99, cited in Pies 1979, p. 140).

8 The ontological status of disease-kinds has been controversial ever since. Usually two models are distinguished, one is often called physiological and the other ontological. The ontological model presumes that there is something like a disease entity which could be discovered. The physiological model, on the other hand, regards disease-kinds as names for phenomena without any clear nature. For this see e.g. Nordenfelt 1987, Appendix, Pies 1979, Reznek 1987, Sadegh-Zadeh 1977.

This view does not seem to hold true for mental diseases. If no underlying pathology can be found, this outcome appears to have no grave significance on the part of the psychiatrists. Even worse, often the mere presumption of mental illness, e.g. in the case of particular symptoms, is regarded as sufficient for inclusion in nosological systems.

> (...) this is the inescapable consequence of confusing discovering diseases with inventing them: the enterprise of trying to discover bodily diseases, constrained by fixed criteria and the requirements of empirical evidence, *cannot* eventuate in the conclusion that every phenomenon observed by the investigator is a disease; but the enterprise of inventing mental diseases, unconstrained by fixed criteria or the requirements of empirical evidence, *must* eventuate in the conclusion that any phenomenon studied by the observer may be defined as a disease. (Szasz 1974, p. 13).

But we can object to Szasz's statement that even with the "discovery" of somatic disease, no such clear criteria prevail. It has been established that there are obvious examples of pathology constituting disease. But there are also cases regarded as a disease for good reasons, although there are no clear pathological evidences, e.g. migraine. Accordingly, one can presume a pathological basis for mental illness too, although to date, this remains to a large extent unclarified. Regarding the probably most frequently investigated kind of mental illness – schizophrenia – it was found that there are alterations in the functioning of neurotransmitters in the brain. To be sure, this is not an empirical evidence which Szasz seems to have in mind. But even if the somatic basis of mental illness cannot be found, it does not seem mandatory to hold such a restricted view of pathology. For him, pathology seems to refer only to evidences, which can be sensually perceived and grasped, i.e. alterations of bodily structure, and therefore regarded as "discoveries" (Szasz 1974, p. 12). In my opinion, this is far too narrow a criterion for the attribution of illness. If one maintains a wider definition of pathology, mental illness will gain plausibility despite the fact that no somatic basis has yet been discovered. Admittedly, this assertion is in need of further justification and Szasz is absolutely right in indicating the neglect of this task in some medical approaches.

To recapitulate: Szasz failed to show a discrepancy between somatic and mental illness regarding the specific concepts of mental illness, i.e. disease-kinds. Concerning the general concept of illness he suggested a difference only by maintaining a restricted criterion of pathology, which seems implausible, because it rules out even some somatic illnesses which are usually included for valid reasons. Nevertheless, one needs to find a plausible criterion for the attribution of mental illness which maintains the analogy to somatic illness, in order to reject this argumentation completely. This task cannot be fulfilled in this essay.[9]

9 But see Schramme 2003.

b) Objective – Subjective

The second form of divergence between somatic and mental illness is related to the first although it does not refer to a criterion underlying illness but to its symptoms. It is claimed that somatic illness is diagnosed on the basis of objective signs while mental illness is attributed merely on subjective complaints i.e. symptoms. Szasz claimed that one form of evidence for this can be seen in the fact that there is no asymptomatic mental illness. In contrast, asymptomatic somatic disease is relatively frequent, e.g. cancer of an early stage or haemophilia without bleeding that would expose the disease. "(...) [M]ental diseases manifest themselves in only one way, by symptoms, and can accordingly be identified in only one way, from symptoms." (Szasz 1987, p. 92)

This variation of the first objection provokes a similar reproach. Firstly, it does not refer to differences between conditions of somatic and mental illness, but to differences in the *indications* of mental and somatic illness. As already noted on this level, illness is just a presumption and even if a sign is objectively identifiable e.g. by means of sounds of heartbeat, that alone would not guarantee a valid diagnosis. In some cases, a result below the norm may not be due to an illness at all, e.g. in cases of overexertion. Hence, this argumentation fails to show a principled difference between somatic and mental illness. Even if somatic illness would be suspected exclusively by means of objective (e.g. measurable) procedures and mental illness exclusively by means of subjective complaints, there would be no rejection, in general, to a possible analogy with regard to the causes of these indications, namely, pathological states or processes.

But Szasz further claims that mental illness is *identified* with symptoms:

> In psychiatry, not only is the word illness used metaphorically and interpreted literally, but also is the word symptom. This is crystal clear from the way we use what we call the two classic *symptoms of psychosis*, namely *hallucinations* and *delusions*. For example, unlike precordial pain, which may or may not point to coronary insufficiency, hallucinations and delusions *do not point* to psychosis; they are (the same as) psychosis. (...) The reason for this lies in the *prejudgments* that words such as *hallucination* and *delusion* carry with them. (Szasz 1987, p. 95)

But Szasz's assertion is plainly incorrect. Even if some psychiatrists would infer mental illness from symptoms like hallucinations in all cases, I, personally, would presume none of them would maintain that these *are* the diagnosed mental illness (and if they did, it would be false). To most of them, it would be quite clear that these symptoms alone cannot justify an illness-attribution, because hallucinations or delusions can also be caused by drug abuse or exhaustion. Szasz's argument therefore stops at the level of indications of alleged illness.

Besides, a diagnosis of somatic illness usually starts from subjective complaints, too (cf. Ausubel 1961, p. 71). A patient feels bad, is feeble, suffers from pain etc. A physician can examine her, maybe with additional help from technical instruments, e.g. he may measure her temperature, perform an electrocardiogram or X-ray pictures. So symptoms and signs together lead to a presumption of illness, which can result in further examinations. Contrary to Szasz's thesis, we do not depend merely on subjective claims in cases of mental illness. For example, orientation in space and time, the ability to reasoning etc. can be examined in an interview. This may even come up with some measurable results, e.g. by means of psychological tests. Of course, we cannot refer to these data as objective as, for example, the data we get from taking someone's temperature. But for my purposes it suffices to say that even a diagnosis of mental illness does not have to be founded on claims of the patient alone and hence, no discrepancy to somatic illness exists in principle.

Probably Szasz would object at this point that the mentioned methods are still subjective, since he seem to accept only bodily signs as objective. "Symptoms are verbal communications or claims; signs are objective measurements of bodily structures or functions, or publicly verifiable observations about the body" (Szasz 1987, p. 94, cf. p. 92, Szasz 1974, pp. 84f., 1978, pp. 461f.). But even if one accepts this restriction of the notion 'sign', it still holds true that psychiatrists do not depend on subjective complaints only when they diagnose mental illness. The simple dichotomy between a symptom as a subjective complaint, on the one hand, and a sign as an objectively recognizable lesion is not convincing. That is why asymptomatic mental illnesses may even be imagined, contrary to the explicit opinion of Szasz, although this in fact may be rare. For example, a phobia might be detected in a psychological interview without any explicit complaint or suffering of the patient.

A variation of this sceptical argument was raised in a study by David Rosenhan (Rosenhan 1973). Together with some collaborators, he simulated common symptoms of mental illness, i.e. hallucinations, confusion as to one's own identity etc. Thereupon they were diagnosed with schizophrenia and sent to a psychiatric clinic. According to Rosenhan, this experiment proves the general differences between a diagnosis of mental illness in contrast to somatic illness.

But in fact this is not shown at all. The possibility of pretending also exists in case of somatic illness and may be discovered fairly easily. The stated differences in diagnosis seem to be due to the limited results in the exploration of mental illness up to date. We should not forget that not long ago it was also difficult to distinguish between "real" illness and malingering in the case of somatic illness.

In summary: both subjective and objective factors play a part in the diagnosis of somatic as well as mental illness. So far the claimed discrepancy is restricted to the still prevailing ignorance whether indicators of illness are really founded on a pathological basis in the case of mental illness. Further investigations and research are essential for better clarification. But the same problem applies also to some somatic illnesses, even today. Hence, a principled disparity cannot be shown by opposing allegedly objective indicators of somatic disease to merely subjective ones, as in the case of mental illness.

c) Illness – Metaphorical Illness

The third difference follows when the concept of illness is defined and then proved that mental phenomena do not apply to it. Szasz points to the fact, correctly in my opinion, that we cannot discuss adequately what mental illness really entails unless we are able to reflect on what illness is in general (Szasz 1987, p. 9). This is often neglected. I myself have not discussed or proposed any explicit definition of illness either, but in order to answer the leading question of this essay, i.e. whether there is such a thing as mental illness, it is essential to have some preliminary comprehension. For a complete rejection of the sceptical arguments we need a plausible conception of the notion 'mental illness'.

> Psychiatrists and all those steeped in the psychiatric ideology take the decisive initial step of omitting to define illness in general, or bodily illness in particular, and instead *define mental illness* (whatever they mean by it) *as a member of the class called illness*. I reject this approach. Instead of accepting the phenomena called mental illnesses as diseases, the decisive initial step I take is to *define illness as the pathologist defines it – as a structural or functional abnormality of cells, tissues, organs, or bodies*. If the phenomena called mental illnesses manifest themselves as such structural or functional abnormalities, then they are *diseases*; if they do not, they are *not*. (Szasz 1987, p. 12)

Szasz could be reproached for defining illness in such a way that leaves no space for mental illness from the outset, because his definition refers to the body only (e.g. Roth and Kroll 1986, Ausubel 1961). However, illness would be synonymous to X, with X determined in a way that again secures the possibility of genuine mental illness. This mere opposition of a different definition does not seem to be a reasonable defence, irrespective of whether it excludes mental illness or not.

However, there is no reason to outrightly reject the cited definition as on preliminary comprehension it does not seem unreasonable at all. But there are still grounds to reject Szasz's conclusion that there is no mental illness. As he himself admits in the second part of the quotation above, there could be mental illness if the phenomena were based on structural or functional abnormalities of cells, tissues, organs or bodies. Since Szasz does not believe that the phenomena, regarded as mental illness, are based on a bodily abnormality (e.g. Szasz 1987, p. 49ff.), there is, in his opinion, no (non-metaphorical) way of referring to mental illness. He counters an obvious objection, namely, that mental illness is brain disease and therefore included in his definition, with the contention that in this case, there would be no reason to call it *mental* illness: "However, diseases of the brain are brain diseases; it is confusing, misleading, and unnecessary to call them mental illness." (Szasz 1987, p. 49)

This contention is not easily rejected either. If we want to speak of *mental* illness, we seem to imply an unpopular mind-body dualism. Even the editors of the DSM, the American classificatory system of mental disorders, believe in this implication.[10] But these doubts are without grounding. One can surely postulate a bodily basis of mental phenomena, but still talk of mental illness. This possibility would be ruled out only if mental phenomena could be exhaustively explained by the underlying bodily processes, i.e. reduced to brain disease. Although I am unable to deal with the mind-body problem in this article, it suffices to state that even if mental illness has a bodily basis, it will not follow necessarily that referral to mental illness will be confusing, misleading and unnecessary. Nevertheless, Szasz's definition of illness applies to phenomena only appearing along a bodily abnormality. This somatic basis has not been proved for many of the conditions regarded now as mental illness, though it is not unlikely that at least for some of them this is going to happen someday.[11]

One further objection could be made against Szasz: If we take for granted that body and mind form a unit in human beings, i.e. that the mind comes into being inside an organism, then we are able to speak of functional abnormalities of minds and, therefore, – on the basis of Szasz's own definition – of mental illness, despite the ignorance of corresponding physiological or neurological processes. To be sure, there would still be the need to demonstrate exactly what mental functions might be. Despite this, even on the basis of his own conceptualization of illness, Szasz fails to deny the existence of mental illness in principle.

In conclusion: The third argument works with an explicit definition of illness in order to show that it does not apply to *mental* illness and that the phenomena in question can only be referred to as illness in a metaphorical way. But even if one accepts the proposed definition, the conclusion would not be a convincing one without any further support. Mental illness could be integrated into the definition. Admittedly, this assertion is in need of some more argumentation, e.g. that body and mind are united and that mental processes are not entirely explicable by bodily processes.

---

10 "Mental disorder. This could not be a more unfortunate term, preserving as it does an outdated mind-body duality." Frances et al. 1991, p. 409, see also DSM-IV, p. XXI.

11 Ausubel (1961) also points to the difference between the assertion that there is a physiological *basis* of disordered mental functioning and the stronger thesis that one could explain the particular nature of a patient's disorder by definite lesions of the nervous system. Szasz supposes that the second thesis is necessary in order to maintain the concept of mental illness, however, at the same time lose its independence by the reduction.

d) Bodily – Mental

The fourth argument deals directly with the relation between body and mind. Szasz suggests that the concept of illness cannot refer to mental phenomena, because 'body' and 'mind' belong to different logical categories. If one speaks of mental illness, one would use this concept only as a metaphor.

With this argument, Szasz refers explicitly to the British philosopher, Gilbert Ryle, who attacked the "official doctrine" of Cartesianism in his book *The Concept of Mind*. Cartesian dualism states that every human being has a body and a mind, both of which exist distinctly. Ryle also refers to this assertion as the "dogma of the ghost in the machine". It was his intention to refute it by proving that it relies on a so-called category mistake. Szasz makes use of Ryle's argumentation in order to show that the "official doctrine" of psychiatry, i.e. that there is both bodily and mental illness, is a category mistake as well. The mistake consists in the dubious assertion that both body and mind could be affected by a disease. To understand Szasz's thesis correctly, we first need to comprehend how the category mistake argument works. (Ryle 1949, ch. 1)

Ryle explains the concept of category mistake by means of examples. Let us suppose a foreign student comes to Oxford for the first time in his life. There, he is introduced to various colleges, libraries, administration offices etc. After the tour he says: "I now know the colleges and where the books are kept. I have also seen where the administrators work, but now I want to see the university." Of course, this request cannot be fulfilled, since the colleges, libraries etc. *are* the university. There is no further object of interest called university. Obviously, the student is unaware that 'university' belongs to a different category than 'New College', 'Bodleian Library' etc. A similar mistake would be made if, for instance, someone, after becoming familiar with the functions of a defender, forward, goal-keeper etc. would ask whose function it would be to contribute the team spirit.

The mistake of Cartesianism is based, in Ryle's opinion, in combining the categories, namely, by putting 'mind' into the same category as 'body'. Thereby it is possible to assert that human beings have both a body and a mind. But one can combine terms in a conjunction only if they belong to the same category. Hence we cannot say, "I have seen New College, Bodleian Library *and* the University." It is not Ryle's intention to suggest that minds do not exist. But if this is asserted, then 'exist' is used with a different meaning than in the statement that bodies exist. Because mind and body belong to different categories it is incorrect to state that mind *and* body exist in the same way. Similarly, one cannot say that *either* mind *or* body exist because the disjunction is also not valid for terms belonging to different categories. To claim: "Either I have seen New College, Bodleian Library etc. or the University" is clearly a ridiculous statement.

Szasz does not clarify in what way he wishes to make use of the category mistake argument for his rejection of the concept of mental illness. For example, in *The Myth of Mental Illness* he writes: "For my part, I prefer the view of those contemporary philosophers who suggest that we regard the relationship between body and mind as similar to that between a football team and its team spirit." (Szasz 174, p. 87). In the following footnote he refers to Ryle's *The Concept of Mind*. But *this* is not what Ryle said. His team spirit example is just an example for a category mistake and has nothing to do with the relation between mind and body. It seems rather as if Ryle wishes to reject any indication of a relation between mind and body as such, since they cannot exist both in the same way.

In another passage Szasz writes:

> However, if we place bodily diseases and mental diseases in the same class, we build a category without a clear or carefully defined criterion for membership in it, on the basis that its members *look alike*. Diabetes and depression are both diseases because they both cause suffering; eagles and bats are both birds because they both fly. The logical error of making such a *category mistake*, as the British philosopher Gilbert Ryle called it, is clear enough. (Szasz 1987, p. 168)

This appears to be a weaker argument as there could be mental illness in the case that one finds a clearly defined criterion for membership in the class of illness. Szasz not only sees little hope for bringing about such a criterion, but also emphasizes that because mind and body belong to different categories, there cannot be mental illness in principle. This thesis and its basis, i.e. the category mistake argument, is very important for Szasz's approach and is featured on various occasions, also without explicit reference to Ryle, e.g. when he says, an illness could only affect a body. Therefore I shall scrutinize it briefly.

Firstly, Ryle's category mistake argument aims, as mentioned, at the "official doctrine", which prevails since Descartes and which postulates two entities: mind and body. The peculiar characteristic of Ryle's argument, compared to other objections to dualism, is his assertion that the very question for the relation between body and mind is flawed. But even if we take this view for granted, it does not support Szasz's thesis, since the claim that 'body' and 'mind' belong to different logical categories does not imply that mental illness cannot exist. The argument does not indicate whether or not mental phenomena exist but merely rejects Cartesianism.

Nevertheless, there is still some persuasive power in Szasz's reasoning, based on the implausibility of *substance* dualism, i.e. Cartesianism.[12] The

---

12 Different theories on the relation of mind and body are often united under the label "dualism". If it has been proved that it is not plausible to postulate an instance called 'mind',

concept of mental illness seems to imply that there is a substance, which exists independently from the body and can be affected by a disease just like the body (cf. Leifer 1982, p. 401). But this appears impossible. What weird substance is a mind supposed to be? It is obviously something immaterial, but then, how could it be affected by a virus or another pathogenic agent in the same way as a body?

With regards to this argument, it can be claimed that its plausibility is owed mainly to a proposition, which has been previously criticized i.e. that a disease is an entity, existing independently from an organism, which creeps into the body and, in turn, somehow affects a substance, called "mind". That, of course, is not true. Disease does not exhibit independently from organisms. If one is rid of this belief, then the postulation of mental illness would no longer be implausible, because the claim is not that the mind *has* a disease, but, as believed, a disorder of mental abilities *is* a mental illness. For this, we need not postulate a separation of mind and body. So substance-dualism is not necessary for maintaining the concept of mental illness. Therefore, Szasz fails to show an absurdity in principle of the concept of mental illness by means of his critique of the Cartesian dichotomy between mind and body.

e) Value-neutral – Value-laden

The fifth and last objection to the concept of mental illness consists in showing a difference between the norms leading to the respective attributions of illness. In the case of somatic illness, it is argued that the diagnosis based on biological norms is applied approximately in the same way. But the attribution of mental illness is guided by interest-laden, moral or cultural norms which lead to different cultural and communal interpretations of mental illness. What is regarded as an illness in one culture may be a social distinction in the other. Sometimes this is formulated by the claim that the concept of somatic illness is value-neutral or descriptive, whilst the concept of mental illness is value-laden or prescriptive.

> The concept of illness, whether bodily or mental, implies *deviation from some clearly defined norm*. In the case of physical illness, the norm is the structural and functional integrity of the body. Thus, although the desirability of physical health, as such, is an ethical value, what health *is* can be stated in anatomical and physi-

---

which exists distinctly (but maybe not independently) from the body, then it is assumed that dualism is rejected. But this is too simple, since not *all* dualistic approaches are rejected by this kind of reasoning, apart from substance dualism (not e.g. property dualism). The confusion about dualism which prevails in the debate on the concept of mental illness, exemplifies in the constant reproach addressed to Szasz that he is a dualist (cf. e.g. Gage 1991, p. 184, Roth and Kroll 1986, p. 26), while Szasz and his followers retort with the same accusation (s. Leifer 1982, cf. Svensson 1995).

> ological terms. What is the norm deviation from which it is regarded as mental illness? This question cannot be easily answered. But whatever this norm might be, we can be certain of only one thing: namely, that it is a norm that must be stated in terms of *psychosocial, ethical, and legal* concepts. (Szasz 1960, p. 21)

This form of argument raised a high degree of controversy in the debate on the concept of mental illness. It has been opposed in two ways. One defence of the concept of mental illness is as follows: It is indeed true that mental illness is often attributed because of political interests or moral values, e.g. in several countries political dissidents or "trouble-makers" are diagnosed as mentally ill in order to have them locked up in psychiatric hospitals. But these abuses do not oppose the concept of mental illness in general, rather they are examples for the need of a better definition. And if we define this concept in a reasonable way, we will find that it can also be based on value-neutral norms. Just like in the case of somatic illness, there are criteria for mental illness which are independent of cultures and politics. Just like a human being is provided with natural bodily abilities, so there are natural mental capabilities which can be affected in a similar way and, therefore, justify an illness-attribution. This approach often referred to as naturalism or neutralism, denies the difference concerning mental illness and postulates an analogous value-neutral concept of illness.

The second defence starts conversely with the somatic concept of illness and denies Szasz's other premise, namely, that the concept of somatic illness is value-neutral. This again can be done by different strategies. For example, it can be said that the concept of illness is value-laden because illness is a condition which is disvalued. Nobody wants to be ill, therefore 'illness' is not a neutral concept. It may also be asserted that the concept of somatic illness is value-laden just like the concept of mental illness because it is determined by cultural ideas of what abilities one should possess as a human being. Only in cases where a culturally valued ability is affected, does an illness-attribution follow. The same condition may be assessed in a different way in a different culture.

This kind of reasoning, which defends the concept of mental illness by showing the value-ladenness of both illness-concepts, is usually called normativism. To give a sufficient answer to the question raised here, whether there is such an affliction as mental illness, both naturalistic and normativistic theories have still to be clarified in more detail. But unless it is shown that the somatic concept of illness is value-neutral and the mental concept of illness is value-laden, the fifth argument can be rejected. Szasz would have to either reject the existing naturalistic theories or else prove that only the concept of mental illness is value-laden. The conclusion to be drawn is that a further and intensified discussion of the concept of mental illness is necessary.[13]

---

13 For a more comprehensice account see Schramme 2003. For more on naturalism and normativism see also the Introduction to this anthology.

My aim in this paper was to scrutinize in detail the sceptical thesis that mental illness does not exist. While I have tried to show that this radical claim is unfounded, it also became clear that sceptical psychiatry nevertheless serves an important task by challenging psychiatric theories in their sometimes apodictic attitude. There are many sound reasons to support the fact that the concept of mental illness remains still a contested concept.

References

Ausubel, D. 1961. "Personality Disorder *is* Disease", *American Psychologist*, 16: 69-74.

Basaglia, F. (ed.) 1971. *Die negierte Institution*, Frankfurt/M: Suhrkamp.

Blankenburg, W. 1989."Der Krankheitsbegriff in der Psychiatrie", in: Kisker, K.P. et al. (eds.) *Psychiatrie der Gegenwart* 9, 3. Auflage, Brennpunkte der Psychiatrie, Berlin etc.: Springer-Verlag, 119-145.

Bopp, J. 1980. *Antipsychiatrie. Theorien, Therapien, Politik*, Frankfurt/M: Syndikat.

Cooper, D. 1967. *Psychiatry and Antipsychiatry*, Tavistock Publications: London.

Cooper, D. 1978. *The Language of Madness*, London: Allen Lane.

Dörner, K. 1975. "Der gesellschaftliche Nutzen und Schaden des Krankheitsbegriffs", in *Diagnosen der Psychiatrie*, Frankfurt/M: Campus.

Edwards, R.B. 1981. "Mental Health as Rational Autonomy", *Journal of Medicine and Philosophy*, 6: 309-322.

Foucault, M. 1967. *Madness and Civilisation*, London: Routledge.

Foucault, M. 1976. *Mikrophysik der Macht*, Berlin: Merve.

Foucault, M. 1978. *Mental Illness and Psychology*, University of California Press.

Frances, A. et al. 1991. "An A to Z Guide to *DSM-IV* Conundrums", *Journal of Abnormal Psychology*, Vol.100 No.3: 407-412.

Gage, B.C. 1991. "Review of: Thomas Szasz: *Insanity*", *Theoretical Medicine*, 12: 183-188.

Gert, B. 1990. "Irrationality and the DSM-III-R Definition of Mental Disorder", *Analyse & Kritik*, 12: 34-46.

Goffman, E. 1961. *Asylums: Essays on the Social Situation of Mental Patients and Other Inmates*, New York: Doubleday Anchor.

Häfner, H. 1981. "Der Krankheitsbegriff in der Psychiatrie", in: Degkwitz, R., Siedow, H. (eds.) *Standorte der Psychiatrie*, Band 2: Zum umstrittenen psychiatrischen Krankheitsbegriff, München etc.: Urban & Schwarzenberg.

Häfner, H. 1989. "The Concept of Mental Illness", *Psychological Developments*, 2: 159-170.

Illich, I. 1976. *Limits to Medicine*, New York: Pantheon.

Jervis, G. 1979. *Die offene Institution. Über Psychiatrie und Politik*, Frankfurt/M: Syndikat.

Kick, H. 1990. "Antipsychiatrie und die Krise im Selbstverständnis der Psychiatrie", *Fortschritte der Neurologie und Psychiatrie*, 58: 367-374.

Kisker, K.P. 1979. "Antipsychiatie", in Kisker, K.P. et al. (eds.) *Psychiatrie der Gegenwart*. Forschung und Praxis, 2.Auflage, Band I, Grundlagen und Methoden der Psychiatrie Teil 1, Berlin etc.: Springer-Verlag, 811-825.

Laing, R.D. 1960. *The Divided Self. An Existential Study in Sanity and Madness*, London: Tavistock Publ. 1969[2].

Laing, R.D. 1967. *The Politics of Experience*, London: Routledge & Kegan Paul.
Leifer, R. 1982. "Psychiatry, Language and Freedom", *Metamedicine*, 3: 397-415.
Margolis, J. 1980. "The Concept of Mental Illness: A Philosophical Examination", in Brody, B., Engelhardt, T. (eds.) *Mental Illness: Law and Public Policy*, Dordrecht: Reidel Publ. Co.
Moore, M. 1975. "Some Myths about Mental Illness", *Archives of General Psychiatry*, 32: 1483-1497.
Mullan, B. 1995. *Mad to be Normal. Conversations with R.D. Laing*, London: Free Association Books.
Nordenfelt, L. 1987. *On the Nature of Health. An Action-Theoretic Approach*, Dordrecht: Reidel Publishing Company.
Pies, R. 1979. "On Myths and Countermyths", *Archives of General Psychiatry*, 36: 139-144.
Reznek, L. 1987. *The Nature of Disease*, London and New York: Routledge.
Reznek, L. 1991. *The Philosophical Defence of Psychiatry*, London and New York: Routledge.
Rosenhan, D.L. 1973. "On Being Sane in Insane Places", *Science*, 179: 250-258.
Roth, J. 1972. "Psychiatrie und Praxis des Sozialistischen Patientenkollektivs", *Kursbuch*, 28, (Das Elend mit der Psyche. I Psychiatrie).
Roth, M., Kroll, J. 1986. *The Reality of Mental Illness*, Cambridge: Cambridge U.P.
Ryle, G. 1949. *The Concept of Mind*, London: Hutchinson.
Sadegh-Zadeh, K. 1977. "Krankheitsbegriffe und nosologische Systeme", *Metamed*, 1: 4-41.
Sadler, J.Z., Wiggins, O.P., Schwartz, M.A. 1994. *Philosophical Perspectives on Psychiatric Diagnostic Issues*, Baltimore, MD: Johns Hopkins U.P.
Scheff, T. 1966. *Being Mentally Ill*, Chicago: Aldine Publ.
Scheff, T. 1984. *Being Mentally Ill*, Second Edition, New York: Aldine/de Gruyter.
Schramme, T. 2003. *Psychische Krankheit aus philosophischer Sicht*, Gießen: Psychosozial-Verlag.
Svensson, T. 1995. *On the Notion of Mental Illness*, Avebury Series in Philosophy.
Szasz, T.S. 1960. "The Myth of Mental Illness", *American Psychologist*, 15: 113-118.
Szasz, T.S. 1974. *The Myth of Mental Illness*, Revised Edition, New York: Harper & Row 1974.
Szasz, T.S. 1978. "The Concept of Mental Illness: Explanation or Justification?" in: Engelhardt, T., Spicker, S. (eds.) *Mental Health. Philosophical Perspectives*, Dordrecht 1978, 235-250.
Szasz, T.S. 1977. *The Theology of Medicine*, New York: Harper & Row.
Szasz, T.S. 1987. *Insanity. The Idea and its Consequences*, New York etc.: John Wiley and Sons 1987.
Wakefield, J.C. 1992. "The Concept of Mental Disorder. On the Boundary Between Biological Facts and Social Values", *American Psychologist*, 47: 373-388.

Archaic Concepts for Explaining Disorders

Hans-Jörg Assion

Throughout the history of mankind and the several differing cultures the concepts and the interaction of human body, soul and mind have included numerous religious magical, mystical and animistic elements. In accordance with this, explanations and concepts have been proven and are still present world-wide. Testimonies at the time of the Babylonians as well as reports in Greek literature and from the age of Rome point to shamanic practices. Likewise, references have been found in medieval writings. The belief in the power of magical actions has been established throughout the world. Several reports arising from a large variety of cultures have been discovered leading up to modern times (Lehmann 1925). Stoll wrote: "The belief in the power of magical acts is widespread throughout the whole of world" (Stoll 1904). Accordingly, magical beliefs and practices are also to be found in Europe as well as several contributions relating to popular ideas for the explanation of sicknesses and disease assumed to have originated from Germany (Schmidt 1956).

Shamans were already active in prehistoric times and had many different functions. They were the hunter's helpers, advisors, soothsayers, predictors and healers. The term Shaman comes from the language of the Siberian Tunguse, derived from the word *saman* meaning "somebody, who provokes moves or raises". An alternative explanation traces the term Shaman back to an old Indian word meaning "to arouse" or "chastise" oneself.

The diversity of abundant ritual acts is impressive. They include techniques involving consciousness, trances, physical contact through touching or extraction, engrossment in song and dance with drumming and beating, rituals and magic practices using masks and amulets as well as the administration of medicinal plants. Tobacco traps are believed to lure and catch spirits. An attempt is undertaken to transfer upon oneself the patient's pain or suffering by projecting oneself into the ill person or, in other words, by becoming the patient through a ritual action. Lommel describes Shamanic practices as a psychic technology aim to render ideas conscious. Conflicts are solved by fashioning pictures and playing them against each other. Emotional participation and other effects stand in the foreground resulting in less of an explanatory and intellectual approach imparting insight into reasons for the conflict (Devereux 1982, Stumpfe 1983).

The Shamanic practices are frequently accomplished in order to achieve an expulsion or a reconciliation of evil forces. The concept of demonology belongs to one of the oldest attempts to draw up an explanatory model for the symptoms and causes of illnesses. Alterations in diseases, with no external recognizable cause, are traced back to these concepts relating to influences on supernatural beings, demons or ghosts. If a human is possessed by such a demon, the simple extortion of the demon will, in the end, bring about a healing process. This idea has survived right up till today and is known to be practised in civilized countries (e.g. witch-extortion ritual performed by the bishop of Mainz/Germany in 2000). Up into the twenty-first century, the archaic belief in Shaman power is certainly still dominant worldwide. An estimated 100 million people are staunch believers in these principles (Landy 1977, Deininger 1998).

People with magical explanations for their suffering, illnesses and complaints are rather reluctant about disclosing their philosophy and social surroundings, for fear of being ridiculed or misunderstood. Supernatural causes are employed as an explanatory concept for environmental influences of bodily functions or illnesses and are seen in connection with the breaking of taboos or, in a ritual sense, with impure behaviour. In contrast to the symptom-related disorder-concepts of modern-medicine there exists the traditional idea that external forces surround the entire body.

Archaic popular concepts for the origin of diseases can be classified in a cultural sense into four main groups; naturalistic, animistic, magical and mystical (Murdock 1978). The "naturalistic" opinion of an illness (nature, weather, climate or nutritional factors) considers elements of the environment responsible for the origin of an illness. Four elements in this model, "air, earth, water and fire", have a special meaning and are held responsible for sicknesses. Illnesses caused through infections, physical or psychic stress, physical impairments, accidents or aggressions triggered by attacks on fellow men, are also included in this category (Ness 1981, Snow 1974).

Other concepts, like magical and mystical ideas are put forward as contrary explanations for diseases originating from supernatural conditions. The "animism" describes the idea of a bustle of nature through personalised, supernatural powers, like spirits, demons, wandering souls, devils or divinities. Deininger writes:

> For the primitive believer (believers in demons) the world exists in an orderless juxtaposition of different spirits. Each hill or mountain, each stone, each animal, each plant, each flash of lightning and crash of thunder, each and every fellow man, including the individual body-limbs are viewed as having an individual soul in which a friendly or hostile demon inhabits (Deininger 1998).

According to animistic ideas there is the belief in the "loss of the soul" as a veritable cause for the appearance of disease. Behind the idea exists the belief that the soul leaves the living body to wander and penetrate into another body, with or without the condition of wizardry, magic or evil intent through another person. Another animistic idea explains an illness through the random punitive or hostile influence of a malicious, miraculous nature. Diseases are viewed as an arbitrary punishment or hostile influence of a malicious supernatural spirit or force of nature. A naturalistic explanation is a distinguishing feature of aggressive or hostile interference manifested in people; intervention comes through supernatural means, which, on behalf of or at the request of another, has a magical explanation and is adversely acted upon.

What understanding or causes can illnesses be bound to in a person under magic influence? How, for example, through envious malevolent human beings who inflict damage through curses, can magic or wizardry be transferred to another individual? This belief was evident to the Greeks and Romans who also engaged in magic rites.

Magic ideas are among the most dispersed of all explanations for illnesses (Maple 1968). By means of sorcery, the health of a human being is disturbed through the influence of another person, a magician, wizard or shaman in command of magic techniques. This happens through spells, incarnations, prayers or curses or by the apparent introduction of a foreign object into the body, also through magic, customs and rituals, whereby a hair or a fingernail of the victim is used. Evidence in the belief in magical strengths and explanations for illnesses can be retraced way back into the history of all known cultures. Other methods include application of damaging substances, poisons with an imaginary effect of sending out a spirit or demon with the intent of taking the soul of the designed victim.

"Witchcraft" was used to explain the presence of an illness, particularly by envious people (witches and warlocks), becoming active with essentially evil abilities. In Southern Italy there is a widespread fascination in the belief in magic. Psychic displays like inhibitions, obstructions and incompetence and an inability to make decisions are connected to a fascination in the theme of magic. For women in particular, the conquest of a man is pursued by a magic power over love (Jaede 1986). This is a reminder of the Voodoo-cult in the Caribbean where needles are symbolically inserted in an object ("attaccatura"). A further form is the "evil eye" assumed by certain persons that can mediate damaging powers through eye contact. These persons are known in Italy as "jettatori" (Murdock 1978).

Under the term "mystical explanations" is the understanding of a power that is based on supernatural influences, like ill-fated feelings or fate. The fateful influences include the belief in astrological constellations, personal predetermination or personified misfortune. Noise, eye contact, or dreams portray the meaning of an ill-fated impression (ominous sensation). This is not only a precursor for an illness, but also as their causation. A further mystical explanation proceeds on the assumption that the touching of an allegedly impure object or an impure person may lead to disease (contagion). This would imply that the blood of a menstruating woman, disease and corpses are impure and a contacting sickness is at work. A further mystical explanation of disease is the mystical retribution, whereby diseases are the consequence of breaking a taboo or of violation of a moral border. To this end the non-observance of orders counts among the nourishment of evil and exists, among sexual rules of conduct, as incest or adultery, and is also seen among hierarchical structures or ritual practices as rules of conduct in the relationship with supernatural forces. Orders exist within foreign property and in connection with poor conduct as, for example, a robbery, false claims or remarks such as blasphemy or other specific words which should not be expressed. These four basic explanation-patterns for the development of illness are spread among the different cultural regions in varying intensity and may partially blend in with one another (Burleigh 1990, Gadit 1998).

The Mexican-American population demonstrate a natural prevailing belief in the magical-mystical ideas of "*curanderismo*" (Kreismann 1975). This original belief combines elements of Catholic, Spanish and traditional Mexican views. The folk-healer was called *curandero* and was sought after by individuals with a different array of personal, social, physical and psychological problems. Especially notable are the beliefs in the "evil eye" (*mal ojo*), witchcraft (*embrujo*), bewitching (*mal puesto*), collapsing of the fontanel in babies (*caida de mollera*), intestinal complaints (*empacho*) and the fear of losing the soul (*susto*) as explanations for the corresponding complaints. The healers (*curanderos*) use magic rituals for healing. They recite prayers and recommend which medicinal herbs should be used. Family members, friends or members of the community may be integrated in these rituals. In rural regions the *curanderos* are the people visited primarily for healing, long before a doctor is consulted (Kiev 1968).

The belief in the obsession with ghosts, witches and overpowering forces has an important meaning in the "Voodoo-Cult". This can be found predominantly in the Caribbean countries and in certain parts of the black population in North America. With this original Haitian superstitious belief, the Voodoo-god, called *Voodoo Loa* is said to take a man's soul and be able to appear in the form of different figures. e.g. a "snake-god", the *Damballa*. In service to God one becomes obsessed by a healer, a *hungan*, or by a god (*Loa*), through a prophesy or healing ritual. In the case of an illness, a traditional healing-priest is consulted for healing the obsessed and, therefore, sick, through an obsession ritual. This service may liberate the evil power or exorcise a witch (Kiev 1961).

In North America there is a version of the Haitian Voodoo belief that also contains elements of Voodoo; the African tribal-culture witchcraft or "root work". This belief holds that a person may impart harm, misfortune, disease or even death ("working roots on someone") upon another person and is motivated by envy or anger by means of "black magic". It is often supposed that friends, colleagues or jealous relatives are to be blamed. Magic imagery is primarily found in rural areas of the southern states of the USA, mainly within the African American population but can also be found among the Caucasian population (Tinling 1967).

Bodily symptoms, such as stomach-aches, nausea or vomiting and psychic symptoms like insanity and lunacy, including misjudgement, hallucination, phobias, uneasiness or mortal anxiety can be traced back to "root-work". Treatment entails a visit to a healer who is called the "root-worker", "root-doctor" or "conjure-doctor". The intensity of the belief in "root work" expresses itself in different ways. It extends from a firm conviction in magical causes up to scepticism by ambivalent individuals who simply consult "root work" under the urging of their family.

There are several reports dealing with the magic ideas of "root work". Snell describes African Americans from Atlanta, Georgia as believers in this form of magic. These beliefs trace psychic symptoms back to the influence of a "witch". Healing through medicaments or psychotherapeutic conversation are not considered in any way as beneficial compared to the help of a "root worker". Based on the fact that the influence of hypnosis achieves successful results, Snell supposes without further verification that a high suggestibility pattern is prevalent in persons with magical explanations (Snell 1967).

Patients are described in another report from Rochester, New York: Medical treatment was administered for a variety of different symptoms. The symptoms were attributed to magical influences, namely "root work". Patients believed they had been bewitched or influenced by a witch and as a result they sought the help of a root doctor (Tinling 1967).

In the initial phase a "root worker" attempts to discover, deduce or reconstruct whether a "witch" or "black magician" is of importance to those being treated. Accordingly, acquaintances, friends and family are also involved. Medicinal herb-tincture is used by applying drops in the eyes or ears and, at the same time, prayers and pleading are verbalised. Orders are then given to be followed for further conduct, for example, when and how often prayers should be recited and what dietary considerations should be observed. Advice is given for the administration of medicinal herbs. Amulets are also distributed and worn as a protection against witches (Ness 1981).

In Puerto-Rico, the belief in a world inhabited by spirits is called spiritualism (espiritismo). Spiritualism unites elements of the Spanish, African and Indian popular beliefs. This popular belief in spirits is said to perform a divine task, namely, the ability to get into the body of a person. Thereby some spirits (causas) are assumed to have, at the same time, the ability to produce bodily complaints. They are held responsible for illnesses as well as psychiatric problems, anxiety attacks, strain and discomfort. A healer (espiritista) tries to bring about a relief of symptoms by appearing at community meetings in order to practice certain rituals. Such an espiritista is regarded as capable of contacting and acting upon spirits.

The multiplicity of popular beliefs of African people can not be presented in entirety due to the extensive complexities. A few reports attempt exemplary explanations for archaic ideas and practices. An investigation carried out some years ago by an institute of primary health care in Harare, capital of Zimbabwe, proved that one fifth of the patients had consulted a popular healer, especially in cases of chronic diseases or in cases involving the conviction of having become a victim of witchery. The investigation included a survey of traditional healers (n´anga) and faith healers (profita) whose explanation patterns were mostly based on "witchcraft" or "too much brooding" (kufungisisa). Unlike investigations some years earlier, there appears to be a decrease in patients who consult traditional healers in comparison with patients visiting a polyclinic or a general practitioner (Patel 1998).

Freeman conducted semi-structural interviews involving the questioning of 114 South African patients in Johannesburg concerning their attitudes to the health care system. One half of all patients had consulted traditional healers for alleviation of their diseases. A quarter of the patients heeded incorporated offers of traditional healing in combination with medical treatment (Freeman 1999). For the Xhosa, South African Bantu-people, more modern traditional practices involving medical authorities and methods are still being practiced today. Herb-healers (ixhwele) recommend various plant extracts and also practice Arabic medicine bloodlettings or burning out of aching body parts with red-hot irons, whereas other healers specialise in the form of bleeding or fleecing, also known as cupping.

Fortune tellers (igqira, witch doctors, magical healers) are said to be able to correspond with the spirit of the deceased. They are regarded as being able to avert damaging "black magic". These healers are consulted for psychological or psychosomatic complaints as well as for love, fertility or blessings for future predictions (Raum 1986).

Maiello reported on the development and education of a South African healer (sangoma). The decision to become a healer is often followed by a certain episode in the life of the individual which is then interpreted as a "vocation". This calling also incorporates features of a psychotic experience. The next step is to get into contact with a practicing healer by living together with that healer for a period of several years. This often leads to difficulties regarding all former obligations and personal relationships. The education includes knowledge of medicinal plants, healing-rituals and ceremonies, predictions, recognition of diseases and preparation for cures. The knowledge imparted often becomes a family tradition (Maiello 1999).

In Europe there are also magical-mystical ideas offered as explanations for concepts for psychological diseases as shown in the following study. A publication in 1997 revealed an investigation by Vlachos in south-western Greece clarifying the meaning of metaphysical and magical-religious explanations for psychosis related deaths of a relative. 85% of the 80 mothers questioned in cases of schizophrenic or bipolar patients assumed a supernatural causation. Explanations like demonic influences, black magic directed against the patient or "evil eye", were blamed for the deaths. More than half of the mothers had visited a church or a convent during the course of their child's illness and one third had visited a traditional healer, fortune teller, astrologer or magician in order to get help for the psychological illness of their child. Vlachos distinguished between the relatives who did not believe in magical causes, relatives with an emphasised religious alignment and relatives with a supernatural explanation pattern. Insanity related deaths had significant and consistent religious or magical elements for children with mothers who believed in supernatural powers (Vlachos 1997).

As is known, the belief in demons is not solely limited to the southern European area. There are reports from Anglo-American countries supporting the belief of "obsession" or so called "possession states". Whitewell described 16 British patients in a psychiatric clinic who were convinced of being possessed by a demon, the devil or an evil ghost. Most of the patients had experienced a strict religious upbringing. Nine of these patients suffered from an affective illness, five from schizophrenia, while two patients were diagnosed as having neurotic disorders. The patients attributed their conviction of being possessed with unchristian attributes, saying prayers to the devil, their relationship to an occult or participation in an exorcism. The need for spiritual help was apparent in all patients. Three of the patients participated in an exorcism, one patient experienced the religious ceremony of laying of the hands, two further patients had their apartments blessed by a priest, one patient consulted a spiritual healer and two further patients had visited a priest who had referred the patients to psychiatric treatment (Whitwell 1980). Contents of religion, obsession and devil's work are again and again related to insanity-issues found in the clinical care of psychiatric patients. Kroll & Sheehan's survey about religious attitude, practice and experience carried out on 52 hospitalised psychiatric patients in Minnesota, USA, revealed that a high number of patients believed in God (95%) or in the devil (67%). Especially schizophrenic patients reported personal, supernatural-religious experiences and verbal communication with God and/or spirits (Kroll 1989). The following case-report from a treatment at the Ruhr-University Bochum offers current examples.

Case-report: "Religious delusion, obsession and witch belief"
The 42-year old patient lives in a home for mentally handicapped people because of her slightly retarded intelligence. Due to her schizophrenia several psychiatric treatments were necessary. She is religious and confesses herself to be a Christian. Currently an "acute psychotic exacerbation" led to hospital admission; meanwhile the patient developed the delusion of being obsessed by the devil. She felt guilty because "she tackled the archangel Gabriel" and therefore feared "being destined to hell" by this angel. During the treatment she repeatedly expressed the fear of "being bewitched by one of the other patients". The patient distanced herself completely from her inner delusions through a pharmacological psycho- and sociotherapeutic treatment and was then discharged.

There is a final further cure known from time immemorial and should not go unmentioned: namely that of "faith-healing" and "healing through religious belief", as described in the following American study. Pattison completed a survey of 43 relatives of different religious sects in Seattle USA, all of whom consulted a "faith-healer" due to a variety of mostly somatic illnesses. He explored their personality-profile, the reasons for consulting such a healer and the question of changes possibly resulting out of their habits. The results indicated distinct personality characteristics without changes in pathological conspicuousness. Their habits did not alter or change. Most of their religious beliefs became stronger through faith-healing (Pattison 1973).

Worth mentioning is a telephone questionnaire of 1539 US-Americans, published in the New England Journal of Medicine in 1993. A third of those interviewed (34%) stated to have applied an unorthodox healing process during the previous year. It can be safely assumed one tenth must have consulted an alternative medical practice and 4% of the interviewed admitted to having participated in faith-healing and, therefore, must have consulted an appropriate healer.

The most frequently named reasons for the implementation of alternative processes of those interviewed were attributed to anxiety attacks, depression, insomnia, headache and back trouble. The survey shows that archaic, alternative or unconventional healing methods are usually of importance in relation to psychic disorders (Eisenberg 1993).

It is estimated that in 1990 there were approximately 61 million Americans engaged in healing rites, constituting an exorbitant sum of 10,3 billion dollars. The amount compares with the same amount paid out for all of the conventional in-patient treatment in America in that particular year (Eisenberg 1993). Considering the current frequent use and various designs of archaic, traditional-medical and unconventional or alternative healing methods it is questionable which motives are the basis for their utilization. The motives are complex. The disorder concepts of modern medicine are extremely complex and not completely understood even by a specialist. This involves not only the complexities that experts use in a technical language, accessible only by a few, but entail as well the limits of the region in which they are in operation. The patient is understood in a limited capacity only for the purposes of scientific explanation and modern therapeutic strategies. This creates concerns and uncertainty in addition to the high costs of modern diagnosis and therapy methods.

In contrast, popular medicine and alternative healing methods have applicable and explicable concepts which are understood and accepted by the person seeking advice. The sought after popular healer also comes from a comparable social environment (Frank 1973). Rappaport noticed the particular kindness and sincerity connected with popular healers and saw therein a decisive difference to procedural medical care. Facing the specialization of modern medicine they convey an impression of a multifaceted approach (Rappaport 1977). In contrast to alternative healing practices, modern medicine is expensive and hardly affordable for the majority of the population in poorer countries. Medical facilities are almost non-existent in some regions. Another point worth mentioning is the fear of side-effects of treatment, as experienced first hand, through descriptions by acquaintances or media reporting. In contrast, alternative healing often appears harmless and without any side-effects. Finally, there is a disappointment in the effectiveness of modern orthodox medicine particularly with patients with chronic symptoms or those aversed to therapy. In cases involving a grim prognosis, alternative methods still produce, at least, temporary hope, comfort and a feeling of being treated seriously and effectively.

References

Assion, H.J., Dana I., Heinemann, F. 1999. "Volksmedizinische Praktiken bei psychiatrischen Patienten türkischer Herkunft in Deutschland", *Fortschr Neurol Psychiat*, 67: 12-20.

Assion, H.J. 2002. "Ethnic Belief and Psychiatry – Patients of Turkish Origin", in: Gottschalk-Batschkus, C.E., Green, J.C. (eds.) *Handbook of Ethnotherapies*. München: Ethnomed.

Assion, H.J. 2004. *Traditionelle Heilpraktiken türkischer Migranten*. Berlin: VWB.

Burleigh, E., Dardano, C., Cruz, J.R. 1990. "Colors, humors and evil eye: Indigenous classification and treatment of childhood diarrhea in highland, Guatemala", *Med Anthropol*, 12: 419-441.

Deininger. R. 1998. *Kultur und Kult in der Medizin: traditionelle Arzneimittel – eine medizinhistorische Betrachtung*. Stuttgart: Fischer.

Devereux, G. 1982. *Normal und anormal. Aufsätze zur allgemeinen Ethnopsychiatrie*. Frankfurt: Suhrkamp.

Eisenberg, D., Kessler, R.C., et al. 1993. "Unconventional medicine in the United States", *N Engl J Med*, 328: 246-252.

Eliade, M. 1975. *Schamanismus und archaische Ekstasetechnik*. Zürich-Stuttgart: Rascher.

Findeisen, H., Gehrts, H. 1983. *Die Schamanen*. Köln: Diederichs.
Frank, J.D., Frank, J.B. 1973. *Persuasion and Healing*. Baltimore and London: Johns Hopkins University Press.
Freeman, M., Lee, T., Vivian, W. 1999. "Evaluation of mental health services in the Free State. Part III. Social outcome and patient perceptions", *S Afr Med J*, 89: 311-315.
Gadit, A. 1998. "Shamanic concepts and treatment of mental illness in Pakistan", *J Coll Phys Surg Pak*, 8: 33-35.
Garrison, V. 1977. "Doctor, espiritista, or psychiatrist? Health-seeking behaviour in a Puerto Rican neighbourhood of New York City", *Med Anthropol*, 1: 65-180.
Harner, M. 1986. *Der Weg des Schamanen. Ein praktischer Führer zu innerer Heilkraft*. Reinbek: Rowohlt.
Harner, M.J. 1973. *Hallucinogens and Shamanism*. New York: Oxford University Press
Jaede, W., Portera, A. 1986. *Ausländerberatung. Kulturspezifische Zugänge in Diagnostik und Therapie*. Freiburg: Lambertus.
Kiev, A. 1968. *Curanderismo: Mexican American Folk Psychiatry*. New York: Free Press.
Kiev, A. 1961. "Spirit possession in Haiti", *Am J Psychiat*, 118: 133-138.
Kleinman, A. 1980. *Patients and Healers in the Context of Culture*. Berkeley: University of California Press.
Kleinman, A., Sung, L.H. 1979. "Why do indigenous practitioners successfully heal?" *Soc Sci Med*, 13B: 7-26.
Kreisman, J.J. 1975. "The curanderos apprentice: A therapeutic integration of folk and medical healing", *Am J Psychiat*, 132: 81-83.
Kroll, J., Sheehan, W. 1989. "Religious beliefs and practices among 52 psychiatric inpatients in Minnesota", *Am J Psychiat*, 146: 67-72.
Landy, D. 1977. *Culture, Disease and Healing. Studies in Medical Anthropology*. New York-London: Collier McMillan.
Lehmann, A. 1925. *Aberglaube und Zauberei. Von den ältesten Zeiten an bis in die Gegenwart*. Stuttgart: Ferdinand Enke.
Lommel, A. 1980. *Schamanen und Medizinmänner. Magie und Mystik früherer Kulturen*. München: Allwey.
Maiello, S. 1999. "Encounter with an African healer. Thinking about the possibilities and limits of cross-cultural psychotherapy", *J Child Psychother*, 25: 217-238.
Maple, E. 1968. *Magic, Medicine, and Quackery*. London: Hale.
Murdock, G.P., Wilson, S., Frederick, V. 1978. "World distribution of theories of illness", *Ethnology*, 17: 449-470.
Murray, R.H., Rubel, A.J. 1992. "Physicians and healers – unwitting partners in health care", *N Engl J Med*, 326: 61-64.
Ness, R., Wintrob, R. 1981. "Folk Healing: A Description and Synthesis", *Am J Psychiat*, 138: 1477-1481.
Patel, V., Todd, C., et al. 1998. "Outcome of common mental disorders in Harare, Zimbabwe", *Br J Psychiat*, 172: 53-57.
Pattison, E.M., Lapins, N.A., Doerr, H.A. 1973. "Faith healing: a study of personality and function", *J Nerv Ment Dis*, 157: 397-409.
Prince, R.H. 1976. "Psychotherapy as the manipulation of indigenous healing mechanisms: a transcultural survey", *Transcult Psychiat Res Rev*, 13: 115-133.
Raum, O.F. 1986. "Die Heiler bei den südafrikanischen Xhosa", *Curare*, S5: 145-165.
Rappaport, H. 1977. "The Tenacity of Folk Psychotherapy. A functional interpretation", *Soc Psychiat*, 12: 127-132.

Scharfetter, C. 1983. "Der Schamane, das Urbild des Therapeuten", *Praxis Psychother Psychosomatik*, 28: 81-89.
Schmidt, P. 1956. *Dunkle Mächte. Ein Buch vom Aberglauben einst und heute.* Frankfurt: Josef Knecht.
Snell, J.E. 1967. "Hypnosis in the Treatment of the 'Hexed' Patient", *Am J Psychiat*, 124: 311-316.
Snow, L.F. 1974. "Folk medical beliefs and their implications for care of patients", *Ann Intern Med*, 81: 82-96.
Stoll, O. 1904. *Suggestion und Hypnotismus in der Völkerpsychologie.* Leipzig: Von Veit & Co.
Stumpfe, K.D. 1983. "Die Heilmethoden der Medizinmänner", *Curare*, 6: 25-31.
Tinling, D.C. 1967. "Voodoo, Rootwork and Medicine", *Psychosom Med*, 29: 483-491.
Vlachos, I.O., Beratis, S., Hartocollis, P. 1997. "Magico-religious beliefs and psychosis", *Psychopathology*, 30: 93-99.
Walsh, R.N. 1990. *The Spirit of Shamanism.* Los Angeles: Tarcher.
Whitwell, F.D., Barker, M.G. 1980. "'Possession' in psychiatric patients in Britain", *Br J Med Psychol*, 53: 287-295.

The Problem of Universalism in Psychiatry

Johannes Thome

1. Introduction

Modern psychiatry shows an increasing tendency to define itself by biological paradigms as definitions, thus fulfilling a crucial posit of an up-to-date scientific medicine. The reason for this development is twofold: Firstly, the application of scientific thinking has brought success and progress to the somatic disciplines of medicine and it is the aim of psychiatry, being placed in the academic setting of medicine, to participate in and to benefit from this trend. Secondly, typical for the psychiatry of the past, there was a tendency to cultivate different schools with often unhelpful dogmatical attitudes and to inhibit progressive developments in psychiatry. By embracing scientific principles and founding psychiatry on neuroscience, many psychiatrists hope to develop a discipline which, thus, cannot be questioned with regard to its fundamental principles, such as its epistemology, nosology or therapeutic strategies.

It is argued that such an empirist psychiatry based merely on science would be an undisputable scientific discipline, its results and findings being generally valid, acceptable and independent of any conceptional issues or cultural background.

By doing so, two assumptions are put forward: (a) the scientific method, which is a unique result of the empirist era of Western philosophy, exhibits a universal validity, (b) the field of psychiatry can be sufficiently reduced to scientific problems which, in turn, can be solved by applying an accordingly appropriate universal scientific method.

2. What is universalism?

Universalism can be defined as an attitude which postulates the general validity of a certain theory, hypothesis, principle or paradigm independent of conceptual or cultural issues. It is, thereby, assumed that a refutation of the theory, hypothesis, principle or paradigm in question would be incompatible with a reasoning so fundamental that it is common to all human beings (rationalism), no matter what their cultural background and biographic experiences are.

In present-day philosophy, the debate on universalism focuses mostly on ethical problems and whether or not it is possible to develop a universally acceptable and generally binding theory of moral acting which would be acceptable to all human beings, no matter what their individual experiences and their cultural, social and historical background are. Representatives of such a moral universalism are Kant or, more recently, Habermas (for review see Johri 1996).

In the field of contemporary psychiatry, it is evident at present that a notion of psychiatry as a medical discipline based on science and empirism, i.e. a Western type of psychiatry[1] founded on the principles of biology and neuroscience, is being internationally propagated. Accordingly, psychiatric research focuses on the pathological alterations of the brain as "somato-morphological correlatives" of mental disorders. Psychiatric diagnosis aims at establishing the use of modern technologies such as brain imaging, biochemical analysis of blood, CSF, biopsies and molecular methods for the assessment of genetic predispositions. Finally, psychiatric therapy involves more and more biological strategies, i.e. the use of psychotropic drugs, ECT and, in the case of psychotherapeutic interventions, those which can be and those which have been evaluated in empirical studies, i.e. mostly therapies based on behaviourist principles.

3. Why is there psychiatric universalism?

A universalist approach in medicine has been proven very useful, especially in disciplines such as surgery and infectiology. Application of the scientific method in somatic medicine led – within a relatively short period of time – to a decrease of infant mortality and an increase of life expectancy unparalleled in human history (Imhof 1981). With the emancipation of psychiatry from religion and mysticism, mental disorders were increasingly interpreted as a medical problem. Until the late 19th century, psychiatry was often considered as part of internal medicine and/or neurology. Later, it became independent and was established as one of many medical disciplines (Ackerknecht 1985). The separation from neurology, however, is an interesting phenomenon: disorders which could not be explained by a pathological alteration of the nervous system were classified as psychiatric disorders in contrast to neurological disorders with a defined and recognisable neural pathophysiology. Paradoxically, psychiatry nevertheless continued to be defined as a medical and empirical science. In a few instances, this led to the discovery of distinctive pathophysiological mechanisms in psychiatric disorders (e.g., Alzheimer's dementia, progressive paralysis). However, this frequently resulted in a shift of disorders with identified pathomechanisms from psychiatry to other "somatic" medical disciplines. Thus, progressive paralysis as a result of a treponema

1 In several cultures, imported Western medicine is often perceived as paternalistic. This is an important issue; however, the paternalism debate shall not be discussed here.

infection is today considered an object of bacteriology and microbiology, whereas Alzheimer's dementia is often treated in neurological rather than in psychiatric departments.

Nonetheless, there are examples for progress in psychiatry manifested in remarkable achievements, such as the development of psychotropic drugs, which considerably improved the outcome of several genuine psychiatric disorders including affective or schizophrenic psychoses.

With the success of somatic medicine in mind, psychiatry was set to use the same principles in order to reveal the supposedly universally valid etiopathogenetic principles of mental disorders and to develop appropriate treatment strategies. Using a strictly scientific and empirist approach, it is assumed that similarly spectacular achievements can be attained in psychiatry as in other medical disciplines.

Presumably, the attempt to help and fight disease by unveiling the fundamental principles of pathophysiology represents the source of universalism in psychiatry rather than an "arrogant (...) need (...) to impose our own cultural categories upon others" leading to a form of European "psychiatric imperialism" (Burton-Bradley 1993).

4. How is universalism propagated in psychiatry?

The universalism of today's academic mainstream psychiatry is characterized by an intellectual framework of strict rationalism and propagated via (a) self-perception and self-interpretation as empirist (medical) science (neuroscience) and (b) widespread use of international classification systems (ICD, DSM).

The research results of modern neuroscience including neuroanatomy, neurophysiology, neurobiochemistry and brain imaging increasingly elucidate the function of neural systems and deepen our knowledge about information processing in the brain on a macroscopical level as well as on the level of cellular and molecular phenomena.

At the same time, this results in an ever better understanding of the pathophysiological principles of mental disorders. Parallely, these insights can be used in order to develop new and promising psychopharmacological therapies and other innovative biological treatment strategies. The fact that mental disorders can be successfully treated with chemical substances, (even if responder rates may vary and adverse effects are relatively common), is a very important argument in favour of a biological psychiatry with its strictly empirist and scientific approach towards mental disorders. This argument is similar to the justification of universalism in somatic medicine by indicating that the Western style scientific approach in medicine leads to effective and efficient diagnostic and therapeutic techniques which are of great benefit to all patients across the different cultures.

However, it remains a paradoxical hallmark of psychiatry that despite all research efforts and the strict application of scientific principles, no consistent nosological concept based on biological parameters with diagnostic relevance has been developed so far. This fact fostered the appearance of several local or national classification systems of psychopathological phenomena with partially considerable conceptional differences and resulting incompatibilities between them. Therefore, so-called international classification systems were developed during the 20th century and introduced worldwide in order to establish a unified psychiatric terminology to facilitate communication and the exchange of ideas between psychiatrists from different countries. According to these manuals, the diagnosis of a specific mental disorder depends on the fullfilment of certain diagnostic criteria. The data necessary for the decision of whether these criteria are fullfilled or not are usually obtained via mental state examination (i.e., behavioural observation and evaluation of case history and self-description of the patient), but not – like in other medical disciplines – via the application of scientific diagnostic tests and tools, because biological markers have not yet been identified which would be pathognomonic for a given psychiatric disorder and, thus, allow an objective diagnosis.

Since the scientific argument cannot be used in order to justify the demand of a general and universal acceptance of international classification systems, the reason for their universality is seen in the fact that they are generated by international consensus conferences of expert committees.

In summary, universalism in psychiatry is propagated by postulating that the principles of science and conventionalism must be generally accepted, an argument which implies an a priori rationalism.

5. Problems of universalist psychiatry

5.1. Transcultural aspects

The benefits of a universalist approach in psychiatry, founded on scientific, empirist and rationalist principles as well as on a conventionalist terminology and classification, become evident in the exciting projects of the international community of researchers and clinicians and in the progress of their work in innovative areas like neurobiochemistry, molecular neuroscience and psychopharmacology. However, tangible limitations of a universalist psychiatry appear when it comes to transcultural issues and issues concerning the individuality of psychiatric patients.

Due to fundamental differences in culture, social structure, language, history and the way of thinking, the Western style of scientific psychiatry may appear less compatible with other traditions than would be necessary for a universally accepted psychiatric framework: The biomedical perspective of ICD and DSM interprets mental disorders as "natural" biological alterations which manifest as dysfunction within individuals; from this it may be concluded that these dysfunctions are similar across culturally and socially different groups and that they are "universal". However, the organisation of "the noetic domains of those groups with different languages" makes it difficult to sustain "the notion of a universal consensual science" (Burton-Bradley 1993, Thakker et al. 1999). In this context latah[2] in Malaysia and susto[3] in Latin-America represent typical culture-bound behavioural states or syndromes[4], which are difficult to integrate into a psychiatric scheme and which are widely discussed in the literature (Logan 1993, Dein 1997, Weller et al. 2002, Lee and Balick 2003). Interestingly, latah has been interpreted as a "cultural pattern and not a mental disorder as such" (Kenny 1978) and it was, thus, hypothesized that latah could be "a social construction of Western-trained universalist scientists" (Bartholomew 1994). This illustrates the problems of medical universalism and ethnocentrism in psychiatry which could be possibly counteracted by a certain cultural relativism (Lin 1986). Critics maintain that a universalist theoretical perspective "tends to obscure the role of local interpretations in the phenomenology of psychiatric illness" (O'Nell 1989) or mental health.

5.2. Pseudo-universalist terminology

Despite the cultural differences, however, it makes sense, of course, to accept certain principles of Western scientific thinking, because it leads not only to an ever deeper understanding of man and nature, but also enables us to use this knowledge for developing specific techniques to alter the world we live in and to improve our life conditions; thus, scientific knowledge of human biology makes it possible to develop modern medical methods and treatment strategies. Although scientific thinking may have its origins in a specific context of Western history, its applicability as technology has made this interpretation of reality universally accepted in a pragmatist and utilitarist sense. This is especially true when it comes to biology, chemistry, physiology, pharmacology and similar scientific disciplines which exhibit great potential for application in medicine. The use of scientific principles has led to Western medicine being a most successful approach to elevate human suffering, a success which can be

2 Simons (1980) gives the following description of latah: "Persons exhibiting the Latah syndrome respond to minimal stimuli with exaggerated startles, often exclaiming normally inhibited sexually denotative words. Sometimes Latahs after being startled obey the commands or imitate the actions of persons about them. Most episodes of Latah are intentionally provoked for the amusement of onlookers".

3 A belief in the loss of the soul.

4 Further examples for culture bound syndromes are amok (Malaysia), pibloktoq (Inuits), shin-byung (Korea).

measured and quantified by undisputable facts such as significantly reduced infant mortality, increased life expectancy and increasingly available options for the treatment of severe and rare disorders which, in former times, could not be treated.[5]

Thus, progress in neurobiology has led to considerably improved preventive, diagnostic and therapeutic possibilities in neurology and neurosurgery. With respect to psychiatry, however, this transition from science to medicine, i.e. from neurobiology to psychiatry, is difficult because it can create terminological confusion and ultimately lead to a pseudo-universalist terminology: While neurobiological terms such as brain, neuron, glia cell, synapse, transmitter, receptor, G-protein, transcription factor, DNA etc. are generally acceptable to a universal scientific community for the above mentioned reasons, specific psychopathological terms such as psychosis, delusion, paranoia, self, thought disorder, emotion etc. are, for the main part, not. However, the combined use of neurobiological and psychopathological terminology, often used in so-called "biological psychiatry", suggests that the step from neuron to schizophrenia is similar to the step from moto-neuron to polio. This is, however, not the case. While the term polio, which determines a viral infection of the moto-neuron, directly depends on the term moto-neuron, the terms neuron and schizophrenia originate from two totally distinct terminologies. Although it might be that schizophrenia has something to do with neurons, this term primarily does not depend on any neurobiological term, but represents a typical psychopathological term which means that it can be used as a descriptive instrument, without being a scientific (empirical) term in the strict sense of a neurobiological term. This means that psychiatry may claim a certain degree of universality, as elaborated above, as long as it operates in the field of pure neurobiology and uses the appropriate terminology. However, where non-biological (e.g., psychopathological) terminology is introduced and used, the field of pure natural sciences is abandoned, and, thus, any universal claim becomes problematical. Terms like self, psychiatric disorder, thought disturbance etc. must be clarified in a discourse which is not restricted solely to the science of neurobiology. If this aspect is neglected and neurobiological and psychopathological terms are confused, the result will be a pseudo-universalist terminology.

5.3. The individual in the clinical situation

With respect to the individual human being suffering from a psychiatric disorder, a universalist approach may also be problematical and become a cause for aporia situations in the interaction between psychiatrist and patient.

---

5 The fact that modern medicine, despite its successes, has created new problems, especially, when it comes to ethics, is not to be discussed here.

Mental disorders mainly interpreted as brain disorders require the application of sophisticated diagnostic techniques such as MRI, endocrinological analysis, psychometric tests and of biological treatment strategies such as the prescription of psychotropic drugs. A patient exposed to these procedures is endangered to become an object of medico-technical measures. Such a patient will increasingly lose the specific attributes of his or her personality and be transformed from a subject with its own individuality to an object classified according to international classification manuals. In such a situation, the ability for empathic understanding of the personal needs of each single patient is systematically reduced as well as the possibilities of a satisfying communication between patient and psychiatrists. Modern diagnostic criteria focus more on the form of a certain symptom and less on its actual content. For example, acoustic hallucinations ("hearing voices") and paranoia are important diagnostic criteria for schizophrenia, but the words these voices say or the exact paranoic system with its specific thoughts which preoccupy the patient are considered less relevant for "diagnosis-making" than the mere fact whether or not hallucinations and paranoia are, in fact, present. From the patient's perspective, however, the content of the thoughts experienced and the voices heard have a considerable impact on his or her mental wellbeing or suffering which, of course, are exclusively subjective feelings. In contrast to other (somatic) medical disciplines, in the field of psychiatry it is often of no help if the physician tries to explain his or her scientific interpretation of the disorder, in order to convince the patient to adopt the same opinion regarding the interpretation of their disorder. It is a characteristic feature of many psychiatric disorders that they imply a loss of freedom of choice of interpretations for the patient. Due to this inability to choose the most appropriate (i.e. rational) interpretation of his or her disorder, the scientific interpretation loses its relevance for the patient concerned. In order to understand the individual suffering of every single patient, it is necessary to listen to their subjective experiences and not to confront them with a "scientific and objective" concept of mental disorders they cannot identify with.[6] Thus, in the daily clinical work, individualism, subjectivism and relativism can be of more benefit for the interaction with patients than universalist theories.

---

6 This does not preclude, of course, the possibility to discuss with the patient the assumed neurobiological background of the disorder and to explain the mechanisms of action of the prescribed (pharmaco)therapies.

6. Discussion and conclusion

The problem of universalism is a typical example how philosophical aspects considerably affect present-day psychiatry. With respect to the interaction of the clinician with the patient as well as to the situation of a psychiatric researcher who wishes to help the patient and is therefore concerned to what extent the patients' suffering relates to neurobiology, these aspects prove not only to be of theoretical interest but also of considerable practical relevance. Thus, Wallace et al. (1997) believe that the exclusion of philosophy would be disastrous for psychiatry, because "if we are not clearly conscious of our philosophy we shall mix it up with our scientific thinking quite unawares and bring about a scientific and philosophic confusion". Furthermore, "since in psychopathology in particular the scientific knowledge is not all of one kind, we have to distinguish the different modes of knowing and clarify our methods, the meaning and validity of our statements and the criteria of tests", all this being possible functions of a philosophy of psychiatry.

The question of universalism elucidates a typical dilemma of modern psychiatry: Whereas neurobiological research activities require the universalist principles of science, the daily clinical work and interaction with patients require a sensitivity to the cultural background and personal beliefs of each patient. Especially as long as the clinical applicability of neurobiological knowledge, despite its continuous increase, is limited in psychiatry, a strictly reductionist and universalist approach would probably be more often than not a disadvantage to the patient.

Emphasis on the scientific neurobiological aspects of psychiatry may lead to biological determinism, the role of which is yet to be defined in the sociocultural context (Brody 1990). However, instead of abolishing the project of a scientific psychiatry as a medical discipline founded on the principles of neurobiology[7], it has been proposed to modify the universalist concepts of psychiatry:

> Advances in the social and cultural sciences have underscored ways in which assumptions of reductionism and universalism need to be chastened with an appreciation of human differences and humane considerations as these relate to mental health problems. The science of psychiatry of the 21st century will have to accommodate to this new creolized world of ethnic pluralism, cultural differences and clashing perspectives between the traditional and the modern. The boundaries, categories, and the conceits governing the closed neurobiologic international program and agenda will need to be modified and broadened by the addition, sensitivity to and appreciation of cultural differences (Fabrega 2001).

---

7 This was and is postulated by different initiatives and ideologies such as the anti-psychiatry movement which was relatively strongly supported by the general population in the sixties and seventies of the 20th century and still finds its supporters today.

It is clear that psychiatry has to respond to the challenges of the present-day world:

> Migration and transnational communication and awareness of cultural differences are changing the character of communities around the world. These changes considered in the context of worldwide political economic factors are bringing into close physical and symbolic juxtaposition persons from distinct nations and ethnic groups. Clashes in world views, attitudes, spiritual orientation and general philosophic and moral outlook are becoming ever-present realities of urban centers around the world. In traditional contexts and among persons who do not physically migrate, the power of communications media manages to psychologically migrate them" (Fabrega 2001).

Therefore, a "responsive international cultural psychiatry (...) based on a blending and integration of all facets of knowledge of the behavioural sciences, from biology, pharmacology, genetics on through sociology and cultural anthropology" is called for: "In a new idiom it seeks to provide all communities of the globe the best that the science of psychiatry has to offer in the areas of prevention, diagnosis and treatment. The best psychiatry possible translates as providing expert scientific diagnosis and therapy in light of an appreciation of the role played by cultural factors in shaping human behaviour" (Fabrega 2001).

However, this enthusiastic approach is difficult to concretize and, thus, to realize. Despite the limitations and drawbacks of modern nosological systems, the development of cultural adaptations is seen by some as a "step backward" (Lopez-Ibor 2003). It has been noted frequently that the symptoms across the different cultures are not so very different and that to "put too much emphasis on local symptoms bears the risk of yielding to social and cultural pressure" (Lopez-Ibor 2003) which would neither be justified nor lead to any improvement in the patients' condition.

Perhaps, it would prove necessary to accept a certain dualism in psychiatry without putting too much effort in reconciling both: On the one hand, rationalism and universalism are needed in order to achieve scientific progress, on the other hand, individualism and relativism cannot be abandoned due to the requirements of daily clinical practice where empathy and understanding is required in the interaction between psychiatrist and patient.

In this context, Jaspers's (1920) fundamental distinction between "understanding" and "explaining" of psychopathological symptoms may actually prove to be highly relevant for modern psychiatry and could be a cue to solve the predicament of universalism.

References

Ackerknecht, E.H. 1985. *Kurze Geschichte der Psychiatrie.* 3rd ed. Stuttgart: Enke.
Bartholomew, R.E. 1994. "Disease, disorder, or deception? Latah as habit in a Malay extended family", *J Nerv Ment Dis,* 182: 331-341.
Brody, E.B. 1990. "The new biological determinism in socio-cultural context", *Aust N Z J Psychiatry,* 24: 464-469.
Burton-Bradley, B.G. 1993. "Culture and psychiatry", *P N G Med J,* 36: 33-40.
Dein, S. 1997. "ABC of mental health: Mental health in a multiethnic society", *B M J,* 315: 473-476.
Fabrega, H. Jr. 2001. "Cultural psychiatry: international perspectives. Epilogue", *Psychiatr Clin North Am,* 24: 595-608.
Imhof, A.E. 1981. *Die gewonnenen Jahre.* München: Beck.
Jaspers, K. 1920. *Allgemeine Psychopathologie.* 2nd ed. Berlin: Springer.
Johri, M. 1996. *On the universality of Habermas's discourse ethics.* Diss. Montreal: McGill University.
Kenny, M.G. 1978. "Latah: the symbolism of a putative mental disorder", *Cult Med Psychiatry,* 2: 209-231.
Lee, R., Balick, M.J. 2003. "Stealing the soul, soumwahu en naniak, and susto: understanding culturally-specific illnesses, their origins and treatment", *Altern Ther Health Med,* 9: 106-109.
Lin, T.Y. 1986. "Multiculturalism and Canadian psychiatry: opportunities and challenges", *Can J Psychiatry,* 31: 681-690.
Logan, M.H. 1993. "New lines of inquiry on the illness of susto", *Med Anthropol,* 15: 189-200.
Lopez-Ibor, J.J. 2003. "Cultural adaptations of current psychiatric classifications: are they the solution?", *Psychopathology,* 36: 114-119.
O'Nell, T.D. 1989. "Psychiatric investigations among American Indians and Alaska natives: a critical review", *Cult Med Psychiatry,* 13: 51-87.
Simons, R.C. 1980. "The resolution of the Latah paradox". *J Nerv Ment Dis,* 168: 195-206.
Thakker, J., Ward, T., Strongman, K.T. 1999. "Mental disorder and cross-cultural psychology: a constructivist perspective", *Clin Psychol Rev,* 19: 843-874.
Wallace, E., Radden, J., Sadler, J.Z. 1997. "The philosophy of psychiatry: who needs it?" *J Nerv Ment Dis,* 185: 67-73.
Weller, S.C., Baer, R.D., de Alba Garcia, J.G., Glazer, M., Trotter, R., Pachter, L., Klein, R.E. 2002. "Regional variation in Latino descriptions of susto", *Cult Med Psychiatry,* 26: 449-472.

Lacan and Psychiatry

Aisling Campbell

In 1964 Jacques Lacan moved his seminar to the *Ecole pratique des Hautes Etudes*, having been excommunicated, as he put it, from the International Psychoanalytical Association, because of his theoretical differences with the main body of the Association. His seminar changed, not only in terms of its venue but also in terms of its audience who were no longer largely clinicians but a more varied group comprising philosophers, linguists and mathematicians. The seminar was *The Four Fundamental Concepts of Psychoanalysis* (Lacan 1964-5); its title, and indeed its availability as a paperback in the English-speaking world (unlike many other of the seminars up to recently) means that it is often the novice's first introduction to Lacan. Ironically, it is also one of the most difficult of Lacan's seminars and may therefore seem to have little or no relevance to the clinician. Not only for this reason, but also because of the general difficulty of the language and concepts used by Lacan, he is unknown to most psychiatrists (at least in Britain, Ireland and the US) and those that have some limited exposure to his work will often dismiss it (along with the entire psychoanalytic enterprise) as unscientific, and inapplicable to clinical problems. In my view, this is an unfair criticism. There is no doubt that many psychoanalytic theories are less based on clinical reality than the desire for their own internal consistency. Psychoanalysis is popularly described as outmoded and irrelevant in the light of advances in the neurosciences as applied to mental illness. However, Lacan brought a rigour of thought to the clinical questions posed to him in his practice, and seriously addressed some of the crucial problems within psychoanalysis; that is, the nature of the human subject, specifically the subject of the unconscious, the relationship between symptoms and clinical structures, the ethics (in the broadest sense) of psychoanalysis, the relationship between theory and practice and the question of whether or not psychoanalysis can be considered a science. Although some of these issues may be of concern mainly to psychoanalysts, his attempts to elucidate the specific structure of the human subject may offer a research framework for a neuropsychoanalysis, a psychoanalytic theory which informs and is informed by neuroscience. Recent thinking on the neuroscientific basis for behaviour embraces the idea of self-organization, for example, and as will be discussed below, Lacan's conceptualization of the subject seems to have a theoretical "fit" with this idea.

It must be commented that Lacan himself had very little time for neurobiological concepts as having any application to the particularities of the subject;

however, when his seminar began in the 1950s, neurosciences were very much in their infancy. Even toward the end of his seminar in the 1970s, psychiatry was dominated by psychoanalysis and pharmacological treatments for mental disorder were relatively primitive. (Nonetheless ego psychology and object relations probably had the greatest influence on the psychiatry of the time, and were and still are entirely different in theoretical terms from Lacan). In Lacan, there is virtually no reference to brain biology, in contrast to Freud, who always hoped that one day biology would explain mental phenomena.[1] Lacan lifts the relatively concrete, apparently almost biological concepts of Freud (for example, the ego, the superego) to another, less tangible plane. However, in doing so he gives greater coherence to the concepts and provides a theoretical framework that has clinical relevance. However, it is difficult for psychiatrists to approach his work because he was always suspicious of reliance on the symptom – as Jacques-Alain Miller put it, psychiatry is a clinic of the symptom while psychoanalysis is a clinic of the phantasy (Miller, 1996). To a Lacanian analyst, it is not the empirically measured symptom but how the analysand relates to his own spoken word (or how he "is spoken") that is diagnostic. Put simply, psychoanalysts might be better at diagnosis than psychiatrists!

Lacan's theory evolved to a considerable degree throughout his lifetime.[2] He trained initially as a psychiatrist and then as a psychoanalyst – paradoxically, he undertook his analysis with Rudolf Loewenstein, one of the ego psychologists whose theories he was later to reject vehemently. His doctoral thesis, on the case of Aimée, a psychotic woman, was the first faint echo of his later view that identity did not automatically come conferred with the physical body. For Lacan, the infant has no innate sense of his own completeness but rather experiences his body as fragmented – a number of disparate parts lacking any unity. This idea of fragmentation at the heart of the subject is a key one, which is elaborated in late Lacan away from its earlier apparently developmental origins; Lacan never considered the subject to have even a potential wholeness (unlike the wholeness that is the currency of counselling and pop psychology). In his paper on the mirror phase (Lacan 1949) comments that the infant of four months looks at his image as though it were a stranger, whereas the infant of six months will smile at his own image and

1 For instance Freud's *Project for a Scientific Psychology* (Freud 1950) is often read by scholars to indicate that Freud hankered after a neurobiological basis to psychic phenomena; Lacan reads the Project as revealing the Real, the elusive Thing that is at the heart of our being, that resists explanation and symbolisation. See Geerardyn (1997) for a full exposition on this subject.

2 The theory is not a static one, laid down as in the gospels; Lacan pointed out that unfortunately it must be reinvented by each analyst in the course of his own training.

then at that of the adult holding him. However, he is unable to see the one as representing the other, attributing to them both a separate reality. Gradually he starts to see the image as complete in itself and gains a way of representing his own body to himself. The task is to get a sense of unity of his own body – however much of a mirage that might be – but to do so he must subvert his experiences into representation. This is what for Lacan leads to the constitution of the ego – it is a device, an imaginary but essential imposition which necessitates a distance from the essence of the direct experience.[3] There is a third stage wherein the infant sees the dependence of the image on reality; for Lacan this confirms his thesis that there is something inherently alienatory in the development of the ego. The infant is captivated by his own image – the illusory wholeness is the ideal ego, an attempt to overcome the lack (of wholeness) that is at the heart of his being, but is also separated from something essential about himself. This formation of the ego however, gives the world consistency – it is the condition which allows us to perceive reality and to live in geometric, Euclidean space. As we will see, however, subjective space, for Lacan, is topological rather than geometric.

This conceptualization is radically different from that of the ego psychologists, who according to Jacques-Alain Miller (Miller 1995) took Freud's second topography of the id, ego and superego as superseding the first topography of unconscious, preconscious and conscious. The ego psychology view – which has been taken up by many forms of psychotherapy and counselling – is of a geometric subject, the subject with an inside and outside, a container. The id (in the reading of Freud according to the ego psychology school) was seen as the "instincts", the boiling cauldron of primitive sexual and aggressive urges which had to be controlled by the ego and superego. In analysis the analyst "lent" his own ego, which could provide a model by which the analysand would gradually learn to adapt to his milieu. Lacan points out, however, that mistranslations (and therefore misreadings) of Freud were at least partly responsible for what he saw a departure from Freud. Strachey translates the word *Trieb* as "instinct"; Lacan suggests that *Trieb* is more accurately translated as "drive" which does not have the implicit meaning of animal urges as does instinct (*Instinkt*), but implies something altogether more human. The drive is established when parts of the infant's body take on a significance in the context of the infant's relationship with the parents. For instance the mouth becomes more than just a biological orifice, and is implicated in feeding as an interaction between child and parent. For Lacan the idea of barely contained animal urges is simply an artefact of the symbolic order, the laws

---

3 The ego therefore has an inherent falsity which must be recognized as such by the analyst in the context of psychoanalytic practice. The error of the ego psychology school was to mistake the ego for the subject.

of language that make us human subjects. The symbolic rules which govern our relationships with the world give the impression that there is something primitive underneath – Lacan gives it a perspective twist in suggesting that this primitive "thing" is in fact an artefact of the symbolic order and has no ontological consistency in itself. Lacan calls this unsymbolizable "thing" the Real. While the early Lacan seems to give primacy to the symbolic order over the imaginary order of the image, the late Lacan is preoccupied with the tension between the symbolic and the real.

The symbolic order is one of the areas which seem to offer possibilities for psychiatric research, as it is concerned with the more tangible phenomenon of language. Lacan points out that the infant is born into a world where relationships have a symbolic structure, that is, there are certain rules which govern relationships. The core of these rules is that of sexual difference. For Lacan this symbolic order is what structures the subject and the unconscious[4] and the subject's relation to it is what is diagnostic. Hence psychoanalysis is the "talking cure" – speech is its medium and its only rule is that of free association – to speak without censorship.

The distinction between signifier and signified is central to Lacan's thesis, borrowing from the work of Ferdinand de Saussure. The chain of signifiers has its own life, as it were, and is not directly correlated with the signified, the world of things. The subject emerges through the chain of signifiers (the Other) which frame reality but also distance us from it. Hence we are divided subjects cut off from knowledge about ourselves (that is, subjects of repression), bound by the laws of language and prohibition, castrated subjects.[5] Lacan, in his return to Freud, takes the whole scenario of castration away from the Theban play to a more complex level. Freud used the Oedipus myth to introduce the operation of the symbolic order in the form of the father – not the real father, Lacan emphasizes, but the father insofar as he represents something beyond the child, for the mother (Lacan 1953). It is the symbolic aspect of paternity that is important – something as simple as a surname indicates to some extent the subject's symbolic place. For Lacan, the paternal function is to metaphorize the mother's desire – to put a metaphor in place of the mother's lack. Instead of trying to make up this lack for the mother, the child can move out of an imaginary identification with her lack and can enter into the world of signifiers and a symbolic identity that is more than just his image. The mother refers, through her speech, to some aspect of the symbolic paternal function (there does not necessarily have to be a real father around). The name of the

4 Hence the Lacanian dictum that "the unconscious is structured as a language"; Lacan pointed out that Freud emphasized the linguistic components of symptoms and dreams.

5 Lacan's matheme, or symbol, for the divided subject is the S barred – the first element of his algebra of the subject.

father (which in French has a resonance of its function in prohibiting the child from solving the mother's lack; "*le non/nom du père*") is substituted for the desire of the mother, a signifying function. This is how Lacan reads Freud's reference to the castrating father in the Oedipus – not as the real father, but at the symbolic level. It is helpful clinically to think of the castrating father as not the vengeful father of myth, but as a necessary substitute for a much more frightening, engulfing mother. Hence Lacan's choice of "*le père ou pire*", the father or worse; it is a question of your money or life (Lacan 1971-2). It is in other words, no choice at all – as in the old highwayman story, if you have to give up all your money you might as well be dead anyway. The "choice" is between (on the one hand) subjectivity,[6] and the loss of access to *jouissance*, and (on the other hand) access to *jouissance* (or pure enjoyment) and thereby the loss of subjectivity. This is symbolic castration and underpins Lacan's basic clinical structures of neurosis, psychosis and perversion.[7]

A Lacanian diagnostics, therefore, would rely on how the relationship with the signifier, with castration, emerges.[8] For example, in psychosis, the name-of-the-father does not operate symbolically – there is a foreclosure of the paternal metaphor (*Verwerfung*) – and what is foreclosed returns in the real (a dramatic example would be a patient who was deluded that his penis was shrinking – a real and graphic example).[9] Likewise perversion, for Lacan, is not diagnosed on the basis of behaviour, but rather on the subject's ambivalent relation to castration. The perverse subject, for Lacan, might not engage in any behaviour that would be considered perverse by the lay person, but might indicate in analysis that the laws of language apply only to others and not to himself. The pervert is one to whom the law of prohibition does not apply – put bluntly, he wants to believe that the mother still has an imaginary phallus under her skirt. Both Lacan and Freud call this a disavowal (*Verleugnung*) of castration. An example would be an analysand who says to his analyst "feel free to say whatever you like, say whatever comes into your head..." in a reversal of the analytic rule of free association that is the analyst's usual instruction to the analysand! Unlike the usual forensic method of diagnosis (in which perversion would be diagnosed on the basis of unconventional sexual behaviours) perversion is seen as a structural category;

6 That is, division by the signifying chain, repression.

7 I have elaborated very little on the phallus, the signifier of sexual difference, as it is beyond the scope of this paper. However it is a key element in Lacan's exposition of the Oedipus complex and in his diagnostics.

8 Strictly speaking this is only possible in the context of psychoanalysis, where speech itself is the medium.

9 The psychotic patient's difficulties with symbolisation is not news to psychiatrists; for instance tests of abstract and concrete thinking are a commonplace part of psychiatric assessment.

it has been suggested for example that many patients with a DSM diagnosis of post-traumatic stress disorder may in fact have a perverse structure in the Lacanian sense (Verhaeghe 2001). In terms of neurosis, Lacan speaks largely of hysteria and obsessional neurosis, but postulates repression (*Verdrängung*) as the core mechanism, that operates in relation to the name-of-the-father; that is, the subject submits to symbolic castration and in the process becomes a subject divided from knowledge of himself.

In this way, a Lacanian diagnostics would be based not so much on the symptom or syndrome, than on a clinical structure which may or may not result in the expression of a symptom, given the right set of circumstances; it is possible only in a setting where the subject's relation to the signifier is apprehended. However, one of the difficulties with the clinical structures is that they appear to offer an easy understanding of patients or analysands (and Lacan warned to beware of understanding); just apply the matheme[10] and away you go. A superficial reading of the structures may suggest that the "cause" of clinical problems can be elucidated, which is no improvement on biological reductionism which suggests that clinical syndromes can be understood if only the gene or the neurotransmitter responsible can be found. The Lacanian conceptualization of the subject as divided by castration, separated from knowledge of himself, and prohibited from pure enjoyment means that attempts to reduce clinical phenomena to their cause, be it biological (as in the case of biological reductionism) or historical (in the sense that the subject is seen as a the result of traumas which befell him) are not satisfactory. The tension between symbolic and real, in particular, shows that historicity is the opposite of psychoanalysis. Nowhere is this more apposite than in the field of trauma, that aspect of experience that defies symbolization.

If the real is the leftover, the bit that the symbolic order cannot grasp, it is also what is lost in the acquisition of subjectivity and desire. The subject's relation to this real is the basis of the unconscious phantasy, hence the matheme already commented on (footnote 10). This notion was introduced by Freud in *Beyond the Pleasure Principle* (Freud 1920), somewhat controversially – Freud shows that the aim of all life is death and relates this to the clinical problem that people do not necessarily operate in terms of the pleasure principle, but are often quite masochistic in the repetition of traumatic experiences. Freud describes the *fort-da* game of his young grandson who throws his reel away and pulls it back, over and over again. The game is repetitive because there is something that resists the symbolization of the word. It is the thing that does

---

10 Lacan described many of the elements of the subject in relation to the Other and the lack in terms of symbolic devices known as mathemes – for instance the divided subject's relation to the petit objet a is described as $\$ \diamond a$, which nicely demonstrates the tension between the symbolic order and the real.

not make sense, the thing that "sticks out", both from the symbolic order[11], indeed for many this notion of the death drive (a function of the real, for Lacan) is what does not seem to fit in Freud's theory. There is in fact a whole debate about the existence or otherwise, of the death drive![12] For Lacan, of course, it is of central importance; man is dominated by the death drive and is derailed by his attachment to it, ever in discord with his own appetites; nonetheless the traumatic real has no consistency in itself but emerges (retrospectively) as the traumatic cause which apparently precedes the symbolic order. It has an artefactual effect of cause – it is the trauma in the past which seems to have caused the subject of today although it only achieves its substance through the inadequacy of the symbolic field. This interdependency of symbolic and real is obviously very different from a *psychological* understanding of trauma, in which trauma is assumed (simply because it appears to be so) to be the cause. The psychological understanding clearly owes much to an ego-psychology based view of the subject. However, rather than the Euclidean, geometrical structure of the subject implied by such theories, Lacan suggests that the structure of the subject is topological – as Žižek puts it "in order to apprehend this paradox of the traumatic object cause, a topological model is needed in which the limit that separates Inside from Outside coincides with its internal limit."(Žižek 1994, p. 31).

What can such a topological model be but a Moebius strip? This is precisely the model that Lacan uses, and moreover he says that it is not a metaphor, but how the subject is in fact structured. The Moebius strip describes the subject's folding back on itself, the coincidence of inside and outside and the obliteration of any simple opposition between container and contained. It is witness to the emptiness of the subject, the fact that the unconscious speaks in the gaps of conscious discourse, the uncanniness of your own face if you stare at it for too long, the inherent decentring at the heart of the subject – what Miller calls *extimité*. The alien that might erupt from the stomach is in fact native to oneself.[13]

---

11 Like the skull at the base of Hans Holbein's famous painting "The Ambassadors", it perturbs the apparently normal world of reality when it is seen from a particular perspective, but is simply a blind spot when the world of reality is apprehended.

12 This failure of the symbolic order is reformulated by Lacan in his assertion that "there is no Other of the Other" (there is no guarantor of the symbolic order, such as the God that Descartes has to invoke to guarantee the *cogito*), "there is Sexual relationship" (there is no perfect fit between man and woman), and by Freud in his assertion that "there is no psychoanalytic *Weltanschauung*".

13 Freud pointed out in *The Uncanny* that the German terms *heimlich* and *unheimlich* can actually mean the same thing – they are not necessarily opposites at all. Lacan rereads Freud's famous aphorism "*Wo Es war, soll Ich* werden" – not (as Strachey would have it) "where id was there ego shall be", but "where it (the Thing, the most intimate kernel of my being) was, there I shall become".

Lacan therefore provides a conceptual bridge between conscious and cognitive processes, and unconscious ones, in that the conscious and unconscious are not really separate (as some other theories would seem to suggest) but intertwined and inseparable.[14] The conscious is essentially the result of repression, of the division of the subject; if there were no "bar", no division by language, then we would be beings rather than subjects. Nonetheless the unconscious is constantly "spoken" within conscious discourse. Subjectivity is clearly linked with the idea of narrative – symbolic castration crystallizes prior events and gives them an apparent meaning, as well as a subjective sense of having been caused, of having an historical continuity. There are certain childhood events that "stick out" in memory; our personal history seems to us to be a linearly progressive development, which is shaped in one direction or another by these happenings. Lacan, of course, perturbs this comfortable historicity in underlining its imaginary nature and taking an entirely different perspective on this "traumatic cause". It is obvious that in a Lacanian perspective, memories are rewritten in the context of later events (the prime example of this being castration), that memories cannot be considered to represent objective truth, and that repression is a necessary condition of subjectivity.[15]

This analytical, as opposed to an historical (read reductionist), perspective on causation, has a broader relevance than simply within a psychoanalytical context. Current thinking on biological axes of behaviour is also at odds with the traditional reductionist viewpoint. Reductionism tends to ignore psychic processes as a focus for consideration because they cannot be measured in an objective way; the reductionistic approach assumes that only data obtained by objective empirical means has validity. From this perspective, reductionism, where psychopathological phenomena are seen as caused by measurable neurobiological correlates, is seen as existing in opposition to hermeneutics, where psychopathology is seen as the individual's solipsistic attempt to put meaning in his experiences. Will (1986) has pointed out that empirical reductionism and hermeneutics are founded on the same mistake. Both assume that knowledge obtained in the natural sciences by objective empirical means has a different ontological value from that obtained in the human sciences. In other words the former is a more accurate measure of human reality. In fact the two forms of knowledge differ only in terms of epistemology – in terms

14 It is notable that there is no Freudian paper entitled "The Conscious".

15 The Royal College of Psychiatrists published a document in response to so-called "recovered memory therapy" (Royal College of Psychiatrists' Working Group 1997) debunking the notion of repression and the possibility that memories could be recovered through therapy. Both this view, and the opposing view, that all memories recovered in psychotherapy must be true, are based on a misunderstanding of the nature of the unconscious. In fact, all memories recovered in psychotherapy are false – they are always distorted by subsequent events. Freud called this phenomenon *Nachträglichkeit* – deferred action.

of the method by which they are obtained – and not in terms of inherent value or ontology. Biological reductionism produces what Parnas & Bovet (1995) call RCVMs – Representational Computational Views of the Mind. Hermeneutics, applied to psychopathology, assumes that there are no general theories, no models, only the individual's interpretation of events; there can therefore be no concept of structure at either a biological, systems, or psychic level. This is the basis of anti-psychiatry where mental illness is seen as simply a construct that has no inherent consistency. Lacan's theory is radically different from hermeneutics (and is not a form of anti-psychiatry) in that it offers a structural theory of the subject, which nonetheless is non-deterministic. The inconsistency of the symbolic order, and the structural necessity of the real, which escapes meaning, allow for an element of choice – man is not merely determined by the Other, but makes his choices about what position he takes up in relation to castration. Furthermore, Lacan is clear that that position has certain consequences and that there are real differences between the psychotic and the perverse clinical structure, for example.[16] His theoretical rigour (and not necessarily rigidity) might lend itself better to generating hypotheses that "fit" with current non-reductionistic thinking in the biosciences that depart from traditional lesion-based, cause-and-effect models of illness.

An example of such a conceptualization would be self-organization. This is discussed by Parnas & Bovet (1995) in the context of immunology. Until the 1950s it was assumed that a foreign molecule "instructed" the combining site of the antibody molecule, thus prescribing the nature of the antibody. However, it now appears that the organism already has a vast number of antibody molecules before any contact with foreign molecules. An antigen simply binds to whatever lymphocyte produces the best-fitting antigen, provoking proliferation of that lymphocyte without actually specifying its characteristics. From a systems theory point-of-view, the immune system maintains organization while exposed to certain molecules, although such molecules bring about structural changes because of the system's tendency to self-organize. Symptoms that may be observed in the patient are a reflection of self-organization rather than a direct result of a pathogen. The same authors compare the traditional "prescriptive" view of natural selection with the current "proscriptive" concept. The older view was that characteristics that were not compatible with optimal fitness were not "allowed" to persist through generations so that the environment specified every characteristic of the organism. A more current

16 There is, however, a danger that the clinical structures can be seen as a simple classification system, and this leads to generalization. Lacan emphasized that psychoanalysis is concerned with the particularities of the subject, rather than general conditions. He should by no means be read as implying that there is some sort of normative sexuality with which other kinds of sexuality can be compared.

view (and one that is compatible with observed phenomena) is that "what is not forbidden is allowed" so that selection discards only those characteristics that are incompatible with survival and allows other characteristics to persist. Natural selection is not a matter of the impingement of the environment causing a lesion in the organism but of the organism or system's tendency to self-organize around what the authors call the "domain of distinction", the world which carries the possibility of impact on it.

It may be that the human cognitive apparatus has its own domain of significance or distinction. Information from the environment carries the possibility of impact on the cognitive apparatus but this information is not simply inscribed on a blank slate. The infant's cognitive agency is no *tabula rasa* to be programmed with information about reality, nor is it simply the potentiality of pre-existing neural networks which gradually mature. Instead the infant constructs his environment and organizes his experience on the basis of his emerging self-coherence. His attempt at mastery of his environment is predicated on a drive toward self-coherence and wholeness. He selects and constructs his environment – and this includes information from the rest of his body – into a partly narrative form which has "agreement" with his emerging version of self-coherence. Using the example of walking ability, Bushell & Boudreau (1993) suggest that rather than following on from pre-programmed instructions, or maturation of neurones (as in older developmental theories) walking ability emerges out of a combination of adjustments and reorganizations of the interacting components of the motor system as a whole. It should be obvious that a psychoanalytic theory that recognizes the linguistic nature of subjectivity implies that the human subject self-organizes. The mirror stage is a prime example of self-organization and is echoed in the example above (regarding the development of walking ability). In the Lacanian context certain symptoms can be seen as a form of self-organization.[17] For example, in psychosis it has already been commented that there is a failure of the symbolic function, that the name-of-the-father is foreclosed. This is a very different mechanism from repression in that it is a radical pushing away, a refusal of the symbolic. Lacan suggests that the delusion may be a way of filling in the gap that arises in the substance of the subject – a way of copper fastening the subject's hold on reality to such an extent that there is no "give" in reality. The delusional belief must be firmly adhered to or it does not work at all.[18] From

17 Although Lacan never used this term and avoided any terminology that might suggest that there is an inherent or potential wholeness to the individual.

18 The usual function of the symbolic order is to allow the subject to perceive reality from a certain distance – to make it bearable and have a degree of flexibility, to allow the subject an escape from the imaginary of the mirror-image. It could be argued that the aggressivity that this relationship with the image, or counterpart is similar to Klein's paranoid-schizoid position and that her depressive position has echoes of the function of the symbolic order.

this perspective the delusion represents an attempt to hold the subject together – a kind of "self-cure". Likewise, in obsessional neurosis, the obsessional's inability to function, to progress, might be seen by Lacan as an attempt to install a castrating father. The obsessional, at an unconscious level, stands in relation to a father who is not adequate to the castrating function; the obsessional chooses to castrate himself at an imaginary level, in order to maintain himself as a desiring subject. Furthermore, the very structure of the subject in relation to the symbolic and real is a prime example of self-organization; as has already been pointed out, the subject has a sense of having been caused, through the vehicle of language. The subject's relation to the signifier is what creates his own history and his conscious sense of being a product of that history. Those traumatic events that seem to "stick in the mind", that seem to us to be turning points in our life-story, provide us with a sense of continuity and more or less linear, if punctuated, development. The truth is, however, that we have only constructed things as such – we organize ourselves around these events so that they seem to be causative. The very process of self-organization creates the illusion that it itself does not occur. There are echoes of Freud's seduction theory and its abandonment in the epistemological shift within the biosciences. The older perspective, whereby the environment impinges directly and causes a lesion is similar to Freud's early views of sexual trauma as causative of psychic lesions or abscesses. The self-organizational view of neurobiological systems has parallels with Freud's abandonment of the seduction theory for the theory of infantile sexuality, which Lacan takes further by locating trauma as structural rather than directly causative. Although the popular "counselling" approach and the biological reductionistic approach may seem aeons apart, it is notable that both are characterized by a lesion-based model of mental disorder in which either trauma or a biological abnormality are postulated as directly causative. Lacan provides a set of coordinates which allow for clearly different clinical structures and the possibility that similar symptoms may in fact have their basis in different structures. This is not incompatible with everyday clinical psychiatric practice. It might be mere fantasy to suggest that the gap between psychoanalysis and neuroscience is reducible – this would be akin to suggesting that primary repression could be overcome and that there would be no bar to knowledge about the subject. However, the Lacanian unconscious, structured as a language and ethical rather than ontic[19] seems more compatible with existing neuroscientific theories. The unconscious is the underside of the conscious; if we trace from one side of the Moebius strip to another (a temporal operation rather than a static object) we meet our starting point. The analysand does not gain an increased stock of conscious memories

19 In the sense that it emerges in the context of the praxis of psychoanalysis, rather than "existing" as an entity beneath the ego.

in analysis, but in fact forgets much of what was articulated. Psychoanalysis involves a kind of conscious forgetting – it is not concerned with an extension of conscious insight, or with relearning, but rather with a shift in the way the unconscious and therefore the conscious are articulated. Perhaps at a neural level this is reflected in changes in the connections between neurones in memory and language centres. What are unconscious are representations, or signifiers, suggesting that the interface between speech and memory might be a meeting ground for neuroscience and psychoanalysis. The Lacanian assertion that "the unconscious is structured as a language" may allow psychoanalysis to generate clinically relevant, non-reductionistic, neuroscientific hypotheses for psychiatry.

References

Bushell, E. W., Boudreau, J. P. 1993. "Motor development and the mind: the potential role of motor abilities as a determinant of aspects of perceptual development", *Child Development*, 64: 1005–1021.

Freud, S. 1950. *Project for a Scientific Psychology*. S. E., Vol. I. London: The Hogarth Press.

Freud, S. 1920. *Beyond the Pleasure Principle*. S. E., XVIII. London: The Hogarth Press.

Geerardyn, F. 1997. *Freud's Project and the Roots of Psychoanalysis*. London: Rebus Press.

Lacan, J. 1949. "The mirror stage as formative of the function of the I as revealed in psychoanalysis", in *Écrits: A Selection* (Sheridan, A., trans.), London: Tavistock, 1977.

Lacan, J. 1953. "The function and field of speech and language in psychoanalysis", in *Écrits: A Selection* (Sheridan, A., trans.), London: Tavistock, 1977.

Lacan, J. 1964-5. *The Seminar of Jacques Lacan, Book XI, The Four Fundamental Concepts of Psychoanalysis*. (Miller, J-A., ed., Sheridan, A., trans.). London: Penguin Books, 1979.

Lacan, J. 1971-2. *The Seminar of Jacques Lacan, Book XIX, ...Ou pire/...Or worse* (trans.Gallagher, C.). London: Karnac, 2003.

Miller, J.-A. 1995. "Context and Concepts", in *Reading Seminar XI: Lacan's Four Fundamental Concepts of Psychoanalysis* (Feldstein, R., Fink, B., & Jaanus, M., ed.), Albany: SUNY Press.

Miller, J.-A. 1996. "An Introduction to Seminars I and II – Lacan's Orientation Prior to 1953 (II)", in *Reading Seminars I and II: Lacan's Return to Freud* (Feldstein, R., Fink, B., & Jaanus, M.), Albany: SUNY Press.

Parnas, J., Bovet, P. 1995. "Research in psychopathology: epistemological issues", *Comprehensive Psychiatry*, 36: 167–181.

Royal College of Psychiatrists' Working Group on Reported Recovered Memories of Child Sexual Abuse. 1997. "Recommendations for good practice and implications for training, continuing professional development and research", *Psychiatric Bulletin*, 21: 663 – 665.

Verhaeghe, P. 2001. "Perversion II: The Perverse Structure", *The Letter*, Autumn 2001, Vol. 23: 77 – 95.

Will, D. 1986. “Psychoanalysis and the new philosophy of science”, *International Review of Psychoanalysis*, 13: 163 – 173.
Žižek, S. 1994. “Does the Subject have a Cause?” in *The Metastases of Enjoyment: Six Essays on Women and Causality*, London: Verso.

Methodology and Philosophy of Science

Methodological Issues in Psychiatry: Psychiatry as an Empirical Science[1]

Hans-Jürgen Möller

Introduction

Psychiatry deals with mental and emotional disorders, i.e. with current disorders of and habitual deviations from the norm of experience and behaviour that are considered pathological. As a clinical discipline, psychiatry is two-faced, as is the case in all clinical disciplines. On the one hand, it is directed at clinical practice in the sense of helping, and, on the other hand, at knowledge, at intellectual fathoming of the processes at which treatment is aimed. At the same time, it thereby achieves the best prerequisites for the physician's practical, i.e. diagnostic, therapeutic, rehabilitative and prophylactic tasks (Möller 1978).

Hardly anyone doubts that the entry of the modern sciences into medicine has accelerated its progress to such an extent that the difference between the current situation and that of 150 years ago is much more significant than that between the latter and antique medicine. This progress does not appear to be quite so dramatic in psychiatry, and the role of the so-called "scientific methods" to acquire knowledge remains disputed. In this context, critical voices stress the fact that mental and emotional aspects cannot be observed objectively, measured quantitatively or manipulated experimentally in the same way as physical and material aspects. Some authors therefore like to assign psychiatry a place close to the human sciences and reject its positioning in the area of empirical sciences, as demanded by others. Depending on the spirit of the times, the pendulum swings in either one direction or the other. As an example, one can think of the importance of the "Daseinsanalyse" (existential analysis) in German psychiatry immediately after the Second World War and the current dominance of the position of biological psychiatry.

The antimony between these two directions has still not been solved to date. Many view it as a typical conflict in psychiatry, as a characteristic constituent of this field. The balance between human and natural sciences is considered by some to be so essential for psychiatry that any larger deviation in one direction or the other is criticized as an estrangement from the subject.

---

1 Reprinted, with permission, from World J Biol Psychiatry (2001) 2: 38-47.

The principal antinomy outlined here appears in various shades and colours and under various names, however, in the end, the basic matter at hand is always the same polarization. As an example, a few more pairs of opposites relevant in this context will be mentioned briefly here: the contrast between biographical/ideographic orientation and research approaches that search for general rules; the contrast between understanding/hermeneutic and explanatory/nomothetic methods; the contrast between purely speculative (intellectually constructive) and empirical/inductive extraction of knowledge; the contrast between the historical position and that of the "Realwissenschaften" (science of realities); the contrast between the holistic approach and the analytical/reductionistic procedures.

These almost incompatible, antagonistic points of view on basic methodological questions do not only concern psychiatry but can also be demonstrated in other fields that deal with psychosocial matters. This is made clear by the discussion of methods in psychology, sociology and psychotherapy. In this way, psychotherapy based on the theory of learning usually presents itself as an empirical science, whereas psychoanalysis is characterized by many well-known representatives as a hermeneutic science. On the other hand, there are debates within the discussion of psychoanalytical methods as to whether psychoanalytical science has a rather more empirical approach and thus is inadequately characterized as a hermeneutic direction (Katschnig and Simhandl 1987).

Of course, this is not only an intellectual discussion since the principle methodological direction in this context has enormous consequences. It determines what is accepted as scientific "truth" or, better said, as the path to the "truth", and how this can be defended, i.e. what is valid as an adequate form of scientific argumentation. All resulting conclusions are of great relevance for routine clinical care and, in a larger frame of reference, also for health policies. For example, reform movements of great political force, that have also resulted in great problems in psychiatry, have mainly emerged from speculative, ideologically exaggerated positions and would hardly have been thinkable from the view of a sober, empirical procedure, which carefully investigates the individual facts and their implications, before maxims for procedures are declared. For example, one should remember the sociopsychiatric reform movement rung in by Basaglia in Italy, or better said: a revolution that could only derive its political power of persuasion from an unrealistic sociopsychiatric ideology and that evaded perception of the negative effects on psychiatric care in Italy.

The consequences for action that can be derived from the results of an empirical psychiatry do not normally achieve such spectacular political force in such a short time. However, by summation of many smaller steps, the consequences of which have been scientifically investigated, this procedure can be extremely effective in the long run and promising for the future. One could think of the development of psychopharmacotherapy, for example, and the scientific evaluation of this approach to analyse carefully the advantages and disadvantages of this kind of treatment. The positive consequences of this laborious scientific development for the acute and long-term treatment of depression and schizophrenia have completely altered the image of psychiatry to the advantage of the patients.

Some authors propose a combination of nomothetic and idiographic methods as the ideal way, as appears particularly convincing to clinicians in routine daily care: while diagnostic clarification, prognosis and treatment are basically related to general laws, specific features of an individual case and its historic and current circumstances are additionally taken into account and thereby contribute to an individually adapted modification of the general laws on which diagnosis and treatment are based. However, this interpretation should not obscure the fact that the necessity of having general laws is also advocated in this methodological variation.

It must be stressed that there are not only general laws in the scientific field but, as we can be sure of today, also in psychological and sociological fields, i.e. in fields whose range of phenomena is often classified as a human sciences approach, due to the hypostasized immateriality. Furthermore, proposition of general laws is possible not only through strictly experimental methods of evaluation, like in the natural sciences, but also under other conditions.

Empirical Psychiatry as a "Realwissenschaft" (Science of Realities)

Each of us has a certain intuitive pre-understanding of what is generally meant by empirical psychiatry or by an empirical science. This pre-understanding of scientifically active colleagues is probably very strongly influenced by their own special method of research. Most would have difficulties to define the basic methodological principles on which an empirical science is generally based. Furthermore, the attempts at definition would probably only correspond in a central area, if at all. Particularly the analytical theory of science has been occupied with the basic methodological questions of the empirical sciences or "Realwissenschaften". It is specifically based on the most important principles of neorationalism and neopositivism, which have blended in a reciprocal corrective and complementary way. Authors such as Hempel, Oppenheim, Carnap, Popper etc. are to be named here. Stegmüller published a critical synthesis of their positions in his multivolume work (Stegmüller 1973).

I shall not speak of empirical science below, but of "Realwissenschaften". According to the modern analytical theory of science, this term refers to sciences that are concerned with statements about the reality that can be experienced

– statements in the sense of general statements of laws, and explanations of individual phenomena based on these laws (Möller 1976). I should like to briefly present the basic principles that I consider central to the "Realwissenschaften" from the angle of the analytical theory of science. I would like to use these elements to erect some mainstays for explication of the term empirical psychiatry, or psychiatry based on the "Realwissenschaften". For a more detailed discussion of these problems, which also considers critical arguments to a greater extent, please refer to my other publications on this topic (Möller 1976; Möller 1978).

- The Logical Structure of Explanation

The aim of the "Realwissenschaften" is to explain or prognosticate individual events by referral to general laws, in which event A is linked to event B. These general laws can be formulated as general statements (B applies for every A) or as statistical statements (B applies in 70% of cases for A). Knowledge of general laws allows one to influence the phenomena being investigated, if it has been clarified beforehand by experimental or quasi-experimental evaluations that the law formulates a causal relationship and not only an indicative relationship.

The structure of explanation, which is simultaneously the structure of prognosis, is at the centre of the methodology of the "Realwissenschaften". The logically adequate form of explanation was described by Hempel and Oppenheim [Hempel-Oppenheim-(HO) Explanation Scheme]:

Example 1: Logical structure of explanation (HO-Scheme):
General rule (G): All M have the property D
Antecedent (A): K is an M

K has the property D

Other forms of argumentation, e.g. circular types of argumentation (Example 2) are thereby explicitly rejected as inadequate.

Example 2: Example of a circular type of argumentation:
Someone asks: Why is there lightning?
Someone else answers: Because Zeus is angry.
The first person asks: How do you know that Zeus is angry?
The other person answers: Can't you see that there's lightning!

It can be demonstrated that not only natural science explanations in the strict sense, but also psychological argumentations follow the Hempel-Oppenheim scheme of explanation.

Example 3: Psychological argument of explanation:

G: People who were subjected to a strict up-bringing are more intolerant and anxious than others
A: Hans had a strict up-bringing

Hans is more intolerant and anxious than others

In parentheses it should be noted that the "Verstehen" (understanding), which has been attributed a special methodological position since Dilthey and Jaspers, also follows this logical structure of argumentation (Example 4), if it is acknowledged as a methodological peculiarity that a different quality of rules is then being used (e.g. subjective experiences with respect to one's own experience/behaviour or statements about the experience/behaviour of other people gained from one's own life experience).

Example 4: Understanding as an explanation:

G: Whenever I am in the situation S, I feel, think and do R
A1: K is in the situation S
A2: Assume that I am K (experiment of identifying thought)

I feel, think and do R in the situation S

- The Principle of Falsification

According to Popper (1969), the principle of falsification has a special place in the "Realwissenschaften". It states that rules in sciences of reality should be formulated in such a way that they can principally be falsified. When delimiting from a naive empiricalism, which sees the basis of empirical sciences in the pure induction principle, and from metaphysical statements in disciplines that do not belong to the "Realwissenschaften", the principle of falsification is a central marker of methodology in the "Realwissenschaften".

An exemplary presentation may illustrate why this postulation is so important and how easy it is to contravene. In an extreme case, statements that did not confer with the postulation of the ability to be falsified would be tautological statements (Example 5). They do not make any statements about the reality and therefore contradict the basic aim of the "Realwissenschaften".

Example 5: Example of a tautological statement:

When the cockerel crows, the weather will either change or remain as it is.

Popper worked intensively on the manner in which statements of rules must be formulated so that it is principally possible to falsify them, or with the question how one can get around the possibility of falsification for the sake of a planned methodological violation (Table 1). The main aspects hereby are as follows:

a) Formulation of tautological statements
According to their definition, tautological statements are without empirical content (Example 5). For example, statements of rules become tautological when every possible reality that can be described in a theoretical system is described as the cause of a certain disorder.
b) Imprecise terminology
Unclear and inconsistent terms allow falsifications to be avoided by emphasizing that the terms, which occur in the theory investigated, were wrongly interpreted. Imprecise terminology can go so far that completely heterogeneous terms are sub-grouped under one concept.
c) Lacking empirical significance of theoretical terms
Use of theoretical terms that are not associated with the level of observation by rules of assignment and therefore do not have any empirical significance result in statements which cannot be falsified.
d) Use of immunising ad hoc hypotheses
After recording falsifying empirical data, a statement of a rule is modified by additional argumentation in such a way that the falsification is cancelled and a falsification of the complete statement complex even made impossible.

In an earlier publication (Möller 1978), I evaluated statements about psychoanalytical theories under the aspect of the ability to be falsified. I showed, under different aspects, that numerous statements contravene this falsification postulate. Other areas of psychiatry are also not free from such violations of the principle of falsification, as will be mentioned below. The complete adherence to this principle obviously only represents a methodological ideal, which is rarely achieved in the reality of science (see below).

- The Ability to Observe Phenomena

Statements of laws are based on single observations of reality or single observations of the range of phenomena being investigated, which are described in so-called basic or protocol theses. Various demands must be made of these basic theses (Table 2), which have been a particular interest of neopositivism (Carnap 1966). These criteria, which probably appear plausible to most at first sight, sound simple, although it is of great relevance whether or not they are observed:

a) Each basic thesis describes one observable event and should reflect the relevant conditions, e.g. of an experiment, as accurately as possible: all statements of observation should be as precise as possible and formulated in the relevant scientific terminology so that colleagues in the same speciality have no doubt as to the circumstances.

b) It should be possible to test the phenomena described in the basic theses between subjects: it must be possible for different scientists who are trained in the particular specialist area to achieve a consensus whether or not the respective phenomenon exists. Obviously, the simpler the technique of observation, the more easily this methodological ideal can be achieved.

c) The phenomena described in the basic theses should be well-established: the described phenomenon should be found by a method of observation which ensures that the investigator did not carry it into the part of reality being investigated. It is already impossible to completely fulfil this requirement when humans are being investigated. However, this does not mean that one can do without it altogether. It describes a methodological ideal that one should always strive for.

A further central aspect is the differentiation between terms of observation and theoretical terms (constructs). This differentiation arose from the conflict between empirical and rationalistic interpretations of the scientific language. It became apparent that also terms of observation – i.e. terms that refer to things that can be directly observed – do not suffice for a science of realities, but that so-called disposition terms or theoretical terms (constructs) are also required. These can only be defined indirectly as part of a theory by reference to observable phenomena or by terms of observation and theoretical terms (Figure 1). The more this empirical anchorage is reduced, the greater the danger that only a minor reference to reality remains, or even that no statement about reality is made whatsoever. A theory in which the important theoretical terms can no longer be reduced to terms of observation, either directly or indirectly, via other theoretical terms, is a metaphysical theory. According to its definition, such a theory no longer fulfils the requirements of an empirical science and is, of course, from the viewpoint of a metaphysical discipline, not required to fulfil them.

In this context, the relationship between theory and observation should be discussed in more detail. A naive empiricism that is only based on the observation of the range of phenomena being investigated appears unsuitable. Alternatively, according to current opinion, an alternating crossover of theory and observation should be assumed, in the sense that almost every scientific observation is directed in some way or another by a hypothesis. This occurs, among others, in the sense of a focussing on areas of phenomena that are relevant for a particular hypothesis, while other areas are excluded (Figure 2). In this way, the hypothesis or theory is expanded by observations directed by hypotheses, which leads to other theory-related observations, whereby it is important to avoid the danger of a complete circularity between theory and experience. This would be the case if only those circumstances were observed that could confirm the theory, while all other circumstances were ignored.

Further aspects of methodology in the "Realwissenschaften" refer to the axiomatic structures of scientific theories and the differentiation of the value of various theories for a certain range of phenomena. There is no space here to go into this interesting aspect in more detail.

Detailed Aspects of the Methodology of an Empirical Psychiatry

In my opinion, it is obvious that there are areas of scientific psychiatry that feel bound to the basic methodological principles presented here, even though the analytical theory of science is not referred to explicitly, and occasionally not all the methodological criteria given above are considered. The basic principles of methodology in the "Realwissenschaften" are surely contravened even in those areas of psychiatry that are explicitly seen as empirical science. This is not surprising since these scientific, theoretical approaches only represent a methodologically ideal norm that cannot be completely fulfilled in the reality of research, for various reasons. I have referred to attempts in psychiatry to fulfil methods of the "Realwissenschaften" and also to the respective violations with the help of several examples in another publication (Möller 1976).

- Biological Psychiatry and Psychopharmacology

An empirical orientation to research is especially relevant in biological psychiatry, where it lies, so to speak, "in the nature of things", i.e. in the application of knowledge and methods from natural sciences, or rather more from the neuro-sciences, to investigate and influence mental disorders. This does not only apply to basic research but also to clinically-oriented biological psychiatry or psychopharmacology (Möller 1976; Möller and Benkert 1980). Example 6, which in this case is paradigmatic for such approaches, is taken from the field of clinical pharmacology and should indicate that not only efficacy and tolerability aspects can be investigated in clinical psychopharmacology, but also further reaching theoretical aspects (Emrich et al. 1979; Möller et al. 1979).

> Example 6: Experiments to test the hypothesis: ß-adrenergic receptor blockade is antimanic
> Experiment 1: Racemat d/l propranolol (ß blocker) is antimanic
> Experiment 2: Isomer d-propranolol (not a ß blocker) is antimanic
>
> ---
>
> Conclusion: ß blockade is not a relevant antimanic method of action

It is of great importance to differentiate between the level of hypothesis formulation and hypothesis testing. While the formulation of a hypothesis is actually a creative act that does not undergo any significant methodological confinement and can therefore happen on a purely clinical-intuitive basis, for example, testing of a hypothesis must follow various rules of empirical science. These include an adequate formulation of the hypothesis, an adequate composition of the sample, an adequate description of the range of phenomena, the inclusion of all relevant parameters, an adequate sample size (to avoid ß error problems) and adequate procedures of statistical analysis. Wrong conclusions can result if these criteria are not considered. For example, for a long time the problem of a ß error – i.e. the non-recognition of a difference between two groups that is actually present – was not sufficiently considered in clinical psychopharmacology when second generation antidepressants like mianserine or trazodone were being compared to standard antidepressants in clinical studies. This resulted in the hasty conclusion that the new substances had equivalent therapeutic efficacy.

A hypothesis can only provisionally be seen as confirmed when it has been subjected to a hypothesis evaluation, and when the empirical findings concur with the hypothesis. The degree of empirical confirmation increases with further verifications from other investigators testing the hypothesis. This methodological approach has found more and more acceptance in psychiatric research, not only in the natural science fields of specialized basic research but also in clinical research. The evaluation of the dexamethasone suppression test (DST) is a particularly striking example of this point. The hypothesis was formulated that the DST could be used to differentiate between endogenous and non-endogenous depression. This hypothesis appeared to be valid at first. However, many investigators had not sufficiently considered the various influencing factors, some of which were associated with endogenous depression. When better experiments that considered these aspects were later performed, it became apparent that the DST is not suitable for differentiating between endogenous and non-endogenous depression, and that it is completely unspecific with respect to the disorder; the test can also be pathological in schizophrenic and manic patients, for example (Berger and Klein 1984; Greden et al. 1983; Möller et al. 1986).

Violations of the laws can even be observed in biological psychiatry and psychopharmacology, the core areas of empirical methodology, e.g. in the sense that there is often no progress made from the generation of a hypothesis and that no decisive testing of the hypothesis is performed, or falsifying conclusions are avoided during the testing of the hypothesis in that, for example, other statistical approaches are used than were originally specified. Even if several results from various experiments seem to suggest the falsification of the hypothesis or theory, there are occasional attempts to prevent this falsification with immunising ad hoc hypotheses. Such a tendency seems to increase with the hierarchical position of a hypothesis within a theory.

In this context, it should be mentioned that the complex interactions in which, for example, neuronal processes can be seen, limit the analysis by experimental specifications. A further problem is that results from animal models can often only be carried over to a very limited extent to the circumstances being experimentally investigated in humans (e.g. schizophrenia, depression). Furthermore, many questions are left open since it is not possible to perform experimental investigations in humans for fundamental and ethical/legal reasons.

It is therefore not surprising that core theories such as the dopamine hypothesis of schizophrenia or the noradrenaline or serotonin hypothesis of depression (Ackenheil et al. 1978; Davis et al. 1991; Fritze et al. 1992) remain, and that various sub-theories have been developed, although there are a great number of inconsistent findings. In such cases, the contrary findings are obviously insufficient for the researchers to actually come to the conclusion that the theory is falsified; instead, the theory is maintained and newer findings adapted or re-formulated accordingly. The theory is obviously too valuable for the researchers, and does not appear to be completely exhausted in its heuristic content, to allow it to be dismissed. Of course, it is legitimate to maintain a hypothesis under these conditions.

- Diagnosis in Psychiatry

The orientation towards the "Realwissenschaften" is becoming more and more established in the diagnosis of psychiatric disorders, in that approaches are preferably incorporated which primarily originated in empirical psychology. In this way, it is possible to achieve an exact record or description of the observable phenomena of current or habitual psychopathological phenomena. In particular, all attempts to standardize diagnostic terminology and improve its precision, as well as the development of psychopathometric methods according to methods of psychological testing (Table 3), should be named here. Besides valid and, above all, reliable documentation, these approaches also offer the possibility of quantification and thereby of a demanding statistical analysis. In this way, they go well beyond the possibilities of classical descriptive psychopathology. The standardized recording of findings and diagnosis of personality with observer- and self-rating scales, the systematic observation of behaviour and the testing of cognitive abilities should be named here as examples (Möller 1989; Möller 1991; von Zerssen 1979).

Descriptive psychopathology is undoubtedly a great treasure in the tradition of German psychiatry. It allowed the range of phenomena to be grasped with great subtlety of observation and great differentiation of terminology. However, the reliability problems and distortions of perception characteristic for this field of observation – as is the case for any observation of behaviour – were not sufficiently accounted for (Table 4). During the development of the AMDP

(Association for Methodology and Documentation in Psychiatry) system, which was created in the course of standardized procedures of evaluation of psychopathological findings and based on the classical descriptive psychopathology, it became apparent how difficult it is to operationalize adequately traditional terms for symptoms from descriptive psychopathology, and to document with sufficient reliability the psychopathological phenomena described with these terms (Baumann and Stieglitz 1983). The consequence of these attempts at standardization was that a great number of symptoms from traditional psychopathology had to be sacrificed, since it was not possible, despite relevant observer training, to guarantee a sufficiently high inter-observer reliability for these symptoms. In this context, an experienced psychopathologist may object to the mediocrity of the physicians participating in such tests of inter-observer reliability: accordingly, the mediocre standard of the physicians making the diagnosis would determine the limit for the inter-observer reliability. Such an objection cannot be completely discredited since, as far as I know, evaluations of inter-observer reliability have never been performed with highly qualified experts in traditional psychopathology in German-speaking countries. However, the school of training and associated theoretical dependency on certain systems, which are not sufficiently communicable with each other, could well become apparent in such a test.

Despite all the difficulties, an attempt should always be made to include traditional descriptive psychopathology in its complete differentiation in attempts at standardization, so as not to give away too hastily diagnostic accomplishments at the level of a range of phenomena. However, this obviously involves a reliability/validity dilemma: the more subtle the observations, the less approachable they are to inter-subject experience. Critics of extremes could, however, ask whether these highly sensitive descriptions are really more valid. For example, it is known from evaluations of assessment stereotypes performed by diagnosticians that certain phenomena are described or named in completely different ways, depending on the diagnostic presumptions given to the investigators. In this way, the same phenomena can be recorded as apathic symptoms when a schizophrenic disorder is pre-defined, but as depressive symptoms when an endogenous depression is pre-defined (Möller et al. 1978).

In this context, the results of multivariate dimensional analyses of observer-rated data on psychopathological findings, recorded in a standardized manner, are also of interest (Mombour 1972a; Mombour 1972b). They indicate that even the most extravagant observer-rating procedures yield the same dimensional structure time and again. This can be interpreted to the effect that the core statements are not substantially changed in content, however differentiated and multifaceted the symptoms that have been taken into account in an evaluation approach. Aspects that were originally described for the phenomena of the actual psychopathological findings were recently also described for the diagnosis of personality. Here, for example, the same basic dimensions were finally achieved, despite the diversity of the approaches to the pre-morbid personality (von Zerssen and Möller 1980; von Zerssen et al. 1988), e.g. extraversion, neuroticism and rigidity, or the "big five".

On the other hand, it can be derived from such investigations that observer- and self-rating of psychopathological phenomena are incongruent, since self-rating is obviously limited in various aspects and less differentiated. Observer- and self-rating are also subject to different falsification tendencies, as has been shown (von Zerssen 1979; von Zerssen 1986).

Various falsification tendencies (Table 4) can be almost completely avoided, or at least reduced, in the observation of psychopathological phenomena by the use of standardized observation procedures (Möller 1989). The relationship between psychopathological phenomena also allows a comprehensive testing of a hypothesis, as shown by von Zerssen during his evaluations of the primary personality in patients with endogenous psychoses, for example (von Zerssen 1982). The operationalization of names of psychiatric disorders, which has been increasingly introduced over the last decade by the stipulation of clearly defined inclusion and exclusion criteria, represents the basis for reliable diagnosis of disorders. It therefore represents an especially important advancement from the earlier diagnostic traditions, in which a single case was assigned to a very vaguely described clinical picture. Operationalization of nosological diagnosis means that a catalogue of criteria is established for every disorder, and that this catalogue is used to decide whether or not a certain patient has the particular disorder. This is performed according to the following principle: the disorder can be diagnosed if symptoms A, B and C but not D and E are present.

The various descriptions of psychiatric disorders should be conceived as theoretical constructs, which are associated with observable reality by various rules of allocation. Different traditional schools have resulted in varying descriptions of disorders, and have therefore significantly contributed to the diagnostic confusion. In this way, several different schizophrenia terms co-exist in the traditional psychiatry of the 20th century. Under the aspect that these definitions of constructs depend on the school, it could never have been expected that a uniform schizophrenia term would be the result. Each of the diagnostic systems operationalizes the respective disorder by slightly different criteria, according to the respective conceptual ideas. Multidiagnosis seems to be the only solution, since no-one in the scientific field is prepared to do without any of these special conceptualizations (Katschnig and Simhandl 1987). The validity of the individual diagnostic concepts should be proven in further empirical investigations. A multidiagnostic approach that retains the different concepts of certain schools for certain disorders, determined by an optimal operationalization, is probably more suitable than the earlier procedure to lead the extensive knowledge in such constructs by famous authors towards an empirical investigation with modern methods of evaluation and analysis.

Of course, such a colourful variety is unsatisfying for everyday diagnosis, since it leads to confusion of language. For this reason, the American psychiatric diagnosis system (DSM-III, DSM-III-R, DSM-IV) and the internationally binding ICD-10 system have been limited, in the sense of a consensus, to certain operationalizations of individual clinical pictures, whereby the definitions in the categories that correspond with each other are unfortunately incongruent (Möller 1990). It would have been advisable to have first performed further cross-sectional and longitudinal validity studies on the basis of multidiagnostic evaluation approaches – with the inclusion of biological and psychosocial parameters – in order to develop empirically an optimal system of diagnosis. The operationalizations of the diagnostic terms in these new systems of diagnosis have certainly led to an increased reliability of everyday diagnoses. This can be considered a major advancement. Under aspects of validity, however, the compulsory consensus has resulted in solutions of which some appear arbitrary. This is especially the case in the ICD-10, which was developed by an international group of experts. These solutions require improvement on the basis of additional research and discussions. It is also unsatisfactory that the postulated "theory-free" approach, in the sense of a syndrome-oriented classification, was not adhered to. Instead, traditional disorder concepts shine through in various diagnostic groups. The distribution of the severities of depressive episodes is also inconsequent in ICD-10, which actually follows a typological approach and not a psychometric evaluation of intensity.

- Epidemiology

It can be only mentioned in passing that modern psychiatric epidemiology also represents an important field of empirical research (Häfner 1978), and that a great degree of methodological awareness and know-how has developed in this area. In particular, acquirement of an adequate sample size is of relevance, besides aspects of exact diagnosis.

- Treatment Research

The main emphasis of psychiatric therapy research lies in the empirical approaches in pharmacotherapy, which is part of biological psychiatry. It is precisely this therapy that has assisted the breakthrough of the employment of objectifying evaluation procedures and methods of statistical analysis in psychiatry (Möller and Benkert 1980). Nevertheless, principle methodological difficulties can be determined here, for example, the inadequate consideration or non-consideration of the ß error problem for a long time in the evaluation of second generation antidepressants like Mianserine or Trazodone in comparison to standard antidepressants (Möller and Haug 1988; Woggon and Angst 1978). In addition to optimal planning of individual study designs, in the sense of sufficient statistical power (adequate sample size, reliable instruments of measurement, reduction of disturbing influencing factors), a statistical meta-analysis of the results of all studies can help to solve these problems.

An additional important topic of clinical psychopharmacology – "onset" research – also shows how, even in clinical psychopharmacology which is highly developed with respect to methodology, sub-parts can be unsatisfactory with regard to the basic methodology, and, in particular, with regard to the concrete documentation of studies (Möller et al. 1996; Müller and Möller 1998a; Müller and Möller 1998b).

For a long time, psychoanalytical therapy formed a refuge for a rather speculative "research". This was due to the carry-over from the theoretical/speculative super-structure (meta-theory), and the massive resistance of many of its representatives to controlled studies of efficacy. A change is beginning to show in psychotherapy research, however, particularly through the introduction of behavioural therapy and cognitive therapy, towards a more empirical orientation in the verification of the efficacy of psychotherapeutic approaches (Hautzinger 2000; Elkin et al. 1989; von Zerssen and Möller 1980).

- The Relationship Between Theory and Experience in Psychiatry

Of course, the application of empirical methods in psychiatric research assumes sound expert knowledge of the area to be investigated (and in the clinical field that means additional clinical experience), knowledge and critical appreciation of relevant theories, ideally also one's own original ideas, and the ability to formulate relevant questions. It should be possible to investigate these questions with the available arsenal of methods, and at an acceptable outlay of personnel, materials and time. As is the case in other sciences (see above), empirical research in psychiatry is always embedded in a network of foreknowledge, speculations about associations, and comprehensive intellectual constructions to explain observable phenomena.

The relevance of intuition and speculation in the formation of psychiatric theories must be emphasized explicitly in this context. Intuitive observations are the first stage of the formation of every hypothesis, either as a descriptive basis or sometimes as the elements that generate a hypothesis. The results of observation and intuition are further extended by creative, speculative approaches in a more or less farther reaching formation of a hypothesis or theory. The importance of intuition and speculation for an empirical science should therefore not be underrated. On the other hand, on their own they are insufficient for an empirical science; the testing of a hypothesis rather represents the decisive step. When a hypothesis is tested, the relevant facts are analysed according to a fixed system of rules and put in relation to the hypothesis. Falsifications are thereby just as valuable for theoretical knowledge as verification of the hypothesis.

The borders of empirical psychiatry relevant in this context can be found, on the one hand, between a simple psychiatry, based on the science of experience, and, on the other hand a speculative psychiatry. In contrast to an experimental science led by theories, a simple science of experience consists of the mere collection of observable facts without farther-reaching systematic association or theoretical statements. In contrast to empirical scientists directed by theories, speculative researchers form theories by intellectual constructions, which they only want to "test" (mostly to confirm), if at all, in their limited field of experience. They do not, however, systematically investigate the complete range of experience in order to examine their theory.

The less hypothesis-oriented psychiatry is, the more it becomes a science based purely on experience; the less psychiatry helps itself with the empirical examination of hypotheses, the more it becomes a speculative science. The combination of deduction and induction, of speculation, intuition and controlled observation/experimental experience, remains characteristic for an empirical psychiatry and a psychiatry based on the "Realwissenschaften" as defined here. In this context, it is important to warn against pure acceptance of plausibility (this is done again and again). Plausibility says absolutely nothing about the correctness of a theory. The "broken home" theory of disturbed behaviour is a relevant example; although it appears plausible, it has led to a great number of inconsistent results from empirical research and can therefore not be sustained (Welz 1983).

It should be stressed that such an empirical psychiatry is not only able to, but must also include psychological and sociological factors in addition to biological factors, e.g. in the sense of a multifactorial disorder model. Of course, the psychiatry as a "Realwissenschaft" outlined in this way also has drawbacks and carries the risk of wrong developments. The concern of older clinicians (Huber 1976; Janzarik 1989) that an empirical orientation of psychiatry defined in this way could lead to rather superficial findings, and perhaps even to a thoughtless and soulless counting and calculation, cannot be completely rejected, since there are definitely such false developments. However, they are mostly based on poor comprehension of science (e.g. a lack of intuition and creativity), or on plain ignorance of the strength of statements that can be made from the methods employed, e.g. certain statistical procedures.

References

Ackenheil, M., Hippius, H., Matussek, N. 1978. "Findings of biochemical research on schizophrenia", *Nervenarzt*, 49: 634-649.

Baumann, U., Stieglitz, R.D. 1983. Testmanual zum AMDP-System. *Empirische Studien zur Psychopathologie*. Berlin-Heidelberg-New York: Springer.

Berger, M., Klein, H.E. 1984. "Der Dexamethason-Suppressions-Test: Ein biologischer Marker der endogenen Depression?", *Eur Arch Psychiatry Neurol Sci*, 234: 137-146.

Carnap, R. 1966. *Philosophical foundations of physics*. New York-London: Nymphenburger Verlagsbuchhandlung.

Davis, K.L., Kahn, R.S., Ko, G., Davidson, M. 1991. "Dopamine in schizophrenia: a review and reconceptualization", *Am J Psychiatry*, 148: 1474-1486.

Elkin, I., Shea, T., Watkins, J.T., Imber, S.D., Sotsky, S.M., Collins, J.F., Glass, D.R., Pilkonis, P.A., Leber, W.R., Docherty, J.P. et al. 1989. "NIMH treatment of depression collaborative research program", *Arch Gen Psychiatry*, 46: 971-982.

Emrich, H.M., von Zerssen, D., Möller, H.J., Kissling, W., Cording, C., Schietsch, H.J., Riedel, E. 1979. "Action of propranolol in mania: comparison of effects of the d- and the l-stereoisomer", *Pharmakopsychiatr Neuropsychopharmakol*, 12: 295-304.

Fritze, J., Deckert, J., Lanczik, M., Strik, W., Struck, M., Wodarz, N. 1992. "Status of amine hypotheses in depressive disorders", *Nervenarzt*, 63: 3-13.

Greden, J.F., Gardner, R., King, D., Grunhaus, L., Carroll, B.J., Kronfol, Z. 1983. "Dexamethasone suppression tests in antidepressant treatment of melancholia. The process of normalization and test-retest reproducibility", *Arch Gen Psychiatry*, 40: 493-500.

Häfner, H. 1978. "Einführung in die psychiatrische Epidemiologie. Geschichte, Suchfeld, Problemlage", in: Häfner, H. (ed.) *Psychiatrische Epidemiologie*. Berlin-Heidelberg-New York: Springer, 1-56.

Hautzinger, M. 2000. *Kognitive Verhaltenstherapie bei psychischen Störungen*. Weinheim: Beltz.

Huber, G. 1976. "Zur Problematik quantitativer Verlaufbeobachtungen bei Schizophrenen", *Psychopathometrie*, 2: 61-66.

Janzarik, W. 1989. "Anthropologic aspects of science and scientific activity", *Nervenarzt*, 60: 612-618.

Katschnig, H., Simhandl, Ch. 1987. "Neuere Ansätze in der Klassifikation und Diagnostik psychischer Krankheiten", in: Simhandl, Ch., Berner, P., Luccioni, H., Alf, C. (eds.) *Moderne Psychiatrie, Klassifikationsprobleme in der Psychiatrie*. Purkersdorf: Medizinisch-Pharmazeutische Verlagsgesellschaft, 59-85.

Mombour, W. 1972a. «Procedure for the standardization of psychopathological findings», *Psychiatr Clin Basel*, 5: 73-120.

Mombour, W. 1972b. «Procedure for the standardization of psychopathological findings. 2", *Psychiatr Clin Basel*, 5: 137-157.

Möller, H.J. 1976. *Methodische Grundprobleme der Psychiatrie*. Stuttgart: Kohlhammer.

Möller, H.J. 1978. *Psychoanalyse – Erklärende Wissenschaft oder Deutungskunst? Zur Grundlagendiskussion in der Psychowissenschaft*. München: Fink.

Möller, H.J. 1989. "Standardisierte psychiatrische Befunderhebung", in: Kisker, K.P., Lauter, H., Meyer, J.E., Müller, C., Strömgren, E. (eds.) *Brennpunkte der Psychiatrie. Psychiatrie der Gegenwart*. 9. 3 ed. Berlin Heidelberg New York: Springer, 13-45.

Möller, H.J. 1990. "Probleme der Klassifikation und Diagnostik", in: Reinecker, H. (ed.) *Lehrbuch der klinischen Psychologie. Modelle psychischer Störungen*. Göttingen-Toronto-Zürich: Hogrefe 3-24.

Möller, H.J. 1991. "Outcome criteria in antidepressant drug trials: self-rating versus observer-rating scales", *Pharmacopsychiatry*, 24: 71-75.

Möller, H.J., Benkert, O. 1980. "Methoden und Probleme der Beurteilung der Effektivität psychopharmakologischer und psychologischer Therapieverfahren", in: Biefang, S. (ed.) *Evaluationsforschung in der Psychiatrie. Fragestellungen und Methoden*. Stuttgart: Enke, 54-128.

Möller, H.J., Haug, G. 1988. "Secondary and meta-analysis of the efficacy of non-tricyclic antidepressants", *Pharmacopsychiatry*, 21: 363-364.
Möller, H.J., Piree, S., von Zerssen, D. 1978. "Psychiatric classification", *Nervenarzt*, 49: 445-455.
Möller, H.J., von Zerssen, D., Emrich, H.M., Kissling, W., Cording, C., Schietsch, H.J., Riedel, E. 1979. "Action of d-propranolol in manic psychoses", *Arch Psychiatr Nervenkr*, 227: 301-317.
Möller, H.J., Kissling W, Bottermann, P. 1986. "The dexamethasone suppression test in depressive and schizophrenic patients under controlled treatment conditions", *Eur Arch Psychiatry Neurol Sci,* 235: 263-268.
Möller, H.J., Müller, H., Volz, H.P. 1996. "How to assess the onset of antidepressant effect: comparison of global ratings and findings based on depression scales", *Pharmacopsychiat*, 29: 57-62.
Müller, H., Möller, H.J. 1998a. "Methodological problems in the estimation of the onset of the antidepressant effect", *J Affect Disord*, 48: 15-23.
Müller, H., Möller, H.J. 1998b. "A regression analytical approach to estimate the onset of activity of antidepressants", *Eur Psychiatry*, 13: 134-137.
Popper, K.R. 1969. *Logik der Forschung*, 3. Aufl. Tübingen: Mohr.
Stegmüller, W. 1973. *Probleme und Resultate der Wissenschaftstheorie und analytischen Philosophie*. Berlin-Heidelberg-New York: Springer.
von Zerssen, D. 1979. "Klinisch-psychiatrische Selbstbeurteilungs-Fragenbögen", in: Baumann, U., Berbalk, H., Seidenstücker, G. (eds.) *Klinische Psychologie. Trends in Forschung und Praxis*. Bern-Stuttgart-Wien: Huber, 130-159.
von Zerssen, D. 1982. "Personality and affective disorders", in: Paykel, E.S. (ed.). *Handbook of affective disorders*. Edinburgh-London-Melbourne: Churchill Livingstone, 212-28.
von Zerssen, D. 1986. "Clinical self-rating scales (CSRF) of the Munich Psychiatric Information System (PSYHIS München)", in: Sartorius, N., Ban, T.A. (eds.) *Assessment of depression*. Berlin-Heidelberg-New York: Springer, 270-303.
von Zerssen, D., Möller, H.J. 1980. "Psychopathometrische Verfahren in der psychiatrischen Therapieforschung", in: Biefang, S. (ed.) *Evaluationsforschung in der Psychiatrie. Fragestellungen und Methoden*. Stuttgart: Enke, 129-166.
von Zerssen, D., Pfister, H., Koeller, D.M. 1988. "The Munich Personality Test (MPT)--a short questionnaire for self-rating and relatives' rating of personality traits: formal properties and clinical potential", *Eur Arch Psychiatry Neurol Sci*, 238: 73-93.
Welz, R. 1983. *Drogen, Alkohol und Suizid*. Stuttgart: Enke.
Woggon, B., Angst, J. 1978. "Principles and regulations for clinical pilot studies on psycholeptic drugs", *Arzneimittelforschung*, 28: 1257-1259.

Table 1: Possibilities of injuring the requirement for an empirical content of statements of rules

Formulation of tautological statements
Imprecise terminology
Lack of empirical significance of theoretical terms
Use of immunising ad hoc hypotheses

Table 2: Criteria for basic theses

Basic theses must fulfil the following conditions:
Description of singular phenomena
Description of phenomena that can be tested between subjects
Description of well-established phenomena

Table 3: Quality criteria for theoretical tests

Objectivity
Reliability
Validity
Norming
Practicability

Table 4: Systematic falsification of observations

Rosenthal effect	Falsification dependent on the expectation
Halo effect	Falsification dependent on the overall impression
Logical error	Tendency to falsification dependent on a theory
Over-/Undervaluing of degrees of disorder	

Figure 1: Relationship between theoretical terms and terms of observation (from Möller 1978)

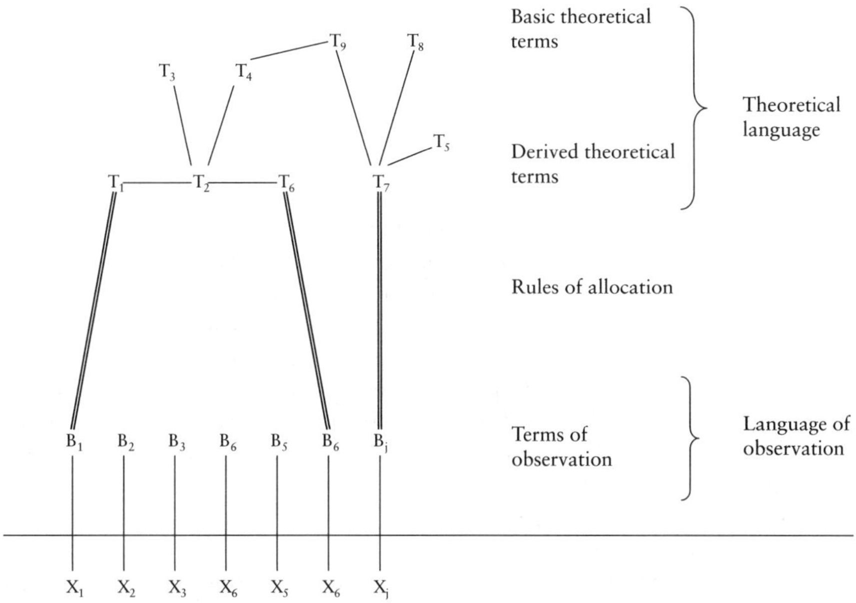

Figure 2: Relationship between the theoretical and observational levels (from Möller 1978)

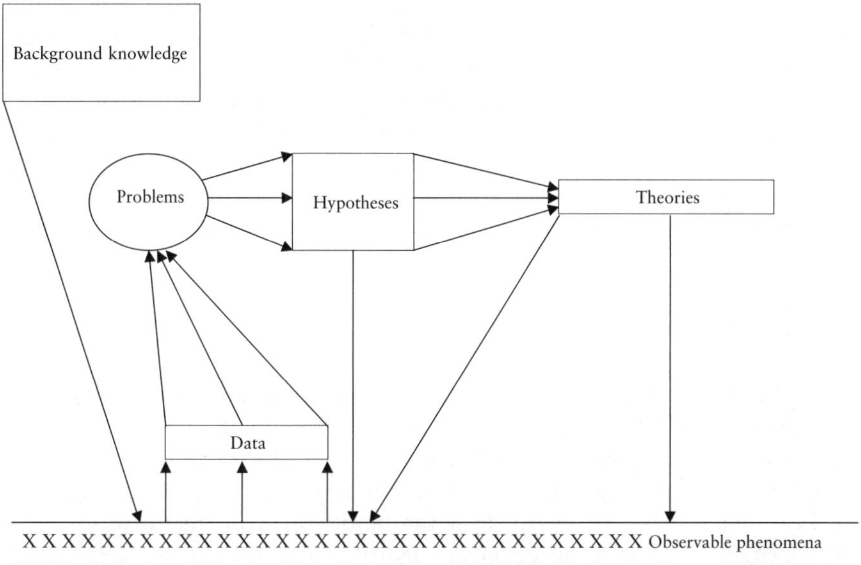

Humanities and Molecular Psychiatry

Johannes Thome

1. Introduction

The segregation between the humanities and the natural sciences during the age of enlightenment represents a fundamental event which has strongly influenced the further development of medicine. In modern times, physicians resolutely embraced the techniques and methods of the natural sciences and, thus, laid down the foundation stone of a scientific medicine with all its achievements and benefits witnessed during the past two decades. Parallely, however, the role of the humanities dwindled away. In the early 19th century, the separation of medicine from the humanities was largely completed. In this process, Kant's disciple, Markus Herz (1747-1803), represents a symbolic figure and can be considered one of the last individuals to be a physician as well as a "humanist" (Davies 1995).

However, with the progress of an engineering-like medicine, its limitations also became evident, especially in the event of a humane and understanding interaction between patient and physician. Presently, there is a renewed recognition of the potentially very positive role which the humanities could play in today's medicine. Recently, the field of "medical humanities" has emerged as an increasingly important discipline which is keenly discussed among health professionals (Evans and Greaves 1999, Dominiczak 2003, Lewis 2003). Although an exact definition of the somewhat vague term "medical humanities" remains to be given (Pattison 2003), it is widely accepted that today's medicine can greatly benefit from the human sciences, since they may help to broaden a sometimes very narrow empirist perspective and to recognize patients' needs beyond a mere biological treatment based on scientific, empirical and rationalist principles. This is especially true for modern psychiatry.

2. Delineation of molecular psychiatry

Molecular psychiatry has greatly increased our knowledge about the neurobiological and cellular processes involved in the aetiopathogenesis of psychiatric disorders. Additionally, it has given new insights into the mechanisms of action of psychotropic drugs such as antipsychotics and antidepressants. For example, it was possible to show that antidepressant treatment not only influences the concentrations of certain neurotransmitters in the synaptic cleft, but that, subsequently, specific signal transduction cascades are induced and, finally, the transcription of certain genes is modulated (Thome et al. 2000). This may lead to profound changes in neural and synaptic plasticity as well as in neurogenesis (Duman et al. 1999), alterations which might ultimately be responsible for behavioural changes observed during treatment with psychotropic drugs.

Furthermore, using tissue-specific transgenic mice (Chen et al. 1998), it was possible to show that the modification of a specific signal-transduction cascade (cAMP-PKA-CREB) leads to considerable changes in behavioural tests representing animal models of human mental disorders (e.g., learned helplessness and depressive disorders) (Newton et al. 2002).

Additionally, molecular psychiatry has identified a panoply of chromosomal loci and gene variants possibly associated with psychiatric disorders (Saunders et al. 1993, Gurling et al. 2001, Liu et al. 2001).

Historically, Alkmaion of Kroton (6th century BC) was the first to attribute psychological processes, such as thinking and feeling, to the brain as an organ. In the following centuries, the Greeks developed the prerequisites for a scientific investigation of the phenomenon psyche, free of any mythological or religious conceptions (Plato, Aristotle). Psyche becomes an object of rational evaluation and investigation and even therapeutical options, i.e. possibilities of influencing psycho-mental functions, are already anticipated (Thome 1995). During the Middle Ages, the Greek traditions were mainly preserved by the Arab culture (Ibn Sina, Ibn Saud) to be later re-discovered in the West during the era of renaissance and enlightenment.

In the vogue of a new humanism, patients suffering from psychiatric disorders are unchained (Pinel), and slowly modern psychiatry began to take form. This form of psychiatry is characterized by a scientific concept of psychological phenomena and psychiatric disorders and by the repudiation of irrational interpretations (Ackerknecht 1985).

With Griesinger's dictum of "psychiatric disorders are brain disorders" (19th century), the rational, biological concept finally dominates psychiatry. In the early 20th century, psychiatry used anatomical and histological research strategies (Kraepelin, Alzheimer). Thus, biological psychiatry as a scientific discipline was born. The development of psychopharmacological compounds further revolutionized psychiatry in the middle of the last century; psychiatric disorders were mainly interpreted as an imbalance between the different neurotransmitter systems. However, doubts about the role of synapses, neurotransmitters and receptors have materialized and biological psychiatry appeared to stagnate when molecular neurobiology gave important new impulses to psychiatry in the mid-eighties and was incorporated into various psychiatric research projects. This proclaimed the beginning of molecular psychiatry.

Based on the promising findings of molecular neurobiology, it is expected that psychiatry will continue to undergo considerable changes, not only concerning its research activities but also with respect to daily clinical practice. Although some of the new developments have already reached a clinical level, especially new developments in psychopharmacology, the impact of molecular psychiatry is presently very much restricted to a research level. Specifically, the following molecular techniques, innovations and new impulses have revolutionized mental health research and signify molecular psychiatry (Thome 2000):

- The finding that classical genetic processes can be explained by processes involving the genetic material, i.e. DNA. Thus, DNA represents the substrate of genetics and this substrate can be modified and analysed by applying certain techniques (e.g., PCR).
- The finding that genetic processes are not solely restricted to hereditary processes in the germline, but that each single gene in every individual organism is continuously regulated (i.e., "switched on and off"). Regulation of gene expression via signal transduction cascades and transcription factors embodies the fundamental principle of functional organisation on the cellular and molecular level.
- The interpretation of mental psychological processes as procedures in the brain, whereby brain is no longer considered as a static organ but rather as a neuroplastic multi-organ unit capable of dynamic processes including neurogenesis, synaptic plasticity and neurocytoarchitectural reorganization.
- An increasing interest in transsynaptic processes including signal transduction, gene transcription and expression as well as the development of applicable molecular biological methods and techniques to study them.
- An increasing interest in combining molecular neurobiology with the analysis of behavioural paradigms in order to elucidate the genetic and neural bases of behavioural biology, or, more specifically, the interaction between molecules and behavioural response or the reciprocity between genes and behaviour.
- The far reaching move from genomics to proteomics which has recently become evident.

3. Non-biological aspects of molecular psychiatry

Molecular psychiatry could be interpreted as a mere extension or further evolution of classical biological psychiatry. But this would perpetuate several shortcomings of the traditional concept of biological psychiatry. In fact, an emerging new medical discipline of molecular psychiatry represents a chance to overcome the strictly reductionist approach favoured in recent decades in order to establish a non-reductionist concept of molecular psychiatry. This would also include non-biological aspects which would probably be more appropriate for the interpretation, also for the medical modulation of such a complex phenomenon as the psychological functioning and malfunctioning of human beings.

Molecular psychiatry as a clinical discipline which focuses on individual suffering must include ethical and anthropological aspects and respect every patient's biographic and cultural background; molecular psychiatry as a research discipline must address, inter alia, epistemological and methodological problems.

Additionally, historical, social, sociological and psychological issues are relevant for a non-reductionist concept of molecular psychiatry. Thus, the humanities have to make considerable contributions to molecular psychiatry as well as to medicine in general.

Although the human sciences include more disciplines than just philosophy, such as, for example, history, sociology and psychology, which are all relevant for molecular psychiatry, in the following, mainly philosophical aspects will be focused, i.e. anthropological, epistemological, methodological and ethical issues; it is crucial for molecular psychiatry as a clinical and scientific discipline to address and clarify such vital issues as moral standards, the idea of man and the mechanisms of knowledge acquisition.

3.1. Anthropology

The idea of man in molecular psychiatry is, not surprisingly, strongly influenced by the natural sciences. Since experience, thinking, feeling, will and consciousness depend on the molecular processes occurring in the brain and since psychological functions are, at least partially, determined by the genetic make-up, man is interpreted as a biological entity which can be explored and investigated using scientific methods in order to generate knowledge about the biological principles of human beings. This knowledge may in turn be used to improve medical techniques including therapies aiming at an improvement of mental disorders. Nevertheless, a reductionist idea of man, which may be useful for mere empirical sciences, is not adequate for the medical discipline of molecular psychiatry because the limitations, especially the limitations of applicability, must be recognized and accounted for when it comes to the treatment of individual patients. Although the theoretical knowledge about anatomy, physiology and pathology of the brain is ever increasing, the spectrum of useful techniques to treat mental disorders is still insufficient.

Confronted with the suffering patient in daily clinical practice and, thus, 'transempirical' phenomena, a responsible molecular psychiatrist cannot accept the limits of empirical sciences. In fact, it is necessary to apply a holistic interpretation of the human beyond the mere biological aspect which is just one of several aspects of the human. In this regard, the anthropological concepts of Binswanger ("phenomenological anthropology"), v. Weizsäcker and v. Gebsattel ("medical anthropology"), Gehlen ("biologically oriented anthropology") and Scheler ("structural analysis") may contribute to a distinct non-reductionist anthropological concept in molecular psychiatry and help to prevent the reification of the human individual and, thus, the loss of humanity (Bräutigam 1980, v. Uexküll and Wesiack 1988).

Molecular psychiatry as a clinical discipline must encompass aspects of natural sciences as well as of social and human sciences because the mentally ill patient is more than just the sum of scientific diagnostic findings; treatment and therapy in psychiatry means more than just the restoration of disturbed physiological balances using scientific methods and techniques (Jacob 1978). Therefore, Karl Jaspers (1920, 1986) opposed "brain-mythology" as well as "psycho-mythology" and distinguished between scientific "explaining" and phenomenological "understanding".

Interestingly, modern molecular neuroscience is beginning to realize the interdependency between biological entities such as genes and social, environmental, cultural and psychological phenomena. Thereby, an earlier strongly deterministic concept of man and human behaviour is becoming more and more relativized. Parallelly, an extensive interindividual genetic variability (gene variants, polymorphisms) is becoming apparent which fosters the rediscovery of the individual, whereas, historically, the strict application of scientific biological principles usually leads to a certain tendency of deindividualization and anonymization. Molecular neuroscience will, thus, considerably alter the idea of man and challenge traditional concepts. Therefore, it is important that the anthropological dimension of molecular psychiatry is reflected in the discourse of modern-day philosophy.

3.2. *Epistemology and methodology*

Epistemology plays a prominent role in the philosophical discourse (Winch 1958) and epistemological and methodological questions constitute a further important issue of molecular psychiatry. These cannot be addressed by empirical techniques of natural sciences but rather represent a subject of human sciences, viz. philosophy (Blankenburg 1981, Marchais 1984, Yonge 1988, Rudnick 1990, Schäfer 1999).

> A failure to recognize both the limitations of empiricism in science and the conceptual richness of alternative formulations that accord more closely with the complexity of psychiatry's domain will result in a naive model of science and inadequate understanding of the limitations of 'evidence' that guide the training, clinical practice and research in our profession. The consequences will be the intellectual, clinical and ethical impoverishment of psychiatry (Harari 2001).

The epistemological aspects of molecular psychiatry including empiricism are based on several principles which have been mainly elucidated by philosophers: In general, processes of the "inner world" of mental and psychological phenomena can be accessed and assessed via similar methods of the natural sciences which are used for the investigation of the outside world (Kant); an increase in knowledge can be achieved by using and applying the principles of logic (Frege, Russell); the planning of experiments should aim at the falsification of theories in order to eliminate incorrect hypotheses (Popper); the way in which science will develop remains open (Feyerabend); from a historical point of view, paradigm shifts represent scientific progress (Kuhn), similarly, the cultural and social framework strongly influences the empirical work of scientists (Laudan, Latour).

Further traditions of the philosophy of science possibly relevant for the epistemology and methodology of molecular psychiatry are hermeneutics (Dilthey, Rickert), structuralism (Lévi-Strauss, Lacan, Foucault, Barthes) and constructivism (Erlangen school).

Interestingly, there is a certain interdependency between the philosophical discipline of epistemology and psychiatry, a discipline which deals with the physiology or pathology, respectively, of the brain, i.e. the organ of information processing and perception:

> When epistemologists address specific questions about how knowledge is actually realized by human beings, their philosophy must be informed by empirical studies of the sort psychiatrists now take up in a variety of forms (...), psychiatrists can likewise improve their understanding of human psychology through a deeper appreciation of philosophical analysis in epistemology (Hundert 1991).

3.3. Ethics

In molecular psychiatry, ethical issues become relevant on several levels: basic research, clinical research and daily patient care including prevention, diagnosis, therapy and rehabilitation.

Ethical questions in basic research are similar to the ethical issues presently discussed in the context of advanced molecular life sciences: the use of foetal tissue, the application of genetic methods which alter the germline and the use of animals to be sacrificed in experiments. Furthermore, it is necessary to reflect the ethical consequences of psychiatric research which may finally lead to techniques to allow the manipulation of human behaviour, thinking, feeling and human will on a molecular level.

Clinical research and clinical trials bring about several further ethical problems (Pichot 1980), especially when it comes to testing new and urgently needed therapeutic strategies in individuals who are unable to give their informed consent (e.g., Alzheimer patients, patients in child psychiatry) (Post 1994, Vitiello et al. 1999).

In daily clinical practice, ethical issues arise if a certain therapy involves restrictions of the patient's self-determination: Forced treatment, restraints, hospitalization against the patient's will authorized by the judge and thereby, loss of autonomy and liberty (Poldinger 1992, Hope 1994, Hell 1998, Jacobs and Thome 2003). Moreover, the treatment of suicidal patients and aggressive psychiatric patients threatening their fellow men always raises fundamental ethical questions which must be addressed (Sakinofsky and Swart 1986, Thome and Riederer 1995). Furthermore, the involvement of psychiatry with the legal system (forensic psychiatry) also creates several specific ethical problems (Appelbaum 1997, Verdun-Jones 2000, Wettstein 2002).

Several of these ethical questions have been under discussion for years. Other ethical issues are newly generated by the progress of molecular psychiatry and research in the field of molecular neuroscience: Conceivable scenarios, which should be put in an ethical context, include genetic and biochemical manipulations of the brain with consecutive alteration of basal psychological functions and the determination of the future risk of psychiatric disorders based on the analysis of a variety of gene variants associated with certain diseases (Hodgkinson et al. 2001).

It is to be applauded that international ethical standards such as the Helsinki declaration have been created and established and that every research project involving human beings must be approved by a competent ethical committee. However, this must not disengage every individual scientist and psychiatrist to reflect and clarify his or her own ethical standpoint. Ethical responsibility cannot be passed on anonymous committees. Especially because modern science may raise ethical questions which cannot be easily answered by traditional ethical thinking, it is important to perpetuate the ethical discourse in molecular psychiatry so that precedence situations may undergo novel ethical evaluation.

Molecular psychiatrists should be aware of the discussion of ethical issues in philosophy and the differentiations evolved from philosophical research: prescriptive (normative) vs. descriptive approaches; meta-ethics as an attempt to identify basic epistemological, ontological and linguistic factors which are involved in the formation of ethical judgements; different ethical principals such as anthropocentric, pathocentric, biocentric, physiocentric and holistic theories; consequentialist vs. deontological attitudes. Furthermore, there is a tendency in modern philosophy to develop ethical sub-specialities addressing different practical needs: For molecular psychiatry the following sub-disciplines are of special interest: medical ethics, bio-ethics, ethics of science, ethics of animals and gene ethics (Kind 1980, Russow 1990, Elliot 1993, Steinberg 1997, Farmer et al. 2000).

Finally, modern neurobiology strongly influences certain philosophers with respect to their ethical theories. With increasing knowledge about the physiology of the brain and the functioning of cognitive processes, several hypotheses discussed in the humanities have been modified accordingly. For example, an ethic of consciousness ("neuro-ethics") has been developed and application has been proposed in order to incorporate the progress of neuroscience and medicine into a cultural context and to assess the consequences of this progress (Metzinger 1996).

Molecular psychiatry can contribute to a better understanding of mental processes and, thus, help to develop an idea of man to recognize the individuality and uniqueness of every single human being, thereby fostering individual freedom. Research in the field of psychiatric genetics gives evidence of the important role of individual genetic variants for the typical personality traits of every man. Molecular psychiatry consequently supports an ethos which prioritizes the individual patient and ensures that the utmost is done to alleviate individual suffering caused by mental disorders.

4. Psychopathology

It seems evident that molecular psychiatry involves several issues which genuinely belong to the humanities. Interestingly, traditional psychiatry has developed an area where such questions central and crucial to psychiatry, representing topics of the human sciences rather than of the natural sciences, can be discussed: psychopathology. By showing that psychopathology signifies more than just description and "classification", Jaspers (1920) established the discipline of psychopathology as an area where methodological and self-critical reflections can take place.

However, this psychopathological tradition is at risk, since psychopathology is increasingly identified with nothing more than the application of standardized classification criteria. But modern molecular psychiatry questions itself in the case that contact to its classical traditions is lost. Psychopathology is a chance to re-integrate humanistic thinking into molecular psychiatry; this is of great significance because modern psychiatry will not be able to cope with the problems and demands imposed if solely restricted to natural sciences. It is important to notice that natural sciences and the human science of psychopathology do not exclude each other, rather they complement one another.

Jaspers's psychopathology was strongly influenced by phenomenology and existentialism. This, however, does not mean that such a conception of psychopathology is necessarily the only possible one. But, unfortunately, alternative concepts of psychopathology qua psychiatric methodology (such as, for example, a structuralist approach (Ey 1965, Luthe 1982)) have barely been undertaken, developed and evaluated or consistently proven.

Nevertheless, the reintegration of psychopathological research is an important and crucial task of present-day molecular psychiatry; there is no humane psychiatry without the humanities. The critical discussion of its theoretical concepts and premises and its practical implications in daily clinical work should be as much an integral part of molecular psychiatry as are neuroscience and neurobiological research.

To understand that the humanities represent an important dimension of molecular psychiatry denotes an important step forward in the development of modern psychiatry and manifests a fundamental distinction from earlier simplistic biologistic and reductionist concepts.

5. Conclusion

The progress of modern molecular neurobiology offers new and unexpected perspectives to the scientific as well as to the clinical aspects of psychiatry. Thus, molecular psychiatry has emerged from an earlier biologically oriented psychiatry and will revolutionize prevention, diagnostics, therapy and research of psychiatric disorders. In this context, the question remains whether or not this new form of psychiatry is conceptualized as applied molecular neurobiology or applies molecular biological approaches without being reducible to nothing more than that.

It has been widely established that the dichotomy between a "brainless" and a "mindless" psychiatry is not acceptable. Both human and natural sciences contribute to psychiatry as a modern clinical discipline which is also involved in research. Therefore, the integration of the humanities in molecular psychiatry prevents reductionist tendencies which have misled the earlier concepts of biological psychiatry exclusively focused on neurobiochemical aspects of psychiatry and neglected the non-biological aspects.

Exemplarily, we have shown that issues of the humanities such as anthropological, epistemological, methodological and ethical questions play a pivotal role in modern molecular psychiatry and must be addressed. One approach would be the reintegration of psychopathological traditions and psychopathological research into today's psychiatry. This would conceptualize psychopathology in a similar way as indicated by Jaspers, thus, bridging the gap between human sciences and natural sciences, both essential constituents of psychiatry.

By accepting the fact that the humanities represent an important dimension of molecular psychiatry, deficits of a simplistic reductionist biological psychiatry may be overcome and a more realistic holistic perspective regained for the benefit of the patients suffering from mental disorders, also for the benefit of the professionals working in this field.

References

Ackerknecht, E.H. 1985. *Kurze Geschichte der Psychiatrie.* 3rd ed. Stuttgart: Enke.

Appelbaum, P.S. 1997. "A theory of ethics for forensic psychiatry", *J Am Acad Psychiatry Law,* 25: 233-247.

Blankenburg, W. 1981. "Nomothetische und idiographische Methodik in der Psychiatrie", *Schweiz Arch Neurol Neurochir Psychiatr,* 128: 13-20.

Bräutigam, W. 1980. *Medizinisch-psychologische Anthropologie.* Darmstadt: Wissenschaftliche Buchgesellschaft.

Carlezon, W.A., Thome, J., Olson, V.G., Lane, S.B., Brodkin, E.S., Hiroi, N., Duman, R.S., Neve, R.L., Nestler, E.J. 1998. "Regulation of cocaine reward by CREB", *Science,* 282: 2272-2275.

Chen, J., Kelz, M.B., Zeng, G., Sakai, N., Steffen, C., Shockett, P.E., Picciotto, M.R., Duman, R.S., Nestler, E.J. "Transgenic animals with inducible, targeted gene expression in brain", *Molecular Pharmacology,* 54: 495-503.

Davies, M.L. 1995. *Identity or history? Marcus Herz and the end of the enlightenment.* Detroit: Wayne State University Press.

Dominiczak, M.H. 2003. "Issues related to humanities are close to core of science", *BMJ,* 327: 1049.

Duman, R.S., Malberg, J., Thome, J. 1999. "Neural plasticity to stress and antidepressant treatment", *Biological Psychiatry,* 46: 1181-1191.

Elliot R. 1993. "Identity and the ethics of gene therapy", *Bioethics,* 7: 27-40.

Evans, M., Greaves, D. 1999. "Exploring the medical humanities", *BMJ,* 319: 1216.

Ey, H. 1965. "La structure des maladies mentales et la delimitation du champ de la psychiatrie", *Acta Psychiatr Scand,* 41: 472-477.

Farmer, A.E., Owen, M.J., McGuffin, P. 2000. "Bioethics and genetic research in psychiatry", *Br J Psychiatry,* 176: 105-108.

Gurling, H.M., Kalsi, G., Brynjolfson, J., Sigmundsson, T., Sherrington, R., Mankoo, B.S., Read, T., Murphy, P., Blaveri, E., McQuillin, A., Petursson, H., Curtis, D. 2001. "Genomewide genetic linkage analysis confirms the presence of susceptibility loci for schizophrenia, on chromosomes 1q32.2, 5q33.2, and 8p21-22 and provides support for linkage to schizophrenia, on chromosomes 11q23.3-24 and 20q12.1-11.23", *American Journal of Human Genetics,* 68: 661-673.

Harari, E. 2001. "Whose evidence? Lessons from the philosophy of science and the epistemology of medicine", *Aust N Z J Psychiatry,* 35: 724-730.

Hell, D. 1998. "Ethik in der Psychiatrie", *Schweiz Rundsch Med Prax,* 87: 34-37.

Hodgkinson, K.A., Murphy, J., O'Neill, S., Brzustowicz, L., Bassett, A.S. 2001. "Genetic counselling for schizophrenia in the era of molecular genetics", *Can J Psychiatry,* 46: 123-130.

Hope, T. 1994. "Ethics of treatment and research in psychiatry", *Curr Opin Psychiatry,* 7: 430-343

Hundert, E.M. 1991. "Thoughts and feelings and things: a new psychiatric epistemology", *Theor Med,* 12: 7-23.

Jacob, W. 1978. *Kranksein und Krankheit. Anthropologische Grundlagen einer Theorie der Medizin.* Heidelberg: Hüthig.

Jacobs, K.A., Thome, J. 2003. "Zur Freiheitskonzeption in Jaspers' Psychopathologie", *Fortschr Neurol Psychiatr,* 71: 509-516.

Jaspers, K. 1920. *Allgemeine Psychopathologie.* 2nd ed. Berlin: Springer.

Jaspers, K. 1986. *Der Arzt im technischen Zeitalter.* München: Piper.

Kind, H. 1980. "Medizinisch-ethische Probleme in der Psychiatrie", *Bull Schweiz Akad Med Wiss,* 36: 367-371.

Lewis, W. 2003. "Medical humanities", *BMJ,* 327: s65-s66.

Liu, C., Badner, J.A., Christian, S.L., Guroff, J.J., Detera-Wadleigh, S.D., Gershon, E.S. 2001. "Fine mapping supports previous linkage evidence for a bipolar disorder susceptibility locus on 13q32", *Am J of Med Genet,* 105: 375-380.

Luthe, R. 1982. *Das strukturale System der Psychopathologie.* Berlin: Springer.

Marchais, P. 1994. "Que peut apporter l'épistémologie en psychiatrie à l'ère des recherches interdisciplinaires?", *Ann Med Psychol,* 142: 1257-1261.

Metzinger, T. 1996. "Hirnforschung, Neurotechnologie, Bewusstseinskultur. Medizinethische, anthropologische und sozialphilosophische Fragen der Zukunft", in: Kaiser, G., Rosenfeld, E., Wetzel, K. (eds.) *Die Zukunft der Medizin – Neue Wege zur Gesundheit?* Frankfurt: Campus: 301-312.

Newton, S.S., Thome, J., Wallace, T.L., Shirayama, Y., Schlesinger, L., Sakai, N., Chen, J., Neve, R., Nestler, E.J., Duman, R.S. 2002. "Inhibition of cAMP response element-binding protein or dynorphin in the nucleus accumbens produces an antidepressant-like effect", *J Neurosci,* 22: 10883-10890.

Pattison, S. 2003. "Medical humanities: a vision and some cautionary notes", *Med Humanit,* 29: 33-36.

Pichot, P. 1980. "The ethics of clinical trials in psychiatry", *Clin Trials J,* 17: 45-50.

Poldinger, W. 1992. "Ethik in der Psychiatrie", *Schweiz Rundsch Med Prax,* 81: 1329-1331.

Post, S.G. 1994. "Alzheimer's disease. Ethics and the progression of dementia", *Clin Geriatr Med,* 10: 379-394.

Rudnick, A. 1990. "Towards a rationalization of biological psychiatry: a study in psychobiological epistemology", *J Med Philos,* 15: 75-96.

Russow, L.M. 1990. "Animals, science, and ethics – Section I. Ethical theory and the moral status of animals", *Hastings Cent Rep,* 20: S4-S7.

Sakinofsky, I., Swart, G.T. 1986. "Suicidal patients and the ethics of medicine", *Can J Psychiatry,* 31: 91-96.

Saunders, A.M., Strittmatter, W.J., Schmechel, D., George-Hyslop, P.H., Pericak-Vance, M.A., Joo, S.H., Rosi, B.L., Gusella, J.F., Crapper-MacLachlan, D.R., Alberts, M.J., Hulette, C., Crain, B., Goldgaber, D., Roses, A.D. 1993. "Association of apolipoprotein E allele e4 with late-onset familial and sporadic Alzheimer's disease", *Neurology,* 43: 1467-1472.

Schäfer, M.L. 1999. "Nomothetic and idiographic methodology in psychiatry: a historical-philosophical analysis", *Med Health Care Philos,* 2: 265-274.

Steinberg, M.D. 1997. "Psychiatry and bioethics. An exploration of the relationship", *Psychosomatics,* 38: 313-320.

Thome, J. 1995. *Psychotherapeutische Aspekte in der Philosophie Platons.* Hildesheim, Zürich, New York: Olms-Weidmann.

Thome, J., Riederer, P. 1995. "Neurobiologie der Aggressivität", in: Nissen, G. (ed.) *Aggressivität und Gewalt. Prävention und Therapie.* Bern: Huber: 29-38.

Thome, J. 2000. "Was ist Molekulare Psychiatrie?", *Fundamenta Psychiatrica,* 16: 48-51.

Thome, J., Sakai, N., Shin, K.H., Steffen, C., Zhang, Y.J., Impey, S., Storm, D.R., Duman, R.S. 2000. "cAMP response element-mediated gene transcription is upregulated by chronic antidepressant treatment", *J Neurosci,* 20: 4030-4036.

v. Uexküll, T., Wesiack, W. 1988. *Theorie der Humanmedizin. Grundlagen ärztlichen Denkens und Handelns.* München, Wien, Baltimore: Urban und Schwarzenberg.

Verdun-Jones, S.N. 2000. "Forensic psychiatry, ethics and protective sentencing: what are the limits of psychiatric participation in the criminal justice process?", *Acta Psychiatr Scand Suppl,* 399: 77-82.

Vitiello, B., Jensen, P.S., Hoagwood, K. 1999. "Integrating science and ethics in child and adolescent psychiatry research", *Biol Psychiatry,* 46: 1044-1049.

Wettstein, R.M. 2002. "Ethics and forensic psychiatry", *Psychiatr Clin North Am,* 25: 623-633.
Winch, P. 1958. *The idea of a social science and its relation to philosophy.* London: Routledge.
Yonge, K.A. 1988. "Reflections on the epistemology of psychiatry", *Can J Psychiatry,* 33: 686-690.

The Challenge of Neuroscience: Psychiatry and Phenomenology Today

Thomas Fuchs

Introduction

The term "phenomenology" is frequently used in psychiatry, but it is still misunderstood as the gathering of "first person data", based on introspective reports, as a raw material for aetiological research (Andreasen 1991, Kaplan et al. 1988, p. 148). However, this "descriptive phenomenology", in the sense of Jaspers, stops half-way; it depicts only catalogues of symptoms and experiences in mental illness (Blankenburg 1991, Wiggins et al. 1992). Instead, phenomenology should be conceived as the methodical effort to describe the basic structures inherent in conscious experience, such as embodiment, spatiality, temporality, intentionality, intersubjectivity, etc., and to analyse their possible deviations and derailments. Thus it starts with first-person accounts, but then arrives at substructures of consciousness such as the formation of perceptual meaning, action planning, temporal continuity or implicit memory. It focusses on the *form* and *building-up* rather than on the *contents* of experience. By analysing the modes in which our world experience is constituted, phenomenology is capable of detecting the critical points where this constitution is vulnerable and open to deviations which appear as psychiatric symptoms. By gaining access to the prereflective dimension of experience, the psychiatrist extends his scope of understanding to include phenomena which could otherwise only be taken as bizarre "secretions of the brain".

In the following I will try to elucidate the role of phenomenology by answering these questions:

(1) Why do we need phenomenology at all in present day psychiatry?
(2) What method has phenomenology to offer to the psychiatrist?
(3) Which areas of psychiatry might benefit optimally from a cooperation of phenomenology and empirical science?

1. Why do we need phenomenology at all in today's psychiatry?

Not long ago, an editorial in *Biological Psychiatry* boldly proclaimed an end of the mind/brain controversy: "Neuroscience has now made it clear that the 'mind' is rooted in the brain"; and: "(...) we can now safely predict that we shall succeed in understanding how the brain functions and how it dysfunctions"

(Marazziti 1997). The biological program with its twin pillars of molecular genetics and neuro-imaging promises to explain the mind either by gene or by brain functions. Biological psychiatrists, neuroscientists, philosophers of mind and eliminative materialists of any provenance smile at seemingly outdated approaches to mental life *via* understanding subjective experience. For present philosophers of mind, such as D. Dennett, there is only a unidirectional relationship between brain mechanisms and personal experience – namely, the latter is entirely produced by the former (Dennett 1991). Consciousness is a by-product of the brain's activity as a symbol-manipulating machine or an information processor. In this view, the riddles of mental illness will soon be explained by identification of localizable brain dysfunctions and transmitter imbalances. There is no longer the need to rack one's brains about subjectivity and to indulge in the hair-splittings of psychopathology.

However, this brave new science suffers some flaws. First, the subjectivity previously excluded returns via the back door. In neurocognitivist accounts of mental functions the brain is often personalized: It "perceives", "learns", "hypothesizes" and "commands" as if it were a living being of its own. Neuronal circuits are attributed intentional and meaningful behaviour, as if they were some kind of homunculi. To a large extent, neuroscience uses an unreflected "as-if" language. This is only the counterpart of its reductionism: reducing personal consciousness to subpersonal mechanisms results in personalizing these mechanisms. Around a hundred years ago Jaspers referred to this kind of science as "brain mythology", and the German psychiatrist Erwin Straus coined a simple sentence which still holds true today: "It is man who thinks, not the brain" (Straus 1956). The person is the proper subject of experience; and meaning is not somewhere in the brain but only in the interaction between the living human being and its natural and social environment (Parnas 1995).

This leads to a second, more serious objection. Cognitive neuroscience still rests on a passive or "mirror" concept of consciousness (Rorty 1979, p. 12; Zahavi 1998): There is an objective world "out there", and it is represented by images produced inside the brain that become conscious to us. But consciousness has the peculiar characteristic of being inseparably linked to what goes on beyond itself. It is not a passive container or a kind of screen on which the world is projected, but an active, self-organizing process of *relating and directing itself to the world*. This dynamic and intentional character of consciousness, however, is not covered by the concept of single 'mental events' that could be translated into corresponding brain states. Therefore the neurocognitive system cannot be grasped separately; it exists only enmeshed in the world in which we move, behave and live with others through our bodily existence. Growing research on neuronal plasticity has made it clear that the brain is not a prefabricated apparatus inserted into the world, but is structured epigenetically by the continuous interaction of organism and environment. *The brain is essentially a historical and social organ*. Thus instead of representationalism with its fixed inside-outside distinction, we need what Varela (1996a, 1996b) termed an "embodied" or "enactive cognitive science" that treats mind and world as mutually overlapping. The recent emergence of a "social cognitive neuroscience" (Ochsner 2001) may be a step in the right direction.

This 'systemic' and 'process' view of mental life has consequences for psychiatry as well. If consciousness is not conceivable on a separate basis, then mental illness cannot be understood in terms of single, circumscribed dysfunctions, but only as a disturbance of the patient's *relation to the world and the others*. A "single-symptoms-view" may be useful for criteriological diagnosis, but it loses the holistic level of experience on which the crises and disorders of the self arise. And this argument necessarily extends also to the neurophysiological level, as Parnas and Bovet pointed out: Unlike neurologic diseases, psychiatric disorders cannot be related to discrete, localized brain dysfunctions, but rather to malfunctioning interconnections between neuronal modules and their interaction with the environment. They have to be explored on the basis of the continuous self-organization of the CNS as a living system (Parnas 1995).

Now if the 'systemic' view of mental illness is indispensable, then we cannot do without thorough analyses of its first-person experience. For subjective experience is not just an epiphenomenal picturing of underlying 'real' processes, but *is itself an essential part of the systemic interaction of organism and environment*. It is only by conscious experience that the organism is able to enter into a relationship with the world on the higher level of *meaning*, of integrated perceptive and cognitive units or 'Gestalten'; and these meaningful units in turn influence the plasticity, structuring and functioning of the brain. So when exploring a breakdown in the meaningful relations of a human being with his environment, where could we better start than with his subjective experience itself? Should we not initially aim at describing the idiosyncratic way the patient experiences and structures his world? What means could better guide us in searching for corresponding neurophysiological dysfunctions than the very sphere in which a meaningful world is originally constituted?

For these reasons, an adequate science of experience is fundamental for psychiatry as well as for cognitive neuroscience. Without exploring the phenomenology of subjectivity we are unable to identify the corresponding subpersonal mechanisms. Cognitive neuroscience will remain blind for its proper subject as long as it operates without an appropriate methodological description of what it attempts to explain. Unless we overcome the present objectivistic, reductionist epistemology in psychiatry, empirical research will be seriously impeded. This leads to my second question:

2. What method has phenomenology to offer to the psychiatrist?

A thorough description of the phenomenological method would be beyond the scope of this paper, therefore, I will only give a short sketch of some of its basic features:

The starting-point of phenomenology as exposed by Husserl is the discovery that our primordial experience is always hidden by habitual beliefs and assumptions. The essence of experience has therefore to be disclosed by the rigorous abstinence from all taken-for-granted convictions, by a suspension of the so called "natural attitude" to reality. We are requested to put in abeyance what we believe we 'should' think or find, and especially any explanation that derives the phenomena from underlying causes not to be found in themselves. By this systematic disengagement or *epoché* as termed by Husserl, the phenomenologist arrives at a "bracketing" even of the primordial belief in the existence of the world. As a result, he is able to turn his thoughts and acts into objects of his awareness, instead of being absorbed by their contents as is usually the case. The direction of thinking is reversed towards the arising of thoughts themselves, towards their transcendental source (Varela 1996b).

This peculiar turn of his attention leads the phenomenologist to a fundamental or *'transcendental consciousness'* which constitutes the world and in all its acts constantly refers to it. The world and all its phenomena become a correlate of this intentional consciousness. Thereafter, the next step in phenomenology is to disclose the *intuition of the essence* of the phenomena by imaginative variations which allow their invariants or essential features to appear. These essences have then to be described and translated into common language by an intersubjective process of mutual understanding in a scientific phenomenologic community. The last step entails that the phenomenologist returns to experience itself – in our case clinical experience – in order to check for the suitability of his findings to the phenomena he encounters. By suspending our commonplace assumptions about reality, this whole process of the so-called 'transcendental reduction' leads to a disclosure of the original underpinnings of our experience. It follows the constitution of self and reality down to the basic structures of corporality, spatiality, temporality, and intersubjectivity.

Now if the psychiatrist undertakes this process of *epoché* and reduction, he arrives at the prereflective dimension of experience which is affected especially in psychotic disorders. For here consciousness loses its ground in the lived body as the seat of taken-for-granted habitualities; it loses its anchoring in temporal continuity and its rootedness in the intersubjective common-sense (Blankenburg 2001). As Blankenburg (1979) pointed out, one could say: What is performed actively by the phenomenologist is suffered passively by the schizophrenic patient, namely, a shaking of the natural attitude, an estrangement from the common and taken-for-granted reality. The framework underlying our everyday experience is itself deranged and laid bare. The schizophrenic person suffers what Laing (1960) called an "ontological insecurity". Therefore the way of phenomenological reduction is, at the same time, the way to pursue as close as possible the disturbed processes of constitution in psychosis. Moreover, even in the erosion of the constitutional processes, the patient still strives for a coherent world view, even though this may only be possible in the form of delusion. Phenomenology also explores the modes through which the patient tries to make sense of the basic disturbances and to reestablish some form of coherence (Schwartz et al. 1992).

This brief outline of the phenomenologic method has indicated its special affinity to the core of psychiatric disorders. The resulting mutual dependence between phenomenology and empirical research is one of the hot topics in today's debate in psychopathology (Gallagher 1997, Sadler 1992, Varela 1996a). This leads to my third question:

3. Which areas of psychiatry might benefit optimally from a cooperation of phenomenology and empirical science?

In the following I will try to illustrate this fruitfulness in three areas: (a) embodiment, (b) time-consciousness, and (c) interpersonality.

a) Embodiment

Phenomenologists such as Merleau-Ponty (1962), Straus (1956) or Schmitz (1965) have shown how our embodiment tacitly permeates all our experiences and bestows on them a sense of 'mineness'. Conscious experiences are thus essentially characterized by having a subjective 'feel' to them, a quality of 'what it is like' to have them (Nagel 1974). This holds true not only for bodily experience itself, but for emotions, mood or even perceptions as well: what it is like to taste an apple, to feel the sand of a beach, to hear the rhythmic sound of a drum. Infant research has shown that the child's perception is permeated with bodily feelings and dominated by felt similarities of rhythm, intensity or tone. There is a primordial layer of a 'bodily felt sense', a "*sensus communis*" that precedes the separation of proprioception, perception and emotion (Fuchs 2001).

This sense is also the phenomenal basis of interpersonal perception: We experience a similitude or resonance between the outward expressivity of others and our own bodily expressivity which, in turn, is in resonance with our emotional states. The body works as a "felt mirror" of the others. It elicits a non-inferential process of empathic perception which Merleau-Ponty called "transfer of the corporeal schema" and attributed to a primordial sphere of "intercorporality" (Merleau-Ponty 1988). Infant research has confirmed this view by showing that even new-born babies are able to imitate the facial expressions of others (Meltzoff et al. 1977, 1989). By the mimetic capacity of their body, they are able to transpose the seen gestures and mimics of others into their own feelings. There is a sphere of embodied sensibility and mutual resonance which we all share from the beginning with others as embodied subjects.

This bodily mirroring is now supported by neurophysiology and its discovery of so called "mirror neurons" in the premotor cortex. These neurons discharge both when someone performs an action and when he observes a similar action by another individual (Rizzolatti et al. 1996, 1998). They seem to represent a system that matches observed events to similar, internally generated actions and, in this way, forms a link between the observer and the actor. This points to a neurobiological basis of mutual understanding, namely, by mimetic or resonance behaviour, be it actual or only virtual.

These converging results from different research approaches are also highly important for psychiatric disorders, especially for schizophrenia. Growing evidence from phenomenologic as well as empirical research signifies that the schizophrenic patient suffers from what may be called a *disembodiment* of experience (Brewer 1998, Eilan et al. 1998, Parnas 2000). He no longer 'inhabits' his body in the sense of using its habits or automatic performances as taken-for-granted in order to participate in the world. The tacit 'mineness' of experience is undermined and an alienation of perception and action results. As Sass writes, "(...) the sense of self withdraws from what it had previously inhabited, and what had previous functioned as the very medium of our selfhood, comes to be experienced as external objects or alien objects rather than as the medium of our existence" (Sass 2000). In a similar way, Ronald Laing described what he called the 'disembodied self' in schizophrenia:

> Such a divorce of self from body deprives the unembodied self from direct participation in any aspect of the life or the world, which is mediated exclusively through the body's perceptions, feelings, and movements (...) The unembodied self, as onlooker at all the body does, engages in nothing directly. Its functions come to be observation, control, criticism *vis-à-vis* what the body is experiencing and doing, and those operations which are usually spoken of as purely 'mental'. The unembodied self becomes hyper-conscious (Laing 1960, p. 71).

In order to compensate for the loss of automatic bodily performance, the patients have to prepare and release each single action consciously and deliberately, in a way that could be called a "Cartesian" action of the soul on the body. It is no wonder that they often speak of a split between their mind and their body, of feeling void, like a marionette or a robot; for the sense of being alive depends on being an incarnated subject with integrated bodily performances at one's disposal. In the same line, we find a disembodiment of perception in schizophrenia: Instead of simply perceiving the world, the subject, as it were, becomes witness to his own perception, hence the artificial or stage-like character of the environment in early schizophrenia (Bovet et al. 1993, pp. 587f.).

This has consequences for interpersonal perception as well: There is a correlation between the disturbance of bodily self-perception and perception of expressive signals from others. Schizophrenic patients have marked difficulties in recognizing faces and in understanding facial expression and gestures, as has been shown in interaction analyses (Berndl 1986, Steimer-Krause 1990). At the same time, they often show a strong impairment of self-actualization in bodily expression. The alienation of the intercorporal sphere that precedes any thematic verbal exchange led Kimura (1975) to view schizophrenia in the last analysis as a disturbance of the "between" or the interpersonal atmosphere. It may also be tempting to speculate on, and search for, a neurobiological basis of this disturbance, concerning neuronal mirroring or resonance behaviour, and its link to the bodily felt sense of self.

As we can see, phenomenology allows access to a deeper layer of experience, here embodiment, that is disturbed in mental illness. My next example is:

b) Time Consciousness

The basic temporal structure of consciousness was described by Husserl as an interweaving of *retentions* (= what has just taken place and still remains at the margin of the present experience), of *presentations* (= what is immediately present) and of *protentions* (= what is expected to be presented). Varela (1996b) has searched for neurological underpinnings of this subjective time-experience in nonlinear, dynamic systems theory; he used it as an example of the necessary cooperation of phenomenology and cognitive neuroscience, or of what he termed "neurophenomenology". I wish to point to a possible application of Husserl's model to psychotic experiences, though here I can only touch briefly on this issue (cf. Fuchs 2000, pp. 144ff.).

The retentional-protentional structure of consciousness is essential for the temporal integration of the sequence of moments into "intentional arcs" (Merleau-Ponty 1962, pp. 135f.): e.g. to speak a meaningful sentence as well as to understand it depends on the continuous awareness of the words just spoken and on the anticipation of the words to come. The span of the intentional arc structures my field of awareness; it helps me to keep my speech along the right track and to prevent intrusion of unfitting ideas or words. At the same time, this temporal integration of single moments is the presupposition for the sense of one's own continuity or identity over a period of time. I am not only aware of the sentence I speak but also of myself speaking it and meaning what I say. There is *a sense of mineness and of agency* built into the retentional-protentional structure of consciousness. It is the carrier of the unity of the self over time.

Now let us assume a weakening or intermittent failure of this retentional-protentional function in schizophrenia, i.e. a *sudden discontinuity of consciousness*. Then the constant intertwining of succeeding moments is cut off. All of a sudden, the anticipated goal of thoughts has vanished; for a moment, even the possibility of any future is abolished. This may be experienced as a kind of "blackout" or, in the patient's language, as a thought withdrawal. However, as a result of this weakening or discontinuity of the intentional arc, the inhibition of unintended thoughts also fails. Associations and ideas appear "out of the blue" and interrupt any line of thoughts that the patient tried to draw. A thought occurring at this moment of discontinuity lacks the sense of mineness and agency. The intentional arc normally bestowing this sense on the thoughts is broken. Such unbidden thoughts intruding into one's mental activity are experienced as alien and inserted, or even as "voices". The same may apply to motor impulses: A movement of my body that I did not anticipate appears as if it were caused by someone else.

Schizophrenic experiences of reference, persecution and control may thus be conceived as an *"inversion of intentionality":* With the weakening and intermittent paralysis of the patient's own intentional activity, the direction of mental events to emerge is reversed and turned against him, as if coming from the outside. For thoughts or actions that cannot adapt into one's own intentional field, but remain as fragments, must appear to be derived from an alien, superior intentional power. The same applies to perception: since the schizophrenic patient may not actively and intentionally direct himself outwardly to the world, everything in turn seems to be aimed at him. He becomes the passive centre of the world: Instead of actively perceiving, thinking and acting, he is being perceived, 'being thought', and acted upon by others.

Thus from a phenomenological point of view, so-called "first rank symptoms" of schizophrenia may be derived from a disturbance of the temporal integration of consciousness, from a discontinuity of the self. Of course this is a very short outline of a theory that would have to be explained extensively and underpinned by evidence. A number of results from experimental psychopathology could be integrated into such a model. Thus Spitzer et al. (1994), working with the semantic priming paradigm in schizophrenic patients with formal thought disorder, found a dopaminergic disinhibition of semantic networks with an extended scope of associations; that means, the patient's attention was not focused on a normal range of obvious associations, but highly distractable ones. This corresponds to a weakening of the intentional arc which allows unfitting ideas to intrude in the line of thoughts. Impairment of the attentional span, disturbances of working memory or executive control functions, mainly located in the prefrontal cortex, may also be interpreted as contributing to a disintegration of the temporal unity of consciousness (Vogeley et al. 2002).

As we can see, phenomenology may provide a framework for the integration of cognitive research results into higher order concepts. On the other hand, it also puts a constraint against attempts to explain the psychotic experience only "bottom-up", i.e. by a simple increase of so-called basic disturbances that finally overburden the brain's capacity of information processing. Phenomenology, for its part, emphasizes the "transcendental" source of the psychotic alienation, namely, in the highest and most complex functions of human consciousness.

c) Interpersonality

My final example concerns phenomena associated with perspective-taking in the interpersonal sphere. Laing (Laing et al. 1966) explored this sphere thoroughly and coined the term of "self-other-metaperspective", i.e. the ability to imagine another person's mental states, thoughts or feelings – today commonly put under the heading "theory of mind" (Frith 1992, Vogeley et al. 2002). Laing also showed how this perspective-taking may spiral up to increasingly higher levels of complexity, according to the following pattern:

I am aware of you.
I am aware of your being aware of me.
I am aware of your being aware of me looking at you, etc.

Now this level of complexity apparently overburdens many psychotic patients. They may say for example:

> The consciousness of others intrudes upon me and lets my self vanish (Kant 1927).

> When I look at somebody my own personality is in danger. I am undergoing a transformation and my self is beginning to disappear (Chapman 1966).

So instead of establishing a mutual understanding, the reciprocity of perspectives threatens the schizophrenic patient with a loss of his self. How can we explain this? First we have to take into account that this metaperspective is only a virtual one. Of course, when I am aware of your being aware of me, I do not become you; I do not lose my embodied being. Interpersonal perception implies a continuous oscillation between the central, embodied perspective on the one hand, and the decentred or virtual perspective on the other. The German philosopher Plessner (1975) coined the apposite term of man's "excentric position", meaning the dialectical integration of both perspectives.

This integration requires the fundamental ability of *pretending*, or in other words, a *symbolizing* or *"as-if"-function* that appears to be a central characteristic of the human mind. This function allows us to suspend the validity of the immediate experience, and to take it to be something other than itself: e.g.

a mirror image, a map of the town, a traffic sign, etc. The "as-if-function" is also necessary for perspective-taking and mutual understanding: I have to put my body-centred existence into brackets and for a moment pretend to place myself in the other's position. However, in order not to lose myself in this oscillation, it is also necessary to keep up the tension and the difference between the embodied and the virtual perspective. Although this happens in every conversation, it is nevertheless a complex task requiring a high intentional effort.

A failure of the symbolizing function can be found in autistic children: They are usually impaired in representing mental states of others and in understanding pretend play (e.g. her mother using a banana as a telephone); they also confuse the personal pronouns which require a change of perspective (they may e.g. say: "you want biscuit" when they actually mean "I want a biscuit" (Frith et al. 1991, Leslie et al. 1995)). Moreover, autistic children are highly impaired in non-verbal understanding, i.e. in their bodily mirroring of others (cf. above). This, however, is the basis for the development of a "theory of mind" and the ability of perspective-taking. A person who is not able to use his body for imitating, mirroring and thus understanding another person's behaviour will also have difficulties on a symbolic level of understanding. Thus autism illustrates the narrow connection between bodily mirroring, development of the "as-if"-function and taking the other's perspective.

In schizophrenia, a failure of symbolization becomes apparent mainly in concretism, in the inability to interpret proverbs, or in the concretistic language of delusion. The tension between the symbolic and the concrete level of meaning cannot be maintained, and they are equated. For the same reason, perspective-taking in social situations threatens with loss of the self: The schizophrenic patient is caught in the decentred perspective and cannot preserve his own embodied centre. The perspectives of self and other are confused instead of being integrated. This short-circuit of perspectives may lead to the experience of thought-broadcasting: All the patient's thoughts are known to others; there is no longer any difference between his mental life and that of the others.

It is for this reason that schizophrenia manifests itself often in situations of social exposure and emotional disclosure, when the affirmation of one's own intentionality against the perspective of the others is at stake: e.g. when leaving the parents' home, starting an intimate relationship or entering a working life. In such situations, the patient may lose his embodied perspective and become entangled in an imaginary view of himself from the outside: Everyone seems to look at or spy on him, everything is meant for him; he becomes the defenceless object of anonymous intentions. His intentionality is not strong enough to keep up the tension between the embodied and the virtual perspective. Thus we find again what may be called a *disembodiment*, caused by a loss of self in the dialectical process of interpersonal perception.

Of course, this symbolizing function is the most complex of the human mind, and there is no easy way to explore its neurobiological underpinnings. We may at least assume that different brain regions have to work in interconnection to allow this metarepresentational function to emerge. And one may speculate that it could finally be based on the mirroring function of the felt body in intercorporality which starts when the baby sees his mother for the first time. Interestingly, Vogeley (Vogeley et al. 2001) recently found different correlates of fMRI-activity when the first-person-perspective changes into taking the perspective of another person: Neural activity then changes from the right temporoparietal cortex (which is closely related to the body schema) to the left temporopolar cortex, while the anterior cingulate cortex is activated in both cases. There is also preliminary evidence for a disturbance of these activities in schizophrenic patients (Vogeley et al. 2002). This remains an important question for further research.

Conclusion

In conclusion, I hope to have shown by these examples how the phenomenologic approach may contribute to psychiatric understanding and research. Finally, I wish to quote Laing once again:

> (...) the theory of man as person loses its way if it falls into an account of man as a machine or as an organismic system of it-processes (...) It seems extraordinary that (...) an authentic science of persons has hardly got started by reason of the inveterate tendency to depersonalize or reify persons (Laing et al. 1966, p. 21).

Laing reminds us that psychiatry as a science is always in danger of depersonalizing the patient by viewing his behaviour and utterances only in terms of disturbed neuronal connections, transmitter imbalances etc. Phenomenology may be a possible remedy against this danger: a scientific attitude that takes subjectivity seriously and by the *epoché* seeks to find the common roots of experience that connect the psychiatrist and the patient even when there is a limit to mutual understanding on the symbolic level.

References

Andreasen, N.C. 1991. "Reply to 'Phenomenology or Physicalism?'" *Schiz Bull*, 17: 187-189.

Berndl, K., Cranach, M., Grüsser, O.J. 1986. "Impairment of perception and recognition of faces, mimic expression and gestures in schizophrenic patients", *Eur Arch Psychiat Neurol Sci*, 5: 282-291.

Blankenburg, W. 1979. "Phaenomenologische Epoché und Psychopathologie", in:

Sprondel, W.M., Grathoff, R. (eds.) *Alfred Schuetz und die Idee des Alltags in den Sozialwissenschaften*. Stuttgart: Enke, 125-139.

Blankenburg, W. 1991. "Phänomenologie als Grundlagendisziplin der Psychiatrie", *Fundamenta Psychiat*, 5: 92-101.

Blankenburg, W. 2001. "First steps toward a psychopathology of common sense", *Philosophy, Psychiatry and Psychology*, 8: 303-315.

Bovet, P., Parnas, J. 1993. "Schizophrenic delusions: A phenomenological approach", *Schizophr Bull*, 19: 579-597.

Brewer, B. 1998. "Bodily awareness and the self", in: Bermúdez, J.L., Marcel, A., Eilan, N. (eds.) *The Body and the Self*. Cambridge, Mass.: MIT Press, 291-310.

Chapman, J. 1966. "The early symptoms of schizophrenia", *Brit J Psychiat*, 112: 225-251.

Dennett, D.C. 1991. *Consciousness explained*. New York: Little, Brown.

Eilan, N., Marcel, A., Bermúdez, J.L. 1998. "Self-consciousness and the body: An interdisciplinary introduction", in: Bermúdez, J.L., Marcel, A., Eilan, N. (eds.) *The Body and the Self*. Cambridge, Mass.: MIT Press, 1-28.

Frith, U., Morton, J., Leslie, A.M. 1991. "The cognitive basis of a biological disorder: autism", *Trends Neurosci*, 14: 433-438.

Frith, U. 1992. *The Cognitive Neuropsychology of Schizophrenia*. Hillsdale, NJ: Lawrence Erlbaum Associates.

Fuchs, T. 2000. *Psychopathologie von Leib und Raum. Phaenomenologisch-empirische Untersuchungen zu depressiven und paranoiden Erkrankungen*. Darmstadt: Steinkopff.

Fuchs, T. 2001. "The tacit dimension. Commentary to Wolfgang Blankenburgs 'First Steps Toward a Psychopathology of Common Sense'". *Philosophy, Psychiatry and Psychology*, 8: 323-326.

Gallagher, S. 1997. "Mutual enlightenment: Recent phenomenology in cognitive science", *J Consciousness Studies*, 4: 195-214.

Kant, O. 1927. "Zum Verständnis des schizophrenen Beeinflussungsgefühls", *Z ges Neurol Psychiat*, 111: 433-441.

Kaplan, H.I., Sadock, B.J. 1988. *Synopsis of Psychiatry. 5th ed.* Baltimore and London: Williams & Wilkins.

Kimura, B. 1975. "Schizophrenie als Geschehen des Zwischenseins", *Nervenarzt*, 46: 434-439.

Laing, R.D. 1960. *The Divided Self*. London: Tavistock.

Laing, R.D., Phillipson, H., Lee, A.R. 1966. *Interpersonal Perception*. London: Tavistock.

Leslie, A., German, T.P. 1995. "Knowledge and ability in theory of mind: one-eyed overview of a debate", in: Davies, M., Stone, T. (eds.) *Mental Simulation. Evaluations and Applications*. Oxford: Blackwell, 123-151.

Marazziti, D., Cassano, G.B. 1997. "Neuroscience: Where is it heading?" *Biol Psychiat*, 41: 127-129.

Meltzoff, A., Moore, M.K. 1977. "Imitation of facial and manual gestures by human neonates", *Science*, 198: 75-78.

Meltzoff, A., Moore, M.K. 1989. "Imitation in newborn infants: exploring the range of gestures imitated and the underlying mechanisms", *Developmental Psychol*, 25: 954-962.

Merleau-Ponty, M. 1962. *The Phenomenology of Perception*. Transl. by C. Smith. New York: Routledge & Kegan Paul.

Merleau-Ponty, M. 1988. *Résumé de cours à la Sorbonne 1949-1952*. Grenoble.

Nagel, T. 1974. "What is it like to be a bat?" *The Philosophic Review*, 83: 435-450.

Ochsner, K.N., Lieberman, M.D. 2001. "The emergence of social cognitive neuroscience", *Am Psychol*, 56: 717-34.

Parnas, J. 2000. "The self and intentionality in the pre-psychotic stages of schizophrenia. A phenomenological study", in: Zahavi, D. (ed.) *Exploring the Self*. Amsterdam Philadelphia: John Benjamins, 115-147.

Parnas, J., Bovet, P. 1995. "Research in psychopathology: epistemologic issues", *Compr Psychiat*, 32: 1-15.

Plessner, H. 1975. *Die Stufen des Organischen und der Mensch*. Berlin: De Gruyter.

Rizzolatti, G., Fadiga, L., Gallese, V., Fogassi, L. 1996. "Premotor cortex and the recognition of motor actions", *Brain Res Cogn Brain Res*, 3: 131-141.

Rizzolatti, G., Luppino, G., Matelli, M. 1998. "The organisation of the cortical motor system: new concepts", *Electroencephal Clin Neurophysiol*, 106: 283-296.

Rorty, R. 1979. *Philosophy and the Mirror of Nature*. Princeton Univ. Press.

Sadler, J.Z. 1992. "Eidetic and empirical research: A hermeneutic complementarity", in: Spitzer, M., Uehlein, F.A., Schwartz, M.A., Mundt, C. (eds.) *Phenomenology, Language and Schizophrenia*. Berlin Heidelberg New York: Springer, 103-114.

Sass, L. 2000. "Schizophrenia, self-experience, and the so-called 'negative symptoms'. Reflections on Hyperreflexivity", in: Zahavi, D. (ed.) *Exploring the Self*. Amsterdam Philadelphia: John Benjamins, 149-182.

Schmitz, H. 1965. *System der Philosophie. Vol. II/1: Der Leib*. Bonn: Bouvier.

Schwartz, M.A., Wiggins, O.P. 1992. "The phenomenology of schizophrenic delusions", in: Spitzer, M., Uehlein, F.A., Schwartz, M.A., Mundt, C. (eds.) *Phenomenology, Language and Schizophrenia*, Berlin Heidelberg New York: Springer, 305-318.

Spitzer, M., Weisker, I., Maier, S., Hermle, L., Maher, B.A. 1994. "Semantic and phonological priming in schizophrenia", *J Abnorm Psychol*, 103: 485-494.

Steimer-Krause, E., Krause, R., Wagner, G. 1990. "Interaction regulations used by schizophrenic and psychosomatic patients: studies on facial behavior in dyadic interactions", *Psychiatry*, 53: 209-228.

Straus, E. 1956. *Vom Sinn der Sinne*. Berlin Göttingen Heidelberg: Springer.

Varela, F.J. 1996a. "Neurophenomenology. A methodological remedy for the hard problem", *J Consiousness Studies*, 3: 330-349.

Varela, F.J. 1996b. "The specious present: A neurophenonemology of nowness", in: Petitot, J., Roy, J.M., Pachoud, B., Varela, F.J. (eds.) *Naturalizing Phenomenology: Contemporary Issues in Phenomenology and Cognitive Science*. Stanford Univ. Press, 266-314.

Vogeley, K., Kurthen, M., Falkai, P., Maier, W. 1999. "Essential functions of the human self model are implemented in the prefrontal cortex", *Conscious Cogn*, 8: 343-363.

Vogeley, K., Bergmann, A., Schneider-Axmann, T. et al. 2002. "Neural Correlates of Theory of Mind and Self-Perspective in Schizophrenia" (submitted, personal communication).

Vogeley, K., Bussfeld, P., Newen, A., et al. 2001. "Mind reading: neural mechanisms of theory of mind and self-perspective", *Neuroimage*, 14: 170-81.

Wiggins, O., Schwartz, M.A., Spitzer, M. 1992. "Phenomenological/descriptive psychiatry: The methods of Edmund Husserl and Karl Jaspers", in: Spitzer, M., Uehlein, F.A., Schwartz, M.A., Mundt, C. (eds.) *Phenomenology, Language and Schizophrenia*, Berlin Heidelberg New York: Springer, 46-69.

Zahavi, D., Parnas, J. 1998. "Phenomenal consciousness and self-awareness: A phenomenological critique of representational theory", *J Consciousness Studies*, 5: 687-705.

Diagnosis of Core Schizophrenia as an Example of Applied Analytic Phenomenology

Dieter Sigmund

I. The Problem of Finding a Valid Concept

> Amongst the manifold types of clinical disease, there has over the years emerged a large group of cases whose outcome comprises a characteristic state of mental feebleness. The development of this [feebleness] is not an incidental "secondary" occurrence, but is rather apparently essential in the disease process; thus it is possible to predict this with a certain degree of probability when one is closely acquainted with this disease group.

This is the surprising assertion that stood at the beginning of Kraepelin's lecture concerning "The Diagnosis and Prognosis of Dementia Praecox" (1898), which was to become a classic work in its field. He then went on to point out that it is of no initial consequence whether the patient-group being treated exhibits the same disease process or not. At any rate, his experience led him to the conclusion that dementia praecox, even in its earliest stages, could be distinguished from other forms of mental disturbance.

Kraepelin's "article of faith" can be said to mark both the beginning and the end of a new development, the apparent starting point of which can be found in the establishment of academic psychiatry between 1850 and 1860 (Peters 1990). The scientific-medical disease model was now a fundamental tenet of psychiatric nosological investigation. According to the reasoning behind this model, the diagnosis refers to a definite 'disease entity'. Such a disease entity can only be said to exist when:

1. there is identical aetiology, or
2. the pathogenesis is the same, or
3. identical pathological-anatomical findings are obtained in conjunction with identical phenomenological pictures, disease courses and outcomes (Heggelin and Siegenthaler 1980).

However, aetiology and pathogenesis, especially of those types of disease that are now referred to as endogenous psychoses, remained to be elucidated. Research into such aspects was still at the stage of proposing hypotheses, many of which were strikingly speculative in character. The relative value of pathological-anatomical research with respect to the delineation of psychiatric disease entities was summarized as follows by Kahlbaum, the first to describe catatonia, more than 120 years ago:

> The pathological-anatomical studies that have been undertaken with such great effort and with the most splendid zeal have brought very extensive and valuable material to light, but they have not contributed anything with respect to our essential understanding of the genesis of psychic illnesses or the anatomical basis of their so varied and different forms *in vitam* (...). (Kahlbaum 1874).

It therefore followed that, at least for some time, the idea of a disease entity was to remain a pure fiction in the field of psychiatry.

Yet in order to achieve the closest possible approximation to the ordering principle offered by the concept of disease entities, Kahlbaum suggested the application of the so-called "clinical method" (Kahlbaum 1874), a concept he originally formulated for the field of psychiatry in 1863. The mentally ill patient must be considered as a whole being, and all psychic phenomena must be individually observed and described without prejudice or any attempt to impose preconceived theories upon them (Kahlbaum 1874). By means of "the summation of the most frequently coinciding symptoms that occur and via purely empirical delimitation", new "groups of disease forms" will emerge "by themselves". The identification of these symptom complexes affords the "possibility, from the momentary condition of a patient" (Kahlbaum 1874), to predict the prognosis.

Although Kraepelin initially adhered to the idea of a unitary psychosis (Avenarius 1979), he was to reject this concept as early as 1883 in the first edition of his teaching manual (Kraepelin 1883). Up until the fourth edition of this work in 1893, he had adopted the approach laid down by Kahlbaum, which was further pursued by his student Hecker (Hecker 1871), who was the first to describe hebephrenia. Kraepelin used this approach as the basis of his clinical-nosological research while also further refining it. The delimitation of clinical pictures must take as its starting point "the typical", i.e. those cases known to each psychiatrist, which, in every respect, exhibit quite a remarkable degree of correspondence according to their phenomenology, all the details of the disease picture and the subsequent course (Kraepelin 1899). The strict exclusion of all cases that do not accord in every detail with the first "typical" disease picture initially leads to the formation of numerous small individual groups that, in a next step, via the application of broader criteria, can be collected together in forms and groups (Kraepelin 1927). The importance of individual signs is to be determined in accordance with a particular degree of certainty that allows conclusions to be drawn with respect to the cause and outcome of the particular case of disease in question (Kraepelin 1910). In addition to general phenomena, as every characteristic disease process always exhibits some particular signs, it must, in principle, be possible to determine the underlying disease via the correct interpretation of those features.

Those investigators who principally strive to record those symptoms that occur together in a regular or consistent fashion are more-or-less bound to arrive at the prognosis and cause of the disease. This is the guiding thought behind Kahlbaum's approach. In Kraepelin's work, however, there is a shift of emphasis. His aim is to discover the typological groupings that are consistently associated with the same subsequent course of disease. As an indicator which points to an identical prognosis, i.e. the course of disease and its outcome, the symptom group becomes a specific syndrome. When this approach reveals identical disease states with the same course and outcome, it could then be postulated that their cause is also the same. In this way, symptom(s) and syndrome(s) point not only to the prognosis but also to the cause. The prognosis thereby becomes a crucial criterion for the validation of individual symptom complexes, while monitoring the course of the disease with the help of catamneses thus becomes an important instrument of research.

Kraepelin's concept of incurable dementia praecox leading to final stages and, on the other hand, a manic-depressive insanity with remissions, can hardly have been based on "detailed clinical work of compilation and comparison" (Birnbaum 1928), as described above. A far more decisive factor in this classification would appear to have been the intuitive consideration of appropriate entities (Kraus 1991), with the intention of attaining a convergence of cross-section and course certainly providing the necessary area of tension. However, when he attempted to translate what he intuitively grasped into a clinical symptomatology – i.e. when he attempted a reflexive, rational reconstruction – serious problems arose. In his description, he goes through each and all of the psychic functions known to him and reports whether they are altered or unchanged (Kraepelin 1913, Peters 1980). His lively, direct style though allows entities to arise and demonstrates which grouping is actually meant by the term "dementia praecox". But a series of factors combine to pose enormous difficulties with respect to practical clinical applications: the wealth of observations, the "accumulation of details" (Janzarik 1979), the absence of systematization and, above all, of an assessment of the phenomena, as well as the impossibility of identifying a prognostically valid symptom complex. A reliable delineation of the type referred to is rendered impossible.

As early as 1909, Zendig presented the results of a catamnesis study showing that about 30% of the cases diagnosed as having dementia praecox had been completely cured. These were, without exception, false diagnoses, resulting from the "incorrect assessment of the so-called catatonic symptoms" (Zendig 1909). Zendig's retrospective evaluation concluded that these cases were instances of manic-depressive insanity. Thus the scientific dispute concerning the boundaries between manic-depressive insanity and dementia praecox had begun. Over the years, these boundaries have been adjusted this way and that, but could not be determined (Leonhard 1972). The cases producing the most difficulties in this respect are usually characterized by the fact that no noteworthy defect arises, even though the patients have been diagnosed as suffering from dementia praecox on the basis of the cross-sectional picture. The adjustment of the boundaries remains at the level of signs, those "certain conspicuous disease phenomena" (Kraepelin 1910). It remains impossible to conceive their "characteristic colouring" (Kraepelin 1910).

About 20 years after giving the 'Heidelberg Lecture' cited above, Kraepelin declared:

> No-one with experience in the matter would deny the unpleasantly frequent occurrence of cases for whom, in spite of meticulous observation, it appears to be impossible to achieve a certain assessment. The experience that it is proving impossible to reduce significantly the number of false diagnoses undermines the willingness for clinical work and is one of the main reasons for the widespread view that the continuation of our efforts will prove fruitless (Kraepelin 1920).

In what follows, Kraepelin again expresses his belief that it is of great importance to hold fast to the fundamental differences distinguishing the disease processes themselves. However, it is not inappropriate to ask seriously about the extent to which those signs – upon which an evaluation is usually based – truly provide an insight into the essential nature of the disease process (Kraepelin 1920). We will have to become accustomed to the thought that the distinguishing features of the disease that have been used up to now are simply inadequate. In difficult cases, one will have to explore other ways and means. These may conceivably involve waiting to see the subsequent course of the disease and its outcome, an appreciation of the entire personality of the patient, as well as the investigation of hereditary factors (Kraepelin 1920). The adoption of an independent nosological intermediate region was rejected by Kraepelin so that, in contrast to the direction followed by Wernicke (1900) and Kleist (1928), no attempt at further differentiation was made in this respect except in the cases of paranoia and paraphrenia.

Finally, one might say that it is the grateful adoption of Bleuler's position that has brought the discussion concerning the boundaries between manic-depressive insanity and dementia praecox to a preliminary conclusion; one which has been met with widespread scientific approval. For Bleuler (1911), the prognosis is no longer the essential criterion. Dementia praecox exhibits widely differing disease courses, may be completely cured, come to a standstill at any moment or may also lead to more or less serious defective states. Thus, a diagnosis drawn up according to the cross-sectional state can still be maintained in the event of improvement or cure. Whereas Kraepelin considered dementia praecox a "species", Bleuler saw it as a "genus" for which he proposed in 1911 the term "group of schizophrenias". Bleuler was the first to draw up a systematic compilation of the symptoms. His description was influenced to a considerable degree by theoretical preconceptions, particularly from the fields of association psychology and psychoanalysis so that a great deal of immediacy and proximity is lost to the phenomena under consideration. His introduction of a subdivision between "fundamental symptoms" – especially affective flattening, loosening of associations, ambivalence, and autism – and "accessory symptoms" (Bleuler 1911) is not meant to represent evaluation with respect to a particular prognosis but rather evaluation with regard to the diagnostic assignment of a cross-sectional state to the genus, i.e. "group of schizophrenias". Further differentiation is rendered irrelevant through the removal of prognosis as a criterion.

Against the background of these altered preconditions, the subsequent analyses of psychopathological phenomena are characterized by an increasing abstraction following formal criteria reaching chronologically beyond the so-called Heidelberg Group (Wilmanns, Gruhle, Mayer-Gross, Beringer, etc.), to Kurt Schneider and the diagnostic systems used today. In continuity with the tradition of elemental psychology, psychopathological phenomena are considered in isolation, without any regard for their relation to other altered or unchanged psychic phenomena. The only point of reference is the corresponding, undisturbed psychic basic function: as in the somatic disciplines, syndromes are constituted additively via serial procedures. Whereas, for example, Gruhle (1932) strives for a formal description of the phenomena which differs greatly, Kurt Schneider (1946) attains a level of abstraction that is limited to the basic formal framework of phenomena. Gruhle, for example, describes schizophrenic thought disturbance as follows:

> (...) to cope with several requirements at the same time; to retain a thought in the long-term (to allow a general tendency to be determined over a longer period) without straying from the point; to grasp an idea both directly and symbolically at the same time; in the case of a metaphor, to draw conclusions from the real picture content, which then retrospectively need to be interpreted symbolically once again: these and the like are all, at times, beyond the thought capacity of schizophrenics. The range of thought, the intentional arch (Beringer), is lacking (Gruhle 1932).

Schneider, in contrast, recognizes merely "desultory or distorted thinking", by which he understands "the condition of being unable to follow the connection of a second thought with the first thought, where for the investigator, one thought stands unrelated alongside the other" (Schneider 1946). Schneider's approach implies that the phenomena, which are taken into account preferentially and subjected to analysis, are highly selective and limited to those that are most easily accessible to purely formal observation, especially verbal statements by the patient. If this procedure were applied in clinical practice, a form of diagnostic concretism would be the result.

A second problem with Schneider's approach is its tendency towards mono- or oligo-categorial definitions. Often only a single property, i.e. the most conspicuous one, is linked with a particular term. This represents a category reduction, which has practical consequences in regard to the reciprocity of scope and content of a term, and the associated increase or decrease of its (relative) specificity. According to Frege (1994), the scope of a term corresponds to the sum of those facts/things (designates) it can be used to describe; the content is the sum of the properties embraced by the term. A reduction in the content generally leads to an increase in the scope and vice versa (Nicole and Armand 1662), i.e. to an alteration of the (relative) specificity of the term in question. Thus the signs obtained by Schneider are unable to differentiate types. Furthermore, they can only indicate to a very limited extent (first-rank symptoms; Schneider 1946) the genus "group of schizophrenias", if they are present. Consequently, investigations concerning the prognostic validity of first-rank symptoms have been unable to prove a sufficient correlation (Koehler 1982).

Currently, applied operationalized diagnostics derived from Schneider's approach, e.g. DSM-IV (American Psychiatric Association 1994), further intensify the disadvantages of his psychopathology while blurring its advantages. As a result of the considerable reduction in the number of signs employed – which are inadequately described and appear to have been selected almost arbitrarily –, this approach currently falls well short of its potential. Its much-lauded high degree of reliability is attained at the cost of its uncertain validity. There can surely be few grounds for satisfaction with an approach that ensures that the highest possible number of investigators is making the same diagnosis, while this diagnosis embraces a large number of different clinical pictures, courses and outcome.

A step towards a differentiation within the group of schizophrenias can be seen in the concept of so-called schizoaffective psychoses (Kasanin 1933, Sauer 1990). Unfortunately, their delimitation remains insufficient for the reasons outlined above, with the result that they are beginning "to grow more and more, so that finally they will be destroyed by their own size" (Jaspers 1913). However, even if the schizoaffective grouping is not taken into account, the prognosis of the remaining schizophrenias remains to a great extent different (Marneros et al. 1991).

Today the extreme heterogeneity of schizophrenia, or more clearly termed, the group of schizophrenias, defined as the whole of endogenous psychoses excluding manic-depressive illness, remains a most vexing and limiting problem for efforts (Andreasen and Carpenter 1993), e.g., to identify its underlying mechanisms and causes. There are two general explanatory constructs or models for dealing with this heterogeneity:

1. a single aetiopathologic process leading to diverse manifestations and outcomes, i.e. the traditional assumption of a schizophrenic unitary psychosis;
2. the 'multiple disease entities' approach or the assumption of at least discrete pathophysiologic processes underlying specific symptom domains.

A current concept of the second construct is the negative/positive dichotomy with or without a mixed type (Strauss et al. 1974; Andreasen 1982; Andreasen and Olson 1982; Crow 1985; Carpenter et al. 1985; Andreasen and Flaum

1991; Carpenter et al. 1991). Attempts to validate these concepts by findings of brain imaging (Johnstone et al. 1976, Andreasen 1982; Weinberger 1987; Pogue-Geile and Zubin 1988; Andreasen et al. 1991, Bogerts et al. 1991), as well as its prognostic validity (Liebermann et al. 1991; Deister et al. 1991) and specificity (Andreasen 1979; Pearlson et al. 1984, Pogue-Geile and Zubin 1988; Mundt and Kasper 1989; Minas et al. 1994, Eilason and Ross 1995; Husted et al. 1995) still remain contradictory. The pronounced differences between the various lists of criteria among different authors delineating positive and, above all, negative symptoms reflect a general uncertainty as to what actually comprises the essence of core schizophrenia and its "state of mental feebleness", respectively. The general level of the description of criteria results in an "over-inclusion" of other disorders. Thus particularly the negative symptoms exhibit a wide overlapping with depression, personality disorders, anorexia, somatoform and organic disorders (Häfner et al. 1987).

In conclusion, if one assumes first of all that within the "group of schizophrenias" there are indeed various types (see, for example, Kasanin 1933, Langfeldt 1937, Leonhard 1972) which can be distinguished from one another on the basis of their phenomenological picture, and secondly, that the dementia praecox specified by Kraepelin is merely one of these types, then the development of concepts has indicated various methodological problems with a purely descriptive approach which make it highly likely that the specific distinguishing features of the different types will constantly elude our view:

1. The fluctuating meaning of the term schizophrenia between a bad prognosis disease and a various prognosis group, connected with the intention to bring those aspects to convergence.
2. The lack of methodological feedback to the mechanisms of intuition as a guideline for observation and description.
3. The exclusive application of an atomic-analytical procedure whose axioms can be characterized as follows:

   > In all multiplicities (complexes), the truly real are the simplest individual components (the elements). All complex constructs are 'additive summations' of their simplest components. This means two things: in these accumulations or aggregations, the simplest components are present in an unaltered form like stones in a mosaic: they are blind with respect to each other; within the accumulation, they have no properties that they do not have outside of it as isolated individual formations. At the same time, in the accumulations, no properties are demonstrable except those of the individual components (...) (Metzger 1954).

4. In accordance with this, the initially observed psychopathological manifestations are looked upon as elements in the sense outlined above, but their selection itself poses a methodological problem following unreflected "figure-background rules" (Metzger 1954).

5. The isolation of these elements from their respective context blinds one to the phenomenological interrelationships. All phenomenological properties and thus descriptive categories, existing only within their respective contexts, "drop out of sight".
6. An increasing tendency towards oligo- or monocategorial term definitions with a progressive loss of specificity, and a high degree of generalization, which finally lead to nominal definitions and a "glossary of technical terms" (APA, 1994).
7. Additive construction of syndromes from these depontialized elements, e.g. the paranoid-hallucinatory syndrome.

Psychopathology as a science still faces the challenge to provide delineations and a more holistic approach in order to reduce heterogeneity within the group of schizophrenias. From our point of view, an improved phenomenological methodology reduces the limiting difficulties analysed above. Thus it represents a way towards identification of different types (species), e.g. primary defective, and, in this sense, primary chronic schizophrenia: Kraepelin's dementia praecox.

II. Methodology of an Analytic Phenomenology

Phenomenology has ambiguous connotations (Andreasen 1991, Rotov 1991, Bovet and Parnas 1993). In Anglo-Saxon psychiatry, phenomenology is synonymous with descriptive psychopathology and refers to the description of symptoms and signs in psychiatric illness. In Continental Europe, phenomenology depicts a methodology providing a differentiation of phenomena by the identification of their basic structure (essence). The analytic phenomenology (Sigmund 1994, 1996, 1998 a, 1998 b; Sigmund and Mundt 1999) used in the present study embraces the elements of 'classic' phenomenology as established by the early Husserl (1900, 1913) and introduced in psychopathology by Jaspers (1913), although only in part. On the other hand, our approach includes methodological steps to reduce the problems deriving from an exclusive application of the 'classic' procedure:

1. 'epoché', a stance characterized by the lack of pre-conditions, i.e. the investigator takes a position without explanatory models, beliefs, prejudgements, theories etc.
2. 'eidetic' reduction by
   - 'presentification' of a phenomenon in mind,
   - 'free imaginative variation' layering similar pictures from other but similar patients, and
   - continuing this variation until an invariant structure appears.

However, if we try to 'reduce' a complete type or a complex phenomenon in one step, the results achieved are admittedly interesting but of a very general level and thus not useful for clinical practice and diagnosis. Examples concerning core schizophrenia are 'the loss of natural common sense' (Blankenburg 1971) or 'being as being a hole' (Binswanger 1957). Furthermore, the classic approach leaves the question open as to how we can know that our pictures, which are superposed in imaginative variation, are in fact really similar. Therefore we need:

3. a feedback system and a step involving aesthetic reduction.
   As a feedback system we use intuitive-holistic cognition (Sigmund 1998), which is not a form of inspiration but a pre-reflective perception leading to specific eidetic feelings corresponding to a distinct phenomenon or system of phenomena, i.e. a type, respectively. A well-known example is the praecox-feeling (Rümke 1958) evoked in the investigator by core schizophrenia. These cognitive feelings are methodologically integrated in a step that we call aesthetic reduction. In this aesthetic reduction pictures that evoke the same cognitive feeling are superposed with the aim of answering the question: What phenomena with what properties evoke this distinct, underlying cognitive feeling?
4. Knowledge of the poly-sensory kinaesthetic basis of those cognitive feelings – both in the given phenomena and in its mental representation (Sigmund 1998) – as well as the need to avoid figure-background effects (Metzger 1954) further requires a perspective variation which shifts the view from conspicuous to non-conspicuous parts of the pictures.
5. At this point an eidetic reduction as described in step (2) is possible, which takes on the character of a structural reduction in order to analyse the properties of those phenomena and relationships, identified as being essential by steps (3) and (4).
6. Some phenomena, especially formal thought disorders, resist, at least in part, such a structural reduction. In this case it is useful to apply the strategies of structural analysis (Birnbaum 1920, Peters 1980) in order to identify qualities via video and text registrations.
7. Permanent feedback of the obtained results to clinical observation.

The descriptive reconstruction of the results obtained in steps 1 – 7 should take into consideration the fact that a psychopathological phenomenon – as a "given" (Hofer 1954) and as an object of recognition – can only be defined adequately if our descriptive statements (the "signifiers"; Saussure 1915) encompass four different levels.

1. The phenomenon's macro- or ordering structure. At this level of observation and description, it is not unusual to focus only upon one single quality of the phenomenon – often a particularly striking one – and to define the designatory term exclusively by this quality. As we have seen above, many

of Kurt Schneider's definitions fall into this category. One example is his definition of the term "thought distortion" (*Zerfahrenheit*) on the basis of a single quality: "an incoherence of thought". While such definitions are indeed correct, they are far from adequate when the defining quality is also typical of other phenomena. Thus, definitions based solely on the descriptive level of the ordering structure remain non-specific (Weitbrecht 1957). Such definitions generally fail to encompass anything "referential" (Hofer 1954) in the sense of a symptom. The same also applies to syndromes, which are "additively" defined at this level of description (i.e. A + B + C...). Nonetheless, the importance of these features as points of orientation during the diagnostic process should not be underestimated. The current operationalizations, e.g. of DSM-IV, remain at this descriptive level.

2. Its micro- or essential structure. Ideally, this would involve the use of as many determining properties as necessary in order to make its essential distinctness perfectly evident. This also allows for further differentiation within a group (e.g. Aa, Ab ...Az). For example, "incoherence of thought" (see 1) could be differentiated into associative-analogic incoherence (particularly in the case of hysterical personalities; Sigmund 1994); inhibited and excited thematic incoherence (cycloid type of schizophrenia; Sigmund and Mundt 1999); fluctuating, distractible incoherence (amentia); various forms of paralogia and thought distortion (*Zerfahrenheit*) in a real sense (core schizophrenia).
3. Its immediate reference system, which both determines its structural composition and permeates it.
4. Its underlying reference system (or framework) which influences and 'colours' it.

As an example, let us examine the concept of perplexity. Considered at the level of the 'ordering structure', one can define this state as "racking one's brains, looking for an answer". With regard to its essential structure, it can be seen that this state primarily comprises a tormenting cognitive feeling (not an affect, mood or cognition) to register, comprehend and grasp the meaning of things as well as to resolve the situation. This condition arises as a reaction to the absence or loss of cognition or the cognitive function and is immediately reflected in certain expressive manifestations, e.g. a searching, questioning look. Thus, we only talk of perplexity when a state unmistakably manifests this character of feeling, our assessment being in no way dependent on whether or not the affected person is able to make a reflective statement about this condition (Aa). However, we would not apply the term in the event where the only presenting manifestation is the patient's own opinion or declaration that he is perplexed ("I don't know what to do"), if there was no other trace of perplexity as a cognitive feeling (Ab). However, the assignment of perplexity to a distinct type is only possible when we take the immediate reference system into account. For example, we are able to conclude that this condition has arisen from thought inhibition which displays decreasing incidence of individual thoughts with blocking, "thought vacuums", loss of the comprehension of meaning, as well as thematic incoherence, while the train of thought remains unaffected by external factors. Thus, at least a binary description is necessary, i.e. (1) perplexity in the sense of a sensation of disorder, on the basis of (2) inhibited thematic incoherence. It is possible to attain a very high degree of certainty in the classification of disorders if we take into account the underlying reference system (framework) and – to carry the example of perplexity a step further – if we are able to ascertain that there is an absence of structural deformations, not only of emotional expression and affect, but also of thought and of movement impulses and sequences. Our classification is now of a cycloid type (Sigmund 1998; Sigmund and Mundt 1999). It would be entirely different if we were to observe perplexity as a reaction to incomprehensible illusions, lacking any co-existent, congruent emotion (underlying mood and affect) but exhibiting concomitant structural deformations. The diagnosis now would be core schizophrenia.

If we continue our analysis in the manner outlined above, we would finally arrive at **axial syndromes.** One (e.g. melancholia) or more (e.g. cyclothymia) axial syndromes define a psychopathological type. Thus the term "axial syndrome" does not only refer to a group of correlating symptoms (Hoche 1912, Berner 1992), but above all to the precondition that these syndromes are essential for a certain type in a phenomenological sense, assuming closer relationship to distinct disease processes. A syndrome in the usual sense of the word is established as a diagnostic unity only by statistical correlation of its elements (symptoms). In contrast, an axial syndrome has to grasp something which is included neither exclusively in the single symptoms nor in their sum, i.e. an axial syndrome focuses on properties of relation and connection, on underlying principles which either characterize its symptoms or from which general symptoms (e.g. positive symptoms in core schizophrenia) are 'coloured'.

For instance, major depression can be defined as depressed mood, diminished interest or pleasure, a significant weight loss, insomnia or hypersomnia, fatigue or loss of energy, feelings of worthlessness or guilt, diminished ability to think or concentrate, and recurrent thoughts of death (APA 1994). Although this description is not wrong, it simply illustrates a correlative syndrome, which fits all severe cases of depression, even those triggered by the loss of a beloved person. On the other hand, the essence of melancholia (endogenous depression) as one type of major depression could be characterized as the inhibition of all basic functions of human experience and behaviour with (1) thought inhibition (never incoherence), (2) an inhibition of the ability to generate affects and moods (except anxiety), including an inhibition of aggressive impulses, resulting in a harrowing "feeling of unfeelingness" (Ziehen 1894), a loss of the ability to be impressed by external stimuli, and a death of inner life, (3) a psychomotor inhibition reducing and slackening of all kinds of movements and a "petrifaction" of facial expression, (4) an inhibition of drive, energy, action and social contact, (5) an inhibition of self-esteem, and (6) of intentions. And precisely this is what we refer to as an axial syndrome. Even without a detailed analysis of the structure of each phenomenon, the difference to the first syndrome should now have become clear.

Psychopathological types (species), as defined by one or more such axial syndromes, represent distinct phenomenological entities, not an area or a continuum. Discovering phenomenological entities based on clinical experience is of empirical value, but requires further empirical-statistical confirmation. The results of psychopathological efforts are of course extremely valuable for empirical-statistical research, since an optimal demonstration concerning the differentiation between patients creates the basis for achieving a higher degree of validity in such investigations.

In a further step, a **framework-like condensation** of the analysed phenomena can be obtained, serving as standardized diagnostic criteria based on phenomenological methodology. We propose the use of such criteria as the basis for further investigation. The application of 'reduced' criteria requires a background of their explication. In the following section these "reduced" criteria are written in bold.

III. Result: the Axial Syndromes of Core Schizophrenia

A Structural Deformations[1] of Emotional Expression and Affect

1. **Pronounced rigid parallelism of the visual axes,** i.e. a rigid look with the eyes fixed in a middle position. From the perspective of an investigator, this particular look creates the impression that patients need to turn their head if they want to see something on the left or on the right side. The disturbance is comparable to a supra-nuclear (especially horizontal) ophthalmoplegia; however, affects only spontaneous, not intended eye movements, since intended eye movements seldom occur, but are still possible.
2. **Increased rarity of eye movements, convergence and fixation, with limited and defective visual scanning of surrounding spaces, objects** (cf. Kojmar 1990) **and persons** with whom the patient is conversing, **with insufficient**

---

1 "Structural deformation" refers to "structure", which is an important term in the psychology and psychopathology of Continental Europe. "Structure" (tectonic) means the properties of a phenomenon concerning its inner construction, order, and formation including changes in space and time (Honderich 1995), i.e. dynamic structures, e.g. a melody.

or ineffective eye contact being particularly marked. A less frequently encountered feature is a restless, wandering gaze that is unable to rest on any object.

3. **Rigid Hypomimia,** a pronounced decrease of facial movements and "expressions" (Homburger 1932, Steiner et al 1998), **with marked rigidity of the upper half of the face,** while the mobility of the lower part of the face is noticeably less restricted. This discrepancy is retained even in cases of neuroleptic parkinsonism.
4. **Loss of intonation with a stereotypic monotonic speech melody,** even when the patient is excited and speaking with a loud voice. Characteristic is, for example, a para-rhythmic sequence of quick initial phases of varying lengths, which are succeeded by a second slow phase also of varying length. These sequences are spoken in only one or at the most very few tones, repeated in a monotonous way and lack any relation to content and necessary intonation. The voice is toneless, hoarse or slightly hollow, the flow of air loose or squeezed. The initial phase can give an impression of "shooting in", i.e., the individual words are uttered quickly and spasmodically. The slow phase may be so pronounced that a pause occurs, as if there were to be a new start, followed by the next quick phase.
5. **Decrease of affects** with respect to intensity, abundance, and frequency despite the **ability to generate moods.** The underlying mood is usually fairly steady, being joyless to joyless-morose, cheerful-serene or cheerful-silly.
6. **Parathymia** (Stransky 1904, 1919) **and/or paramimia** (Ziehen 1894). Parathymia consists of an incongruity between thought content and situation on the one hand, and emotion on the other, e.g. a patient talks about his harrowing persecutions and is at the same time smiling and feeling silly (*läppisch*). Paramimia is an incongruity between emotion and emotional expression, e.g. a patient who constantly smiles cheerfully, despite feeling serious and depressed at the same time.

B Structural Deformations of Thought

Preliminary remarks: A term is characterized by a literal core meaning, which is defined by some properties, and a surrounding field of metaphorical meanings. The thought process itself has a starting point and a goal, e.g., induced by a question or task. This goal works as a "determining trend" leading to a questioning and seeking which already contains the information sought after and asked for and finally found in a judgement or conclusion, in a strangely undefined form as an "anticipatory scheme" (Lersch 1958), which guides the train of thought. This anticipatory scheme is associated with an activation and appearance of the more or less relevant complexes of ideas, i.e. of subjects as unities of meaning. Their respective suitable aspects (propositions) are activated, fixed into terms, and their relations reconstructed logically, chronologically or teleologically, becoming a thought in spoken or non-spoken language by an ordering in accordance with grammatical rules. Irrelevant aspects and related but irrelevant ideas, as well as completely heterogenous ideas are suppressed. One of the preconditions of understanding and thinking is the ability to activate simultaneously more than one idea or complex of ideas.

Structural deformations of thought can be tested by (1) asking for the meaning of figurative terms like "letter-head" and abstract terms like "fidelity"; (2) asking for the meaning of certain proverbs like "a bird in the hand is worth two in the bush"; (3) asking for the difference (Leonhard 1972) in pairs of concrete and abstract terms that are similar but not identical (box/basket, stairs/ladder, tree/bush, avarice/austerity, error/lie); and (4) asking the patients to retell a short fable like that of the "salt donkey":

"Once upon a time there was a donkey who was loaded with salt. He went on his way and arrived at a river and wanted to cross over the bridge. The bridge was slippery and he fell into the water. He swam to the other side and while he was swimming the salt dissolved. When he arrived at the opposite side of the bank the donkey was happy to find himself relieved from his burden. The next day the same donkey was loaded with sponges. He went the same way as before and arrived at the same river. He remembered the wonderful experience from the day before, so did not bother using the bridge but tried otherwise to swim to the other side. But the sponges became soaked through with water and became so heavy that the donkey drowned". After retelling the fable, the patients are (5) asked for the meaning behind this story.

For a diagnosis of core schizophrenia the following disturbances are important:

1. **Alterations in the range of meaning of terms, exhibiting a melting down to the literal core meaning; and/or dedifferentiation of closely related terms; and/or agglutination of a single peripheral meaning with the core meaning** (Bleuler 1916, Peters 1977)**; and/or complete loss of meaning with reduction to a meaning of the most general nature; and/or inclusion of a heterogenous meaning in addition to the usual meaning of the term; and/or transposition of the meaning of one term to another term; and/or a neogenesis of terms (neologisms).**

   Melting down to the literal core meaning of a term is the basis of concretism (described later), e.g., "head" is understood only as a physical head but not in a figurative sense as used in "head of family", "letter-head" etc. The agglutination of meaning connects a single peripheral meaning, e.g., "love" with the core meaning, "fire" (Bleuler). Thus, "fire" always has the meaning of "love", or, to give another example, "green" always has the meaning of "sexually inexperienced". The dedifferentiation of closely related terms results in a situation where terms that normally have a different meaning are used as synonyms. Thus, vocabulary is restricted and terms are used to cover a greater range of meaning than they usually encompass. For example, (difference between stairs and ladder?): "Stairs are fixed and a ladder has *poles.*" The complete loss of specific meaning results in a reduction to a vague and general meaning, e.g., "good", "bad" etc. For example, (difference between austerity and avarice?): "Austerity is a virtue. Avarice is no virtue". Examples of an inclusion are: "with this colleague we have lost a bank". "Today I've looked in David's stomach." A transposition would be, for example, the use of the term "version" in the meaning of "relapse" (see below). Examples for neologisms produced by contamination are "occupational station" (occupational therapy and station) or "cross discussion" (crossfire and discussion).

2. **Paragrammatisms,** for example, in the conjugation of adjectives, in the construction of incomplete sentences etc., i.e. paragrammatism is understood as a deformation of the grammatical construction of sentences by false application of grammatical rules. Example (in reference to the proverb about the birds): "Less as more," or (taken from a letter) "That I had many more among such versions, which ended under happy circumstances, my store of luck was drained."

3. **Particularism** as the inability to activate more than one idea at the same time resulting in an inability to compare things and to grasp relations between different ideas through their opposition. This is associated with a loss of categories. Patients with particularism answer a question by giving statements to the individual ideas and elements of the question, and often only to one single word. For example, (in reference to the meaning of the birds proverb): "what you have in your hand, in a figurative sense, a secure job or something like this, makes a secure future".

4. **Deformations in contextual comprehension, with concretism** (Goldstein 1944) **as a loss of the metaphorical level** (Gruhle 1922), i.e., the figurative sense; **and/or loss of the meta-communicative level** (Peters 1973, 1951). Loss of the metaphorical level can be tested by asking for the meaning of proverbs such as the one above. A patient with concretism will answer, for example, "if you are hungry, it is good to have a bird in the hand. You can roast it. In Italy they also catch songbirds". Loss of the meta-communicative level implies that a sentence can only be understood in its concrete meaning, despite a situational context, which lends it a completely different meaning.

5. **Paralogical associations; and/or omissions; and/or condensations (fusions), as well as one of the various forms of paralogical derailment** representing deformations of the train of thought. A paralogical association replaces "thus", "therefore", "because", etc. by a simple and incorrect ranging, i.e. by "and". For example: "I was going to my chief and had trouble with my colleague." Another example of paralogical associations is creating a causal relationship between two independent events or situations, i.e. when a patient causally relates his decreasing social life to a minor surgery that was performed a few years ago.
A paralogical omission links two thoughts in order to come to a conclusion while omitting one or more steps that would have been necessary to guarantee logical coherence. For example, "I am out of work. Therefore I was going down to the cellar to grab a beer", or (regarding the fable of the salt donkey): "Okay, it's a donkey, it has a load on its back and wants to cross the river and it walks over and notices, when it's there, the salt was gone".
With fusions (Mayer-Gross 1932), several, perhaps mutually contradictory thoughts are condensed into one.
Paralogical derailments are understood as gradual deviations of the train of thought missing the original goal and leading nowhere. Every step is only tangentially and vaguely connected with the previous one. Characteristic for derailments is both an insufficient and short-lived determining trend and anticipatory scheme. This is connected with (1) an over-activation of the basic structure of the relevant first, or first few idea(s) (Sigmund 1998), which are more or less altered (over- or under-inclusion); and (2) an insufficiency or lack of suppression, i.e. an activation also of the irrelevant aspects and of related but irrelevant idea complexes. The simultaneous activation of irrelevant aspects and ideas, however, inhibits the delineation of relevant aspects (propositions) and a further progression towards the original goal of thought. The disturbance is associated with insufficient logic and categorical ordering functions. Initially, the determining trend may already be modified by an altered understanding of meaning and change during the thought process according to the activated irrelevant ideas. Different types of derailment can be distinguished.
Type I: short derailments.
Example: what was the result of your final high school examination? "I don't know". You don't know? "I don't know, but it's surely possible to have a look at the individual tests at school."
Type II: parapulsive derailments.
In this type, the train of thought deviates from the goal step by step. For example (regarding the meaning of the proverb, "there is no rose without a thorn): "The rose is actually something beautiful, a beautiful flower, nice colour, that nice red. Thorns, at the same time, on the other hand inju-

rable, that you can prick yourself with them, but a rose without thorns, that there's always difficult roads you have to go down. It won't always be easy, um, to go normally down your path in life, and that there are not always nice sides, there are also definitely those situations which demand a lot from you, which want a lot from you and, um, and then you have to go this way too and have to be ready as well to be committed, to fight and to look ahead."

Type III: perifocal derailments.

The patients make statements to the subject without understanding the task or goal. Example (the difference between box and basket?): "You can make something out of it, you can drive it (meaning a soapbox) – I saw that once on television. In baskets you can put fruit. There's also a basket for shopping."

6. **Thought distortion** (*Zerfahrenheit,* Kraepelin 1899)

Thought distortion is a form of incoherent thinking which is characterized by a loss of the determining trend (the goal of thought), the anticipatory structure, the ability to activate more than one idea simultaneously, the ability to suppress irrelevant aspects of the occurring ideas, and by the appearance of completely heterogeneous ideas.

Typical of thought distortion is a seemingly haphazard mixture of: (1) basically compatible thoughts that lose their purpose and direction because of incorrect positioning; (2) thoughts which are more or less vaguely and indirectly linked with the topic or with single ideas belonging to the topic or even with only one single element of the question that has been asked; and (3) completely heterogeneous thoughts that, in the case of overall arhythmic thought production, usually arise after thought production decreases or after blocking and are often expressed together in one single sentence (contamination). If there are no heterogeneous ideas, it is not possible to speak of a thought distortion.

This entails a loss of direction in the thought process and a further development of thoughts will not take place. Distraction by external stimuli can be observed, since the patient will answer questions with new, distorted thoughts. However, it is also possible that the investigator will suddenly be given a whole range of perfectly ordered answers. The disturbance may only be confined to certain sequences of a conversation, although it will usually increase as the conversation continues. In terms of external aspects the basic structure of communication, e.g., switching from question to answer, will remain the same. Usually sentence construction will also be left unaltered. Patients do not seem to have any doubts about the fact that they are providing meaningful statements.

For example, in response to the question, "Are your thoughts sometimes disturbed?":

"I don't know. I have been a lot more open, I have thought a lot more than before, a lot more than before, I think. And during these seven years (this period of time was mentioned earlier in the conversation) I usually spoke out loud what I was thinking. If I hadn't, I would be completely different, much more powerful, much stronger, much more masculine. You know, I have seen it all. I have really seen it all."

C *Structural Deformations of Movements*

1. **Restriction** (*Gebundenheit*), meaning a stiffness of posture and movements that decrease in frequency and become monotonous. Particularly striking characteristics are the relative immobility of the head and the extremely upright and stiff posture of the back, often with a curious bending of its upper part that is even maintained when the extremities are moved. The underarms are also often unusually bent. Restriction is associated with a loss of expressive movement. The degree of restriction is stable over of a longer period.
2. **Against a background of this inhibition** process, the simultaneous emergence of **psychomotor excitation phenomena** (Homburger 1932, Leonhard 1979); e.g., the emergence of involuntary spontaneous movements like a short swinging of the entire upper body (*Jaktationen*), a brief splaying of the fingers, a shrug of the shoulders, or a similar action.
3. **Parakinesis** is understood as deformations of movement sequences due to a disturbance of agonistic-antagonistic impulses, thus resulting in a two-phase sequence of individual movements. The basic forms can be classified as follows:
   Type 1: a fast first phase followed by an increasingly pronounced slowing of movement;
   Type 2: the antagonistic slowing process is of undulating, oscillating intensity, such that the movement sequences have a flowing, irregular, wave-like quality; and
   Type 3: the slowing phase involves the rotator muscles, with the result that the movement sequences appear "pretentious".
   In all three types, the initial phase can give the impression of suddenly "shooting in" or the slowing process may be so pronounced that the movement is "blocked".
4. **Iterations.** Iterations are monotonous, inexpressive repetitions of a just intended voluntary movement, e.g., a quick repetition of the movement "sitting down" several times.
5. **Movement stereotypy** as automatic, monotonous, and inexpressive repetitions of single movements at different times. Such movement is not connected with the internal state of the patient or the external situation in which it takes place. The patient is not able to say why he makes this movement. Signs of general excitation cannot be observed. Stereotypes do not change over a long period. For example, "After each mouthful of food a patient

opened and closed his eyes three times; another stamped the floor each time before he went through a door".

6. **Para-axial postures** with striking axial positions (Homburger 1932) of joints with respect to the torso, or of joint segments with respect to each other or to the torso. Example: the patient sits on a chair; the upper body points in a different direction as the legs and the head points in a different direction altogether; one arm is slightly twisted.

We take the view that the structural deformations described represent the specific basic symptoms of primary chronic schizophrenia (dementia praecox) occurring with or without delusions, hallucinations, cenesthesia etc., and play a crucial role in the appearance of the "praecox feeling" (Rümke 1958), evoked in investigators by those patients but never by other types in the group of schizophrenias.

The diagnosis of core schizophrenia requires the presence of two points in two regions and at least one point in the other region. The symptoms can be rated positively if they are observable in a state of composure (*Besonnenheit*), by which is meant clear consciousness without any intensive and disturbing affects and moods or signs of general inhibition or excitation, a state of full awareness and orientation, and a condition in which the patient is able to think about a question. Exclusion criteria for the three axial syndromes are (1) relations to any brain injury, and (2) oligophrenia.

If we analyse the underlying principle of these axial syndromes, we find (1) a disconnection, a decoupling between the partial functions of a functional unit and between functional units, and (2) a deregulation and imbalance with a decrease, loss or inhibition of partial functions as well as an excitation of (antagonistic) inhibitory partial functions and an excitation of other (i.e. agonistic) partial functions within one functional unit at the same time. A disconnection is revealed, for example, between spontaneous and voluntary eye movements, the upper and lower parts of the face, speech melody and the content of speech, affect and the ability to generate moods, thought content and affect, emotion and emotional expression, terms and their mental representations, between partial functions of the thought process, between expressive and voluntary movements, thought content and situation on the one hand and movement on the other etc.

The presence of excitation and inhibition within one functional unit at the same time is found, for example, in the rigidity described in parallelism of the visual axes, hypomimia, and restriction, since rigidity is caused by a simultaneous excitation of agonists and antagonists (Scheid 1983), i.e., by excitation and inhibition occurring at the same time. If excitation prevails for a shorter or a longer period, spontaneous involuntary movements arise, e.g., grimacing, a restless gaze, a short splaying of the fingers, etc. or para-axial postures, respectively. A short alternation of excitation results in a swinging of the torso, a short tripping, etc. In parakinesis we have an overactivation and an overinhibition within a single movement, in iterations excitation of the movement impulse and an inhibition of the propulsive aspect of the movement process; in thought derailments there is an overactivation of ideas and an inhibition of the determining trend and the anticipatory scheme etc. Stansky (1904, 1919) was probably referring to this kind of mental disconnection when he spoke about an "intrapsychic ataxia" as a crucial feature of dementia praecox.

IV. Discussion and Conclusions

Analytic phenomenology avoids the methodological problems of pure descriptive approaches. It is a specific way of identifying phenomena essential for a different type and the basic structure of these phenomena and their interrelationships and best fit to generate conceptual models derived from this inquiry. As shown in the present study, from a phenomenological perspective, it is possible to reduce heterogeneity within schizophrenia by the differentiation of a primary chronic type, whose syndromes are demonstrated to be axial syndromes in the above mentioned sense. The conceptualization of structural deformations, never observable in the schizoaffective and cycloid type, but occurring in core schizophrenia with or without "productive" (positive) phenomena, contributes to the actual negative syndrome discussion. It shifts the perspective from a descriptive level with low specificy (e.g. abulia) and great overlap, e.g., with depression, to phenomena of higher specificy that "colours, prevades, and standardizes" (Mayer-Gross 1924) the clinical picture of core schizophrenia.

The identification, of (1) a disconnection between partial functions and (2) an imbalance, i.e. the simultaneous presence of excitation and inhibition within one functional unit, as being the crucial underlying principle of structural deformations, shows that the current positive/negative definitions (Marneros and Andreasen 1991) – "function that is normally not present in an individual" (positive symptoms) and "absence of a function which is usually present in a normal individual" (negative symptoms) – do not cover an essential and central feature of core schizophrenic symptomatology.

As emphasized by Bovet and Parnas (1993), in order to be fruitful, phenomenology must maintain a dialectic exchange with the empirical-statistical approach. Operationalized diagnostic systems are necessary for this approach to establish reliability. Nonetheless, any serious empirical-statistical investigation relating to diagnosis and classification should not ignore the fact that if it includes a phenomenological differentiation (Kraus 1991) then there is a better chance for achieving much more valid and consistent results. The condensation of our phenomenological analysis leads to operationalizations providing the basis for empirical-statistical investigations, e.g., with respect to genetic factors, for results of brain imaging and for prognosis. In our experience, the axial syndromes of core schizophrenia are very useful for an early diagnosis of this type. It should be noted that the patients in our case-by-case observation series who were diagnosed as primary chronic type according to the phenomenological criteria suggested, all developed a characteristic schizophrenic defect, that "characteristic state of mental feebleness" (Kraepelin 1898).

References

American Psychiatric Association. 1994. *Diagnostic and Statistical Manual of Mental Disorders*. 4th ed. Washington, DC: APA.

Andreasen, N.C. 1979. "Affective flattening and criteria for schizophrenia", *American Journal of Psychiatry,* 136: 944-947.

Andreasen, N.C.1982. "Negative symptoms in schizophrenia: Definition and reliability", *Archives of General Psychiatry,* 39: 784-788.

Andreasen, N.C., Olson, S. 1982. "Negative and positive schizophrenia: Definition and validation", *Archives of General Psychiatry,* 39: 789-793.

Andreasen, N.C. 1991. "Reply to 'Phenomenology or Physicalism'", *Schizophrenia Bulletin,* 17: 187-189.

Andreasen, N.C., Flaum, M., Arndt, S., Alliger, R., Swyze, V.W. 1991. "Positive and Negative Symptoms: Assessment and Validity", in: Marneros, A., Andreasen, N.C., Tsuang, M.T. (eds.) *Negative Versus Positive Schizophrenia.* Berlin, Germany: Springer, 28-51.

Andreasen, N.C., Carpenter, W.T. 1993. "Diagnosis and Classification of Schizoprenia", *Schizophrenia Bulletin*, 19: 199-214.

Avenarius, R. 1979. "Emil Kraepelin: seine Persönlichkeit und seine Konzeption", in: Janzarik, W. (ed.) *Psychopathologie als Grundlagenwissenschaft.* Stuttgart: Enke.

Berner, P., Gabriel, E., Katschnig, H., Kieffer, W., Koehler, K., Lenz, G. et al. 1992. *Diagnostic criteria for funtional psychoses.* 2nd ed. Cambridge: Cambridge University Press.

Binswanger, L. 1957. *Schizophrenie.* Pfullingen, Germany: Neske.

Birnbaum, K. 1920. "Die Strukturanalyse als klinisches Forschungsprinzip", *Zeitschrift für die gesamte Neurologie und Psychiatrie,* 53: 121-129.

Birnbaum, K. 1928. "Geschichte der psychiatrischen Wissenschaft", in: Bumke, O., (ed.) *Handbuch der Geisteskrankheiten.* 1st ed., vol. 1. Berlin: Springer.

Blankenburg, W. 1971. *Der Verlust der natürlichen Selbstverständlichkeit.* Stuttgart: Enke.

Bleuler, E. 1916. *Lehrbuch der Psychiatrie.* Berlin: Springer.

Bleuler, E. 1911. "Dementia praecox oder Gruppe der Schizophrenien", in: Aschaffenburg, G. (ed.) *Handbuch der Psychiatrie.* Leipzig: Deuticke. English edition: *Dementia Praecox or the Group of Schizophrenias.* Translated by I. Zinkin. New York, NY: International Universities Press, 1950.

Bogerts, B., Falkai, P., Degreef, G., Lieberman, J.A. 1991. "Neuropathological and Brain Imaging Studies in Positive and Negative Schizophrenia", in: Marneros, A., Andreasen, N.C., Tsuang, M.T. (eds.) *Negative Versus Positive Schizophrenia.* Berlin: Springer, 292-317.

Bovet, P., Parmas, J. 1993. "Schizophrenic Delusions: A Phenomenological Approach", *Schizophrenia Bulletin,* 19: 579-597.
Carpenter, W.T., Buchanan, R.W., Kirkpatrick, B., Thaker, G, and Tamminga, G. 1991. "Negative Symptoms: A Critique of Current Approaches". in: Marneros, A., Andreasen, N.C., Tsuang, M., (eds.) *Negative Versus Positive Schizophrenia.* Berlin: Springer, 126-133.
Carpenter, W.T., Heinrichs, D.W., Alphs, L.D. 1985. "Treatment of negative symptoms", *Schizophrenia Bulletin,* 11: 440-452.
Crow, T.J. 1985. "The two-syndrome concept: Origins and current status", *Schizophrenia Bulletin,* 11: 471-486.
Dreisler, A., Marneros, A., Rhode, A. 1991. "Long-Term Outcome of Patients with a Positive Initial Episode Versus Patients with a Negative Initial Episode", in: Marneros, A., Andreasen, N.C., Tsuang, M.T. (eds.) *Negative Versus Positive Schizophrenia.* Berlin: Springer, 208-218.
Eilason, J.W., Ross, C.A. 1995. "Positive and negative symptoms in dissociative identity disorder and schizophrenia. A comparative analysis", *Journal of Nervous and Mental Disease,* 183: 236-241.
Frege, G. 1994. *Funktion, Begriff, Bedeutung.* 7. Aufl. Göttingen: Vandenhoeck & Ruprecht.
Goldstein, K. 1944. "Methodological approach to the study of schizophrenic thought disorders", in: Kasanin, I.S. (ed.) *Language and Thought in Schizophrenia.* Berkeley, CA: University of California Press, 10–39.
Gruhle, H.W. 1932. "Die Psychopathologie", in: Bumke, O. (ed.) *Handbuch der Geisteskrankheiten.* 1st ed. vol. IX. Berlin: Springer, 135-210.
Häfner, H., Gattaz, W.F., Janzarik, W. (eds.) 1987. *Search for the causes of schizophrenia.* Berlin: Springer.
Hecker, E. 1871. "Die Hebephrenie", *Archiv Virchows für pathologische Anatomie und Psychologie und für klinische Medizin,* 52: 394-429.
Heggelin, R., Siegenthaler, W. 1980. *Differentialdiagnose innerer Krankheiten.* 14th ed. Stuttgart: Thieme.
Hoche, A. 1912. "Die Bedeutung der Symptomenkomplexe in der Psychiatrie", *Zeitschrift für die gesamte Neurologie und Psychiatrie,* 12: 540-551.
Hofer, G. 1954. "Phänomen und Symptom – Zum Gegenstandsaspekt in der Psychopathologie", *Nervenarzt;* 25: 342-344.
Homburger, A. 1932. "Motorik", in: Bumke, O. (ed.) *Handbuch der Geisteskrankheiten.* Vol. 9. Berlin: Springer, 211-264.
Honderich, T. 1995. *The Oxford Companion to Philosophy.* Oxford: Oxford University Press.
Huber, G. 1988. "Langzeituntersuchungen bei Schizophrenien", in: Kaschka, W.P., Joraschky, P., Lungershausen, E. (eds.) *Die Schizophrenien.* Berlin/Heidelberg: Springer, 138-144.
Husserl, E. 1900. *Logische Untersuchungen.* Tübingen: Niemayer. English edition: *Logical Investigations.* Translated by J.N. Findlay. London: Routledge & Kegan Paul, 1970.
Husserl, E. 1913. *Einführung in die Logischen Untersuchungen.* English edition: *Introduction to Logical Investigations.* Translated by P.J. Bossert and C.H. Peters. The Hague, The Netherlands: Nijhoff, 1975.
Husted, J.A., Beiser, M., Lacono, W.G. 1995. "Negative symptoms in the course of first-episode affective psychoses", *Psychiatric Research,* 56: 145-154.
Janzarik, W. 1979. "100 Jahre Heidelberger Psychiatrie", in: Janzarik, W. (ed.) *Psychopathologie als Grundlagenwissenschaft.* Stuttgart: Enke. 1-32.

Jaspers, K. 1913. *Allgemeine Psychopathologie*. Berlin: Springer. English edition: *General Psychopathology*. Translated by J. Hoerin and M.W. Hamilton. Manchester, England: Manchester University Press, 1963.

Johnstone, E.C., Crow, T.J., Fritz, C.D., Husband, J., Kreel, L. 1976. "Cerebral ventricular size and cognitive impairment in chronic schizophrenia", *Lancet,* 2: 924-926.

Kahlbaum, K. 1863. *Gruppierung der psychischen Krankheiten – Versuch zur Anbahnung einer empirisch-naturwissenschaftlichen Grundlage der Psychiatrie als klinische Disziplin*. Habilitationsschrift.

Kahlbaum, K. 1874. *Die Katatonie oder das Spannungsirresein, eine klinische Form psychischer Krankheit*. 1st ed. Berlin: Hirschwald. I-XIII.

Kasanin, J. 1933. "The acute schizo-affective psychoses", *American Journal of Psychiatry,* 13: 97-126.

Kleist, K. 1928. "Über zykloide, paranoide und epileptische Psychosen und über die Frage der Degenerationspsychosen", *Schweizer Archiv für Neurologie und Psychiatrie,* 23: 3-37.

Koehler, K. 1982. "Symptome Ersten Ranges und die Prognose der Schizophrenie" in: Huber, G. (ed.) *Endogene Psychosen: Diagnostik, Basissyndrome und biologische Parameter.* Stuttgart: Schattauer, 97-104.

Kojima, T., Matsushima, E. 1990. "Eye movements in acute, chronic and remitted schizophrenia", *Biological Psychiatry*, 27: 975-989.

Kraepelin, E. 1883. *Psychiatrie.* 1st ed. Leipzig: Abel.

Kraepelin, E. 1893. *Psychiatrie.* 4th ed. Leipzig: Abel.

Kraepelin, E. 1899. "Zur Diagnose und Prognose der Dementia praecox", *Allgemeine Zeitschrift für Psychiatrie,* 56: 254-263.

Kraepelin, E. 1899. *Psychiatrie*. 6th ed., vol. II. Leipzig: Barth.

Kraepelin, E. 1910. *Psychiatrie*. 8th ed., vol. II. Leipzig: Barth.

Kraepelin, E. 1913. *Psychiatrie*. 8th ed., vol III. Leipzig: Barth. Translated in part by Barclay, R. M. *Dementia praecox and Paraphrenia*. Huntington, NY: Robert E. Krieger, 1971.

Kraepelin, E. 1920. "Die Erscheinungsformen des Irreseins", *Zeitschrift für die gesamte Neurologie und Psychiatrie,* 62: 1-29.

Kraepelin, E. 1927. "Klinische Psychiatrie", in: Kraepelin, E., Lange, J. (eds.) *Psychiatrie*. 9th ed., vol. II. Leipzig: Barth.

Kraus, A. 1991. "Phänomenologische und symptomatologisch-kriteriologische Diagnostik", *Fundamenta Psychiatrica,* 5: 102-109.

Langfeldt, G. 1937. "The prognosis in schizophrenia and the factors influencing the course of the disease", *Acta psychiatrica scandinavia*; Suppl 13.

Leonhard, K. 1972. "Aufteilung der endogenen Psychosen in der Forschungsrichtung von Wernicke und Kleist", in: Kisker, K.P., Meyer, J.E., Müller, M., Strömgren, E. (eds.) *Psychiatrie der Gegenwart.* 2nd ed., vol II/1. Berlin/Heidelberg/New York: Springer, 183-212.

Leonhard, K. 1979. *The Classification of Endogenous Psychoses*. 5th ed. Translated by R. Bermann. New York, NY: Halsted.

Liebermann, J.A., Jody, D., Alvia, J.M.J., Borenstein, M., Mayerhoff, D.T., Geisler, S., Szumanski, S., Gonzales, A., Bogerts, B., Ashitari, M. 1991. "Negative Symptoms in Schizophrenia: Relationships to Positive Symptoms and Outcome", in: Marneros, A., Andreasen, N.C., Tsuang, M.T. (eds.) *Negative Versus Positive Schizophrenia.* Berlin: Springer, 109-125.

Marneros, A. 1989. "Definition der schizoaffektiven Psychosen", in: Marneros, A. (ed.) *Schizoaffektive Psychosen.* Berlin/Heidelberg/New York: Springer, 21-28.

Marneros, A., Andreasen, N.C. 1991. "Positive and Negative Symptomatology: The State of Affairs", in: Marneros, A., Andreasen, N.C., Tsuang, M.T. (eds.) *Negative versus Positive Schizophrenia*. Berlin: Springer, 441-460.

Mayer-Gross, W. 1924. "Selbstschilderungen der Verwirrtheit", in: Forster, O., Wilmanns, K. (eds.) *Monographien aus dem Gesamtgebiet der Neurologie und Psychiatrie,* 42. Berlin: Springer.

Mayer-Gross, W. 1932. "Die Klinik", in: Bumke, O. (ed.) *Handbuch der Geisteskrankheiten*. Vol. 9. Berlin: Springer.

Metzger, W. 1954. *Psychologie,* 2nd ed. Darmstadt: Steinkopff.

Mundt, Ch., Kasper, S., Huerkamp, M. 1989. "The diagnostic specificy of negative symptoms and their psychopathological context", *British Journal of Psychiatry,* 155: 32-36.

Pearlson, G.D., Garbacz, D.J., Breackey, W.R. 1984. "Lateral ventricular enlargement associated with persistant unemployment and negative symptoms", *Psychiatric Research,* 12: 1-9.

Peters, U.H. 1977. "Die Struktur schizophrenen Symbolgebrauchs", *Psychiatria Clinica,* 10: 186-198.

Peters, U.H. 1980. "Der Strukturgedanke in der Psychopathologie", in: Peters, U.H. (ed.) *Die Psychologie des 20. Jahrhunderts,* vol. 10. München: Kindler, 93-108.

Peters, U.H. 1980. "Semiologie der Schizophrenie", in: Peters, U.H. (ed.) *Die Psychologie des 20. Jahrhunderts, vol. 10. Ergebnisse für die Medizin* 2. München: Kindler, 381-396.

Peters, U.H. 1990. *Wörterbuch der Psychiatrie und medizinischen Psychologie.* 4th ed., München/Wien/Baltimore: Urban & Schwarzenberg.

Pogue-Geile, M.F., Zubin, J. 1988. "Negative symptomatology and schizophrenia: A conceptual and empirical review", *International Journal of Medical Health,* 16: 3-45.

Rümke, H.C. 1958. "Die klinische Differenzierung innerhalb der Gruppe der Schizophrenien", *Nervenarzt,* 29: 49-53.

Sauer, H. 1990. "Die nosologische Stellung schizoaffektiver Psychosen. Problematik und empirische Befunde", *Nervenarzt,* 61: 3-15.

Saussure de, F. 1967. *Cours de linguistic général*, 2nd German edition. Berlin: de Gruyter.

Scheid, W. 1983. *Lehrbuch der Neurologie.* Stuttgart: Thieme.

Schischkoff, G. 1991. *Philosophisches Wörterbuch*, 22th ed. 22. Stuttgart: Kröner, 554.

Schneider, K. 1946. *Klinische Psychopathologie*. Stuttgart: Thieme.

Sigmund, D., Barnett, W., Mundt, Ch. 1998. "The Hysterical Personality Disorder: A Phenomenological Approach", *Psychopathology*, 31: 318-330.

Sigmund, D. 1996. "Die Aporie der Psychopathologie: Versuch einer Metaanalyse", *Fortschritte der Neurologie und Psychiatrie,* 64; 452-459.

Sigmund, D. 1998. "Die Phänomenologie zykloider Achsensyndrome und ihre Abgrenzung gegen eine schizophrene Kerngruppe", *Nervenarzt,* 69: 228-237.

Sigmund, D. 1998. "Wahn und Intuition", *Nervenarzt,* 65: 390-400.

Sigmund, D., Mundt, Ch. 1999. "The cycloid type and its differentication from core schiozophrenia", *Comprehensive Psychiatry,* 40: 4-18.

Steiner, E., Krause, R., Sänger-Alt, C., Wagner, G. 1988. "Mimisches Verhalten schizophrener Patienten und ihrer Gesprächspartner", *Zeitschrift für klinische Psychologie*, 17: 132-147.

Stransky, E. 1904. "Zur Lehre von der Dementia praecox", *Centralblatt für Nervenheilkunde und Psychiatrie,* 27: 1-19.

Stransky, E. 1919. *Lehrbuch der Allgemeinen und Speziellen Psychiatrie.* Leipzig: Vogel.
Strauss, J.S., Carpenter, W.T., Barrko, J.J. 1974. "The diagnosis and understanding of schizophrenia: part III. Speculations on the process that underlie schizohrenic symptoms and signs", *Schizophrenia Bulletin,* 1 (Experimental Issue No. 11): 61-69.
Weinberger, D.R. 1987. "Implications of normal brain development for the pathogenesis of schizophrenia", *Archives of General Psychiatry,* 44: 660-669.
Weitbrecht, H.J. 1957. "Zur Frage der Spezifität psychopathologischer Syndrome", *Fortschritte der Neurologie und Psychiatrie*, 25: 41-56.
Wernicke, C. 1900. *Grundriss der Psychiatrie in klinischen Vorlesungen.* Leipzig: Thieme.
Zendig, R. 1909. "Beiträge zur Differentialdiagnose des manisch-depressiven Irreseins und der Dementia praecox", *Allgemeine Zeitschrift für Psychiatrie,* 66: 932.
Ziehen, T. 1894. *Psychiatrie.* Berlin: Wreden.

Epistemology

Can We Know What Others Feel? Anthropological and Epistemological Considerations in Emotional Neuroscience

Georg Juckel and Andreas Heinz

Introduction

A series of neuroscience studies was conducted to measure central correlates of emotions elicited by pictures or other affective stimuli. It is often argued that the results of such studies are indicative of the emotions of the probands, independent of whether psychiatric patients or healthy controls are studied. In the last decades, different methods such as evoked potentials, the affect-modulated eye blink startle response or hormone blood levels were used to study emotions. Currently, neuroimaging strategies use functional magnetic resonance imaging (fMRI), positron emission tomography and other imaging methods with sophisticated paradigms to investigate different emotions. These studies may represent a major methodological progress in the field of emotion research, because patterns of neuronal activity can be precisely localized and indicate which brain areas and circuits are associated with the experience of distinct emotions. Most of these so-called "emotion induction" experiments are based on the assumption that a picture with, for example, a sad face will induce a distinct inner state in the viewer that may be recognized as "sadness" or "having sad emotions". In some studies that use standardized stimuli, the pictures have previously elicited sadness or related negative mood states according to the self-report of probands (Lang et al. 1988). The main questions, however, remain unsolved: Can we be sure that we measure what we want to measure? Can we obtain any evidence that other people feel what we have tried to induce? How certain can we be that other people feel as we do?

The Face as the Organ of Expression in Human Beings

A basic assumption in neuroscience suggests that emotions, like all human experiences, possess a biological neuronal base. Emotions such as anxiety, happiness, disgust etc. can be described according to several dimensions. A common approach distinguishes between three dimensions: a) emotion, perceived in introspection, b) cognition, involved in ratings and evaluations, and

c) motivation, which can lead to action. Emotions are expressive – the Latin word "e-movere" means to move out. The expressive dimension of emotions appears especially in the face. Almost all emotions of human beings are accompanied by an involuntary movement in the face, known as facial expressions (Ekman 1993). Every time someone feels happy or angry, we can only believe him if we see a corresponding facial expression. We would feel alienated or interpret it as a psychopathological symptom if the statement "I feel angry" differed significantly from the facial expression of the speaker.

The importance of facial expressions seems to be caused by human phylogeny and ontogeny, which transformed the face and its expressions into the most important organ of inter-individual communication. Darwin (1872) pointed out that facial expressions primarily developed from "useful habits," which were connected to form a system of social communication that translates personal information about inner states to other persons in relation to distinct aspects of the environment. The evolutionary development of facial muscles and their innervation may help us understand how the face became a primary tool for the communication of emotions. Human facial expressions and movements exhibit great similarity to animal reactions. A fearful face in human beings and non-human primates signals the perception of danger and the intention of the organism to flee or to freeze. However, compared to non-human primates, humans possess a more complex behavioural repertoire, and their capacity to demonstrate facial expressions are strongly increased. This increase may reflect the development of specific human abilities, of the requirement to follow and express behavioural rules in complex societies and of the human brain itself (Schiefenhövel 1989, Leonhard 1997).

From an ontogenetic point of view, facial expressions are a focal point for the relationship between mother and child (Bowlby 1975). For a long time during individual development, human infants cannot express their desires and moods in language and rely solely on facial expressions for communication. Facial expressions and vocalizations indicate the infant's inner emotional states, whether it feels good or bad. To understand these facial expressions is extremely important for the person who is most closely related with the infant, be it the mother or any other primary caretaker. The interaction is mutual and babies start early to fixate the face of the mother and to react to "messages" that are transferred by her facial expressions. This reciprocal and long-term interaction creates binding and forms social behaviour.

Assessment of Affective States in Psychiatric Patients and Healthy Subjects

Disturbances of affect and emotions are symptoms that are often decisive for a correct psychiatric diagnosis. For example, depressed patients may report symptoms such as negative mood, sadness, anhedonia, or to feel "like a stone" or dead. In contrast, manic patients in a euphoric state may feel like they could "hug the whole world" and respond enthusiastically to every new idea or person. These different emotional states are not only reported by the patients but also expressed in their psychomotor behaviour, which is often the only source of information about the inner emotional states of psychiatric patients (Juckel 1998). Bleuler (1911) and Kraepelin (1883) were convinced that affects and emotions of psychiatric patients are expressed in psychomotor functions such as facial expressions, gestures, postures, gait, etc. Concerning facial expressions, different emotional states are expressed by the involuntary movements of facial muscles during affective situations (Jaspers 1913). Pictures in Bleuler's textbook of psychiatry show "typical" facial expressions of depressed and manic patients. Faces of depressed patients seem to be void, sad and rigid, as if no emotions exist anymore, while faces of manic patients appear animated and actively orientated to the environment. The facial expression of a depressed patient may look slackened and heavy, unable to express laughing or crying. Facial expressions of manic patients, on the other hand, can be characterized by fast changes, so that euphoric and joking states can rapidly switch into irritated and aggressive expressions.

As a psychomotor phenomenon, facial expressions of psychiatric patients display a motor and an emotional side. In psychiatric and neurological disorders such as schizophrenia, depression, and Parkinson's disease, the motor and the emotional side can be affected in isolation, and it may be difficult to judge which side is primarily affected by the illness. This distinction can have important consequences for the diagnosis, our understanding of the pathophysiology and for the treatment of psychiatric disorders. In Parkinson's disease, we assume that the motor side is primarily affected and therefore treat patients with dopamine agonists to improve extrapyramidal function. In major depression, on the other hand, we normally assume that the motor deficit is the result of the negative mood state, which is then treated by serotonergic or norepinephrinergic antidepressants. The postulated association between psychomotor slowing and negative mood in major depression is, however, increasingly doubtful. Rogers (1992) argued that the psychomotor slowing of cognitive and motor functions in depression is a separate and possibly central disturbance, since the psychomotor dysfunction usually starts earlier than the affective symptoms in a depressive phase and may also last longer. In the view of an "integrative" neuropsychiatry, cognitive slowing in depression shares key aspects with the symptom of bradyphrenia in Parkinson's disease. Phenomenologically, psychomotor and cognitive slowing show similarities in major depression and extrapyramidal disorders such as Parkinson's disease. Reduced facial expressions, a gait with small steps without accompanying movements of the arms, hanging shoulders, bent posture and monotonic voice can be found in Parkinson patients and patients suffering from major depression (Pfau 1994). However, patients with Parkinson's disease may not suffer from depressed mood, while depressed patients report negative mood or a lack of vivid feelings. These considerations indicate that the relationship between feelings and their expression by motor movements may not be trivial.

In the light of these considerations, it is evident that assessment and interpretation of a proband's affect and mood state is crucial to emotional neuroscience. In a wider perspective, our entire interindividual communication and social life is based on an adequate interpretation of other persons' emotional reactions, independent of whether they are communicating verbally or in the modulation of the voice, facial expressions or posture. In turn, we have to answer with corresponding emotional signals using our own "instruments of expression." The human face has a wide and complex range of abilities to express emotions (lifting the eyebrows, contraction of the mouth, etc.), which is comparable with the possibilities of verbal communication. Furthermore, verbal and non-verbal communication occurs simultaneously and the latter may help to transfer additional information. Even interruptions of communication carry a communicative meaning. For example, breaks may take place during verbal communication or at the end of talks, and may indicate a speaker's ambivalent feelings or result from a disturbance in the mutual exchange of ideas and emotions. Such breaks may be misinterpreted if they occur in psychotic patients and result from ego disorders such as thought insertion rather than emotional problems with the communicative partner.

It is obvious that problems in understanding and misinterpretations can occur frequently when a "healthy" person with a "normal" range of feelings and emotions tries to understand and to interpret signals of psychiatric patients. Psychiatric diagnostic work and psychotherapeutic interventions are based on the necessity to correctly assess a patient's inner emotional state and to respond accordingly. If we are not sure about the feelings, emotions and affects of psychiatric patients, we may fail to correctly classify the symptoms and to ascertain an accurate diagnosis which would determine the appropriate treatment. It was this general uncertainty in the classification of a patient's expressions that motivated Schneider (1942) to focus on "first rank symptoms of schizophrenia" that rely on symptoms reported by the patients (such as commenting voices or thought insertion) rather than the clinician's impression of their emotional reaction. Nevertheless, understanding a patient's emotion is necessary both for psychotherapeutic interventions and the selection of adequate medication that affects mood states.

Inner States and External Expressions: Are There No Private Emotions?

With all our clinical and psychological training – are we really able to infer from facial expression the "real feelings", "inner affective states" or the "introspective part" of another person's emotions? The other person may try to deceive us about his or her true inner feelings and to come up with another affect in his face. He or she may also wilfully decide to signify the feeling with a word that does not characterize the "real" feeling. A person may be angry but state that he is sad. Unconscious psychodynamic mechanisms could, on the other hand, prevent that a person exhibits his or her "true feelings", and instead elicit reaction formations that transform anger into sadness or desire into disgust. Such a person would suffer from incongruent feelings and may benefit from psychotherapy. However, to deceive another human being about one's inner feeling is rather difficult. Facial expressions are telling, as the example of smile and laughter shows. In case of an authentic (so-called Duchenne) smile and laughter, the muscles around the eyes, especially the orbicularis muscle, are involuntarily innervated (Ekman et al. 1988). Among persons who often laugh, the frequent contraction of these muscle leads to the well known "crow feet" laterally from the eyes. In case of a non-authentic smile or laughter, the muscles around the mouth are voluntarily innervated, and the mouth opens up, but the eyes remain "mute". This is in correspondence to different EEG patterns during authentic and non-authentic smile and laughter (Ekman et al. 1990). It is also well known that the face muscles contract more asymmetrically the less deeply felt the emotions (Ekman et al. 1981).

From a philosophical point of view, Ludwig Wittgenstein tried to solve the problem of the relationship between inner states and external expression of emotions. With the help of the famous argument against a private language, he tried to show that a solipsistic position ("an inner world of emotions and language exists to which only one person has access; I have no empirical evidence that other people exist and have feelings") has to be rejected. He reasoned that all expressions or terms that we possess and use for intra-subjective feelings are acquired within a social context and community and are, therefore, inter-subjective (Wittgenstein, 1967). Wittgenstein's argument was motivated by doubts about the value of introspective data for scientific purposes. Behaviourists, who criticized the uncertainty and subjective character of introspection, voiced a similar concern. We have only language terms for something that has an inter-subjective meaning ("I feel happy", and I want others to be aware of this), but there is no name for a private thing.

> 'What would it be like if human beings showed no outward sign of pain (did not groan, grimace etc.)? Then it would be impossible to teach a child the use of the word 'tooth-ache'.' Well, let's assume that the child is a genius and itself invents a

> name for the sensation! – But then, of course, he couldn't make himself understood when he used the word. (Wittgenstein 1967, §257).

Wittgenstein suggests that meaningful communication about a feeling requires signification with a term. This term is a part of a language or language game, and the rules of how to use the term are learned like the rules of any other game. In Wittgenstein's view, it is senseless to follow a rule alone, since all rules are embedded within an institutionalized practice (Kripke 1984). A law without a society has no foundation. To follow a rule alone fails to fulfil all criteria for following a rule: learning the rule by others, social control of rules, breaking the rule with consequences (punishment, to lose the game, etc.). Furthermore, private definitions are meaningless, since there is no possibility to communicate the definition, to correct the words and their meaning within a learning process, to question or modify the definition, and so on. All definitions imply or presuppose a public communicative space. If I invent a private language, there is no possibility to prove the use of such private names as incorrect, since I have no criteria to indicate whether or not I use the names correctly (Wittgenstein 1967). Only in communication with others, can my terms be inter-subjectively examined and their correct use objectively controlled. Wittgenstein thus claimed that a set of words or behavioural expressions can be only declared a true language if the use of its terms can independently be examined and justified.

Wittgenstein's ideas can be understood as a strong argument for the reliability of our interpretation of other person's emotional expressions. Whenever I experience a certain feeling, I can refer to this feeling with an expression that was acquired and controlled in a social context. For example, I have learned to use the word "happiness" within my language family from other members of my social community. I have learned to use the word in exactly those contexts in which others approved my previous use of the word. This learning process is based on "directing definitions" of a word; gestures and other devices provide information about the range of situations in which this word can be used to indicate something specific. I may not be able to define a distinct "inner state" that corresponds to the word, but I have learned to use the word in an appropriate context. Compare the situation with other learned behaviours: I may not be able to define what "inner state" elicits a conditioned reaction, but the conditioned stimuli can nevertheless reliably activate a certain behavioural response.

In a similar way, we may have learned to understand and use facial expressions for the expressions of distinct emotions (Zepf et al. 1998). Facial expressions can be understood as a "language" for social communication to enable us to define which emotions other persons express in their faces, and which facial expression or word we have to demonstrate when we wish to be understood by another human being. Therefore, one could argue that the inner state of emotions is necessarily represented in the external state of emotions, i.e. their verbal and behavioural manifestations in words, facial expressions, gestures, postures, etc. Only with the help of facial expressions and other external manifestations can my communication partners and I be sure about inner feelings and react to them accordingly. If I have learned to understand social signals and their correct use in a social context, it is within this social context that I am able to interpret the expressions of others correctly and that others can correct me if my use of a term deviates from the accepted use. As a consequence, social contexts guarantee that the perception and assessment of language and behavioural expressions, be it in everyday life or a research setting, provide sufficient insight into other persons' emotions.

However, in the case of Parkinson's disease or neuroleptic-induced Parkinsonism, a subject's face may express sadness or affective flattening, although there are no negative emotions and the facial expression is caused by extrapyramidal movement disorder rather than affective dysfunction (Heinz et al. 1998). Alternatively, the patient may feel extremely happy but his face is unable to express the emotion. In such situations, should we not rely on the "inner experience" of the person to tell us whether facial expression is indeed in correspondence with the emotional state? A simple answer may be that the subject remembers previous emotional states, which were acquired in social situations in which facial and verbal expressions did not differ due to the motor disorder. So the previous learning experience and not the current social feedback could guarantee the correct labelling of the emotion. However, the situation may be more complex and the patient may well identify his or her feelings correctly based on specific information about his or her "inner state" that he nevertheless learned to identify in social situations. It was Lotze (1882) who tried to explain empathy with the suggestion that observing another person stimulates us to mimic his or her behaviour and thus enables us to feel what the observed person feels and is trying to accomplish. Automatically elicited mirroring of the other person would thus allow us to feel the way he or she feels, and current neuroscience even identified so-called "mirror-neurons" that may be crucial in the performance of externally observed movements (Wohlschläger and Prinz 2003). Such socially evoked intentions to "mirror" the emotional facial movements of other persons may be registered by the patient who suffers from Parkinson's disease, independent of whether his or her motor disorder allows the performance of adequate facial expressions. So the patient who suffers from an extrapyramidal disorder may not have to rely on some mystically correct "inner experience" to describe how he or she "really" feels. At least in social situations, the subject's perception of the intended rather than the performed facial expression may provide crucial information for the labelling of his or her "true" emotion.

Where Are Emotions Localized?

Another related problem of inner states and external expressions of emotions is associated with the question where – if at all – emotions can be localized in the body. Emotions may be localized in the central nervous system, as Cannon (1927) suggested, and if so, the only question to be addressed is which parts and processes of the brain are involved (Panksepp 1998). However, emotions may also be generated in the body's periphery, as James (1884) pointed out. Do the tears lead to the feeling of sadness, or does sadness induce the tears? Both of the two sides are well founded by arguments and empirical results. Some evidence indicates that the two sides of emotions, central nervous processing and external facial expression, are related and interact reciprocally. Inner neuronal processes, for example, elicited by cortex stimulation (Fried 1998), generate emotions and associated facial expressions, but it is also possible to induce emotions with the adequate neuronal correlates by voluntary processes in the body periphery. Levenson et al. (1990) observed that although volunteers were blind about the intended facial expression and the corresponding emotion, the initiation of voluntary movements in the face induced distinct emotions and corresponding changes of heartbeat, skin temperature and skin resistance. Further studies revealed that voluntary facial movements also elicited EEG changes that were characteristic for the intended emotion (Ekman and Davidson 1993). These observations form the background for therapeutic approaches such as laughter therapy, which aims to induce positive emotions in patients by voluntary laughing.

Can Anthropological Models Guide the Understanding of Foreign Emotions?

What if emotional reactions are learned and expressed in a different cultural context? Can we, as members of a certain society understand people with a different cultural background? This seems to be possible, at least in principle. All men are part of any kind of society with few or many members. In all human societies, communication is performed by language, facial expressions etc., i.e. with a set of behavioural and social signs. To understand persons from a foreign culture, these signs have to be translated as accurately as possible. In any culture, the verbal expression "kurzykzki" can refer to an emotion, which we as members of another culture call "sad." In that culture, lifting of the eyebrows may mean "I feel angry," while we, in our culture, contract our eyebrows to indicate a similar emotion. How can we translate or transfer this expression from one to another sign system?

Wittgenstein's answer is: by learning and following the rules in which a word, a facial expression, a gesture is used for something that we are trying to signify (Wittgenstein 1967). In an assumed perfect communication, we can together examine whether or not e.g. a word was correctly used. When I am laughing and say "I am happy" and explain to someone from a foreign culture: see, whenever I laugh and say "happy," I am in a positive mood state in which I feel euphoric or enthusiastic or feel good vibrations, the other could say: "ok, I understand what you mean, we call this 'x5rsf27' and lift our left leg regularly, whenever we are enthused or euphoric, but what do you mean by 'good vibrations'?" Then, I would try to explain "good vibrations" by language or behavioural signs, with which my foreign friend is already acquainted. Thus, the process of communication and understanding proceeds until the two of us are satisfied.

On the other hand, some facial expressions or gestures seem to be common all over the world. It has been observed that facial expressions for happiness or sadness are universal, from Papa-Guinea to New York City (Ekman and Davidson 1994). These so-called primary emotions are therefore easy to understand across the different cultures, since the involuntary movements in the face are so similar in all societies. All over the world, crying represents a sign of sadness and despair. In conclusion, once we have learned the rules about how words, gestures and facial expressions are used in other cultures, we should be able to comprehend better what people from another culture feel.

It can, however, be questioned whether emotions can indeed adequately be "translated" – is there really a set of basic human emotions that are expressed in all societies or does every society teach and express its own set of culturally acceptable emotions? Cross-cultural studies may suggest that some basic dimensions of emotions, such as positive or negative valence and arousal, are expressed in all cultures (Lang et al. 1988). However, is a widespread emotion such as jealousy really sufficiently mapped with these dimensions? Is "jealousy" a satisfactory term to describe emotions elicited by e.g. sexual interactions in a society that sanctions monogamy instead of polygamy? Some anthropological studies tried to identify a basic set of emotions that are closely linked to the brain and its evolution and therefore found in all human cultures. However, anthropological models of the emotional mind have to cope with several methodological pitfalls. Anthropological studies often assume that brain structure reflects evolution and that "higher" and more complex centres are phylogenetically younger and control older, more "primitive" brain centres (Heinz 2002). Since ontogeny is often conceptualized as a recapitulation of phylogeny, children were examined to detect fundamental and simple emotional and cognitive processes. However, while ontogeny may recapture phylogeny during intra-uterine development, there is little empirical evidence that children's beliefs and emotional structures resemble those of presumably "primitive" cultures (Erikson 1965).

Anthropologists and psychoanalysts often studied cognitive and emotional structures of so-called "primitive" people and hoped to achieve clues for the understanding of "primitive" or "prelogic" mentality (Heinz 1997). A major problem of this approach was that contemporary, colonialized people were examined and differences to Western cultures were attributed to "primitivity" rather than to contemporary social hierarchies or the "colonial view" of the missionaries, officers and travellers (Heinz 1998). Moreover, the duration of historical developmental of contemporary, non-Western cultures is of course as long as the history of Western cultures, and in any given society, a "primitive" level of technical development may concur with complex and highly developed social systems or religious beliefs or with an extremely refined and empirical understanding of natural events (Malinowski 1955; Lévi-Strauss 1962; Evans-Pritchard 1965). To date, it is difficult to dissect the complex interplay of cultural differences, colonial history and social prejudice, which can interfere with the identification of "basic" human emotions and the intercultural translation of emotional reactions.

Conclusion: Emotions Are Principally Communicable – Do We Possess Performative Rather Than Propositional Knowledge?

According to Wittgenstein (1967), our day-to-day false belief is that our emotions and the emotions of other persons are only accessible and detectable by introspection. Wittgenstein's main argument is that we always refer to feelings or emotions using a certain language and behavioural terms. We have experienced all these terms during postnatal development by means of education and imitation within our society ("language play" or "language family", Wittgenstein 1980). We have no chance to withdraw ourselves from this mechanism, because in every situation involving feelings, we are building up a referential relationship to this feeling and signifying it with a term that was previously learned. In other words, whenever I feel "something", there is "something" for which I have learned to signify it using a special word, facial expression, posture, gesture, etc. Therefore, our "emotional knowledge" may be performative rather than declarative, it may include behavioural responses and their neural correlates as constitutive parts. Since other members of our society share the process of signifying, we can determine the other facial expressions, gestures and words. Developing a private language for emotions is pointless, since there would be no social control to indicate that the use of terms for "private" emotions refers to any constant "inner" process. I need other people with whom I can share common words, facial expressions etc. to give me feedback on whether I am using e.g. the word "anxiety" correctly or not. If, on the other hand, I stay in this socially constructed language play, I can communicate my feelings and understand the emotions of other human beings.

However, it becomes more and more clear that it may be a rather limited approach to simply show emotional pictures and to hope that they will reliably induce certain feelings in other persons. Whenever I wish for reliable information e.g. about a neurobiological parameter of an emotional reaction, I must be sure that I elicit a certain emotion in the persons that I study with functional brain imaging. What should I do? In our opinion, a promising approach may be to assess specific behavioural parameters that reflect (or in some views even constitute) emotional reactions. One of the best examples for this approach is to measure the contraction around the eyes to indicate the "authentic Duchenne smile", which can be elicited when e.g. a person watches a scene that evokes laughter (Juckel and Polzer 1998, Juckel et al. 1999, Padberg et al. 2001, Juckel 2004, Mergl et al. 2003). Such measures obtained in psychiatric patients and in healthy controls can indicate emotional responses elicited during psychophysiological, neurochemical or neuroimaging experiments. They may also help to identify basic emotions in cross-cultural studies. However, the problem remains how to adequately describe cultural differences in emotional research without simplifying the complex interactions between cultural codes and prejudices, post-colonial hierarchies and a presumably universal "human nature".

References

Bleuler, E. 1911. *Lehrbuch der Psychiatrie*. Heidelberg: Springer.

Bowlby, J. 1975. *Bindung – eine Analyse der Mutter-Kind-Beziehung*. München: Kindler.

Cannon, W.B. 1927. "The James-Lange theory of emotions: A critical examination and an alternative theory", *Am J Psychol*, 39: 106-124.

Darwin, C.R. 1872. *The Expression of Emotions in Man and Animals*. London: John Murray.

Ekman, P. 1993. "Facial expression and emotion", *Am Psychologist*, 48: 384-392.

Ekman, P., Davidson, R.J. 1993. "Voluntary smiling changes regional brain activity", *Psychol Science*, 4: 342-345.

Ekman, P., Davidson, R.J. 1994. *The Nature of Emotion: Fundamental Questions* (Series in Affective Science). Oxford: Oxford University Press.

Ekman, P., Hager, J.C., Friesen, W.V. 1981. "The symmetry of emotional and deliberate facial actions", *Psychophysiology*, 18: 101-106.

Ekman, P., Friesen, W., O´Sullivan, M. 1988. "Smiles when lying", *J Pers Soc Psychol*, 54: 414-420.

Ekman, P., Davidson, R.J., Friesen, W.V. 1990. "The Duchenne smile: Emotional expression and brain physiology II.", *J Pers Soc Psychol*, 58: 342-353.

Erikson, E.H. 1965. *Kindheit und Gesellschaft*. Stuttgart.

Evans-Pritchard, E.E. 1965. *Theories of primitive religion*. Oxford: Oxford University Press.

Fried, I., Wilson. C.L., MacDonald, K.A., Behnke, E.J. 1998. "Electric current stimulates laughter", *Nature*, 391: 650.

Heinz, A., Knable, M.B., Coppola, R., Gorey, J.G., Jones, D.W., Lee, K.S., Weinberger,

D.R. 1998. "Psychomotor slowing, negative symptoms and dopamine receptor availability IBZM SPECT study in neuroleptic-treated and drug-free schizophrenic patients", *Schizophr Res*, 31:19-26.

Heinz, A. 1997. "Savage thought and thoughtful savages – on the context of the evaluation of logic thought by Lévy-Bruhl and Evans-Pritchard", *Anthropos*, 92: 165-173.

Heinz, A. 1998. "Colonial practices in the construction of the schizophrenic patient as primitive man", *Critique Anthropol*, 18: 421-444.

Heinz, A. 2002. "Anthropologische und evolutionäre Modelle in der Schizophrenieforschung", in: Heise, T., Schuler, J. (eds.) *Das transkulturelle Psychoforum*. Verlag für Wissenschaft und Bildung, Berlin.

James, W. 1884. "What is emotion", *Mind* 4: 188-204.

Jaspers, K. 1913. *Allgemeine Psychopathologie*. Heidelberg: Springer.

Juckel, G. 1998. "Motorik", in: Hegerl, U. (ed.) *Neurophysiologische Untersuchungen in der Psychiatrie*. Wien: Springer, 163-189.

Juckel, G., Polzer, U. 1998. "Abnormal facial activity in chronic schizophrenic patients – a pilot study", *German J Psychiatry*, 1: 6-8.

Juckel, G., Präßl, A., Froschmayer, S., Mavrogiorgou, P., Tigges, P., Möller, H.J., Hegerl, U. 1999. "'Im Gesicht lesen lernen' – Mimikanalyse schizophrener Patienten", in: Machleidt, W., Haltenhof, H., Garlipp, P. (eds.) *Schizophrenie – eine affektive Erkrankung ?* Stuttgart: Schattauer, 127-134.

Juckel, G. 2004. "Beeinträchtigungen von Mimik und Emotionsausdruck", in: Jahn, T., Förstl, H. (eds.) *Bewegungsstörungen bei psychischen Erkrankungen*. Heidelberg: Springer (in press).

Kraepelin, E. 1883. *Lehrbuch der Psychiatrie*. Leipzig: Abel.

Kripke, S.A. 1984. *Wittgenstein on rules and private language*. Boston: Harvard University Press.

Lang, P.J., Oehman, A., Vaitl, D. 1988. *The International Affective Picture System. (photographic slides)*. Center for Research in Psychophysiology, University of Florida, Gainsville.

Leonhard, K. 1997. *Der menschliche Ausdruck in Mimik, Gestik und Phonik*. Psychiatrische Klinik, Würzburg.

Levenson, R.W., Ekman, P., Friesen, W.V. 1990. "Voluntary facial action generates emotion-specific autonomic nervous system activity", *Psychophysiology*, 27: 363-384.

Lévi-Strauss, C. 1962. *La pensée sauvage*. Paris: Librairie Plon.

Lotze, H. 1882. *Grundzüge der praktischen Philosophie*. Leipzig: Hirzel, (Reprint: Rodopi, Amsterdam, 1969).

Malinowski, B. 1955. "Rational mastery by man of his surroundings", in: *Magic, science and religion*. New York: Doubleday, 25-35.

Mergl, R., Vogel, M., Mavrogiorgou, P., Göbel, C., Zaudig, M., Hegerl, U., Juckel, G. 2003. "Kinematical analysis of emotionally induced facial expressions in patients with obsessive-compulsive disorder", *Psychol Med*, 33: 1453-1462.

Padberg, F., Juckel, G., Präßl, A., Zwanzger, P., Mavrogiorgou, P., Hegerl, U., Hampel, H., Möller, H.J. 2001. "Prefrontal cortex modulation of mood and emotionally induced facial expressions: A transcranial magnetic stimulation study", *J Neuropsychiat Clin Neurosci*, 13: 206-212.

Panksepp, J. 1998. *Affective Neuroscience. The foundation of human and animal emotions*. New York: Oxford University Press.

Pfau, B. 1994. *Körpersprache der Depression*. Stuttgart: Schattauer.

Rogers, D. 1992. *Motor disorder in psychiatry – Towards a neurological psychiatry*. Wiley, Chichester.

Schiefenhöfel, W. 1989. "Vom physiologischen Reflex zur Botschaft – Über evolutionsbiologische Zwänge und semiotische Entwicklungslinien in der menschlichen Mimik", in: Hippius, H., Rüther, E., Schmauß, M. (eds.) *Katatone und dyskinetische Syndrome*. Berlin: Springer, 27-39.
Schneider, K. 1942. *Psychischer Befund und psychiatrische Diagnose*. Leipzig: Thieme.
Wittgenstein, L. 1967. *Philosophical investigations*. Oxford: Blackwell.
Wohlschläger, A., Prinz, W. 2003. "Handlungssteuerung, Handlungsauswahl und Handlungswahrnehmung", *Neuroforum*, 1: 11-16.
Zepf, S., Ullrich, B., Hartmann, S. 1998. "Affekt und mimisches Verhalten", *Psychother Psychosom Med Psychol*, 48: 156-167.

On Time Experience in Depression – Dominance of the Past

Hinderk M. Emrich and Detlef E. Dietrich

1. Introduction: The Brain as a Time-Machine

"Time is the way in which we perceive the world around us" (Ehlers 2003). This fundamental sentence by Ehlers gives the opportunity to raise the question as to how the brain may act as a "time-machine" to enable this. Indeed one may envisage the brain as containing aspects of a "time-machine" in three different ways as follows:

- Firstly, the brain is a neurobiological physical system like other systems – existing in time – being an object of understanding by physics and biophysics, especially of neurochemical oscillators, and a subject to the concepts of chronobiology.
- Secondly, the human brain is a "time-machine" since it can memorize "stored regularities" and recall them. The brain thus contains aspects of "time-transcendence" – to use here a term employed by the Berlin philosopher Michael Theunissen (1992). Human beings are – in the sense of the phenomenology of Edmund Husserl – able to perform protension, i.e. the conceptualization of the future as well as retention, the recall of the past. Furthermore, we are able to generate the time-experience of the "now", of the time-moment, the "presence within time". One specific problem, however, is how to relate, how to synchronize the "outer", the so called Aristotelian or "physical" time to the "time of inner experience", i.e. the time of Augustinus, and the Bergsonian time. The psychiatric disorders as well as extraordinary experiences of normal life tend to induce problems within this type of coordination, and depression represents a mood-disorder, within which, also experimentally, a disturbance of the inner organization of time in relation to objective time can be demonstrated.
- Thirdly, there is the aspect of a "time-machine" in a Kantian understanding, namely, that the human mind – apparently on the basis of brains – can construe the universals of perception, especially the category of "time".

How are the functions of such a "time-machine" realized within ourselves?

2. Time and Affect: Something About Anxiety

One of the main ideas within the neuropsychological research is that affective changes are great determinants in the construction– (and deconstruction–) processes of cognition and thus of the constitution of consciousness (Emrich 1992). We have demonstrated this in illusion research, in psychosis-research, in the understanding of the action of psychedelic drugs as well as in "synaesthesia", an excellent way for normal probands to construe hyperintegrative inner perceptual worlds (Emrich 1998).

Interestingly, this emotional determination ("emotional tone") behind cognition and self- and world-experience contains fundamental aspects of neurobiology of time as well as philosophy and psychopathology of time. Pöppel (1985) as well as Singer (1990) concerned with physiology and Theunissen (1992) with philosophy have made some remarkable contributions to this theme.

We would like to demonstrate the basic principles of the fundament of a neurobiological theory of anxiety and depression in relation to time, established by the neuropsychologists Gray and Rawlins (1986). An understanding of this concept, however, requires a representation of the basic principles, according to the way in which our brains are functioning.

As the neurophysiologist von der Malsburg (1993; personal communication) stated, the brain – as a machine – represents a "significance-detector"; that means it is able to detect – within an excessively high level of noise – a special event, which incorporates the quality of being "meaningful". To exert this function, the brain is composed – as a multi-systems-parallel-processor – of many more or less independent "modules" which interact in an intricate way. There are systems of conceptualization within the frontal lobe, systems of processing sensory data within the occipital brain and systems of emotionality and of valuation within the inner temporal lobe and limbic system.

These functions can be demonstrated by functional brain imaging, e.g. in PET scans or functional nuclear magnetic imaging. The neuropsychologist Desimone (1995) has proposed a general organization scheme of the flow of processing in such a way that so-called top-down processes are realized from prefrontal to occipital and "bottom-up processes" appear to function from occipital to prefrontal. What does this mean from the point of view of experience of time? Interestingly, we are led to understand that the theory of time starts, so to speak, in the future (in an analogy to Heidegger), from the conceptualization of "what comes next?" It is the world of predictions and desires. The neurobiologist Martin Heisenberg (1989) construes the world of activities of a biological system not from reflex or from reaction to outer changes but from novelty-seeking, a mode of action he refers to as "initial activity". The presence, the "now" is, accordingly, construed from actual sensory data in relation to these conceptualizations, i.e. from bottom-up information in relation to expectations. This is realized within the intermediate part of the brain, namely the temporal lobe. However, it is interesting to note that here the entrance is realized to limbic structures and to memory structures. How do we gain access to the past? How do we enter Marcel Proust's (1993) inner memory-world within his "recherché" as to the "lost past"?

For this we have to go into the physiology of memory, which is a physiology of the hippocampus, as a temporal organizer in relation to cortical feedback-loops.

From these basic principles, we are now able to understand how anxiety is organized within our brains. It is an extreme form of "significance detection" of something that turns out to be aversive. The model is called the "hippocampal comparator system" and represents very clearly the components of the generation of inner time.

Again we start – in the sense of Heisenberg (1989) – in the future, "what comes next?" *The predictions dominate the perception of time.* With regard to the predictions – and we may add: the emotionality, the emotional climate, the "emotional tone" of the predictions, it depends what the "measurement of significance" will disclose within the present situation, according to von der Malsburg (1993, personal communication). These predictions are possible deriving from the special type of actualization of the "stored regularities" of the past only. Here the cortico-cortical loops containing memory traces come into function. Thereafter, from the sensory data of the occipital lobe, the presence, the data of "now", take over the "comparator"-function. Should an unexpected possibly dangerous situation occur, the system will generate an "alarm-signal" which, in turn, activates the limbic system. This input creates "arousal", "motor inhibition" and increased attention via a behavioural inhibiting system. Interestingly, this is where the famous anxiolytic drugs, the benzodiazepines, act, since they can down-regulate the intensity of this internal alarm-signal and thus reduce the anxiety reaction. If there is a malfunction of these binding sites, anxiety and epilepsy can occur.

This concept of constitution of time within our internal "time-machine" is also plausible from another point of view: the neuropsychology of synaesthesia (Emrich 1998). Here an additional intermodal integration is realized within one moment of presence. This integration is apparently manifested by a so-called "limbic bridge", in which the integration of e.g. a digit and a colour is realized in a synthetic "fusing". Whether or not this limbic integration is performed by chronobiological oscillators (Pöppel 1985, Singer 1990) or by a special neurobiological "wiring", this is a problem yet to be solved (Emrich 1998, Singer 1990).

3. Internal Balance of Values

Disturbances of the inner equilibrium of the components of the self which shape identity, brought about by processes of representing by remembering and the consequences brought about by these disturbances elucidate the potential for explanation inherent in a theory of the processes of identity formation, based on the psychology of the self.

It is important to consider the structural principles of forgetting in relation to overvaluation with respect to the stability of "promise contexts". The sociologist Hans-Dieter Gondek (1990) emphasized the specific value of promise contexts in evaluating personal identity which is essential in connection with the problem of forgetting: a forgotten promise, after all, is not really a promise. In other words: how does identity change when forgetfulness takes place? Identity would seem to imply the promise that one is – and will remain – the person one is at the present time, quite the opposite of Nietzsche's "You must become the person you are". Of course, people do not generally behave in this way; they do not accept that they and others are, or can be, only what they manifestly are at the present moment. They do in fact intuitively behave in the way Nietzsche demands; they expect developments in other persons, which they assume would also take place within themselves. We expect to meet the person whom the other person will have become by the time the appointment takes place, that is, if we are sensible. We form an opinion of others according to the available possibilities, according to tendencies rather than to "faculties". Falling back or surpassing oneself can both occur; both must be possible and are indeed necessary. Within the framework of psychoanalytic therapies, but also spontaneously in everyday life, people can in fact take themselves completely by surprise. During the therapeutic process, it may happen – indeed it is the intention – that alien-image and self-image come together or at least interact with one another, something which can lead to the most radical of changes.

From what we have seen so far, it is clear that the formation of identity is always accompanied by complex processes of adjusting the inner balance of values, so that it is to be expected that any disturbance of the processes aimed at restoring such equilibrium will lead to psychopathological phenomena. Disturbances in the internal balance of values normally lead to "coping" processes, i.e. processes of management and increases in performance, which ensure that one's self-demands and one's self-image fit optimally together once more. In cases where this fails or where it cannot succeed, a whole range of changes in behaviour are possible. These range from grieving to processes during which the balance of values is distorted, to processes of denial, of encapsulation or repression. Nietzsche's famous statement (1981) is appropriate here: "'I did this', says my memory. 'I cannot have done it', says my pride, and remains relentless. Ultimately it is my memory which gives in."

4. System Theory and Forgetting

From the perspective of a system theory model how should such a process be conceived, namely, of coping with alteration of the past and thus also of the process of "forgetting"? How does such a system behave in a concrete situation when what is involved is effectuating plans and relating them to the past? Suggestions concerning such decision-making processes can be found in the theory of non-linearly dynamic processes. As Friedrich Cramer (1993) demonstrates in his book on the theory of time, complex systems, which are evolving constantly display successive branching with "the mutual influence of three aspects of dynamic systems, namely, structure, function and fluctuations, leading to unexpected phenomena". If one applies this description of a complex system to the field of physical chemistry as a metaphor for the biographical development of a biological system, one can compose – with Peitgen (1993) – a tree diagram in which it is not possible to predict how the final state of the system will actually turn out. This is because after the evolution of a complex system, a large number of unstable final situations arise, the variety of which can be greatly reduced by impaired development ("trauma"). Instead of sixteen final situations (as shown in Figure 1), only three or four such states can actually be determined.

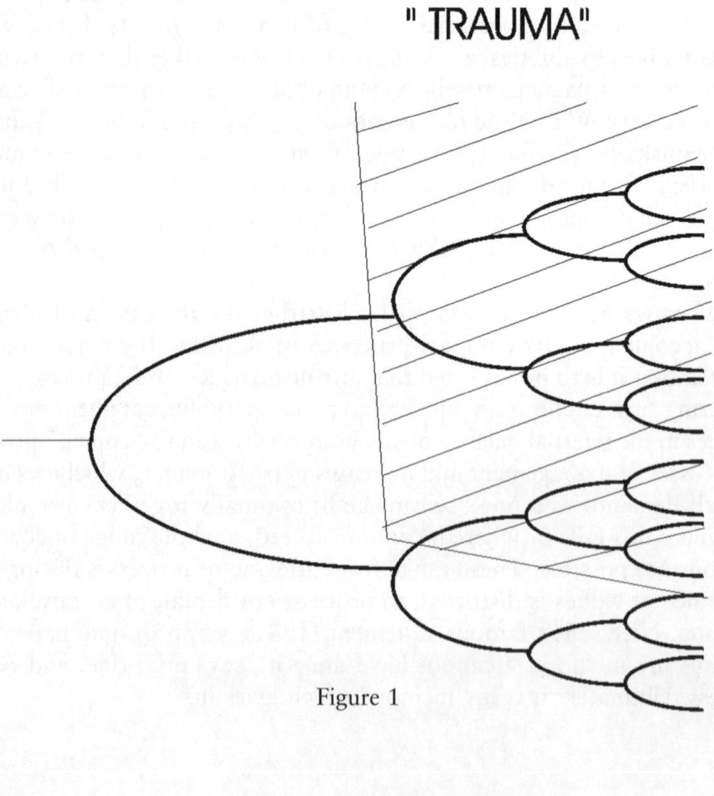

Figure 1

On examining this disturbance chronologically and using the metaphor of the "path travelled", one finds that influences on the system have caused the path to be a specific and an extremely restricted one. The question that arises when looking back is how one should deal with this enforced path in a "coping" manner. If one decides to use this method of description as a metaphor for the reconstruction of the "path" along which an individual develops from a plurivalent initial situation to a final situation moulded by the various factors relevant to development, one can also describe the influences – both favourable and harmful – which have served to determine this path. Early traumas may have had such a powerful negative influence on the available choices in a vulnerable phase of development that these events – which are later generally "forgotten" – entirely determine, modify and restrict the rest of the subject's life. A whole range of options, lives and choices as potential system states have thus been eliminated. There are three ways for the subject to deal with the consequences of this development. The first deals purely with certain points: it is only the outcome as it actually is that is considered: "one must base oneself on the facts." The second possibility is – in Hegel's view – to consider the truth in the context of both the path and the outcome. The third and final viewpoint does not only involve reconstructing the path but also reconstructing the other options, which would have been possible at each given diversion. This way of interpretation might be understood in terms of Proust's (1993) "recherché du temps perdu", as an associative recalling of subliminal truths from the past. It is dealt with at length in Michael Theunissen's book on the "negative theology of time" (1992). Theunissen says that "Proust's 'spontaneous remembering' uncovers, to put it traditionally, the eternal element in the past. What he finally calls 'time regained' is time only as the self's own other."

5. Balance of Values and Forgetting

The interrelationship between forgetting and the internal balance of values may be summarized as follows: the essence of the process of disregard involved in "active" forgetting is disturbance of the "internal balance of values". This means that the internal model of the world is always, at the same time, an internal value model, both of external objects, processes and intentional contents, also with respect to self-esteem. Disturbances in the internal balance of values with respect to self-esteem are usually answered – and this is likely to be their "biological significance" – with a "coping strategy", in other words, with an active compensatory increase in performance. If such an increase in performance is not possible for external and/or internal reasons, the question arises as to how to deal with the internal imbalance of values. Three "active" (but no doubt essentially unconscious) disregard processes are available. The active disregard of past reality is therefore linked to the internal balance of values. It offers denial as a mechanism: here, the internal psychological mechanism consists of removing a fact from the balance of values and more or less "encapsulating" it. The memory material actively committed to the process of forgetting remains present intra-psychologically and basically also accessible; it can thus be remembered but it does not play any role in determining the balance of values because it is "denied". The Israeli philosopher and psychologist Dan Bar-On (1988) demonstrated in a large number of studies that, for the reasons described, Nazi war criminals were able to remember minor offences, indeed they remorsefully accused themselves of them, whereas they denied any feelings of guilt in much more serious matters where both they themselves and others were concerned. Bar-On's deep insights into the structure of the internal balance of values in these persons show that they display "improper forgetting".

Another more energetic means of eliminating memory material from the balance of values lies in the form of repression. According to Heinz Kohut (1973), we need to distinguish between the vertical and horizontal boundaries. In repression, memory material is submerged below the horizontal boundary. This material is no longer accessible to consciousness by means of active remembering, on the contrary, irreversible active forgetting has taken place. However, shocks and psychoanalytic techniques allow this seemingly irreversible process to be reversed. One somewhat caricatured example is to be found in Hitchcock's film "Spellbound". Elimination from the balance of values can, however, have even more radical intra-psychological causes, namely, splits in personality in the sense of the vertical boundary described by Kohut. Here, particularly in "borderline personalities", fracturing and segmentation of the personality take place, with whole components of intra-psychological activity being removed from consciousness while reappearing as intact personality components. Other ways of coping with deficits in the balance of values are to be found in various types of delusions, the essence of which is the appearance of "falsifications" within the balance of values, with the "internal court of judgement" (cf. Kleist's play "The Broken Pitcher") applying various different criteria, enlarging certain positive components while reducing negative ones.

6. Neurobiological Experience

The fact that the dimension of time is an extremely relevant aspect within the experience of depression is indicated by, for example, the time-dependent typical course of the intensity of the symptomatology in endogenous kinds of depression. Therefore, the dimension of time in melancholia was recognized as a dominant factor to perform a special kind of "dominance of time".

Another important aspect, however, regarding the pathogenesis of depressive diseases was also recognized: this involved the impact of the neurophysiology of memory systems. Is depression a type of memory deficit, a lack of forgetting in the sense of Nietzsche? With regards to this point, depression may be suggested as an extreme and rigid adherence to the "facts of the past". As a consequence, this may lead to an intense pressure without any creative possibilities or options of future intentional acting.

We have tried to measure phenomenological aspects of Theunissen's theory of time, using objective neurophysiological parameters. In this way, it should, in addition, be possible to gain more information about a main problem in psychiatry, the coupling between emotional and cognitive processing. How do thoughts and emotions interact? Which part does the memory system play with this in mind?

Therefore, we made use of a continuous word recognition experiment (Rugg 1995) which we modified specifically according to the emotional connotation of the presented words. We presented words with negative, positive and neutral emotional content on a video monitor and, at the same time, measured the electrophysiological activity, the EEG. One method, however, to measure the stimulus related electrical activity, the activity which is related to the presentation of the words, is to record so-called event-related brain potentials (ERPs). ERPs are minute voltage fluctuations, which can be recorded non-invasively from the intact human scalp occurring in response to stimulus events simultaneously to their cognitive processing. These ERPs have been shown to be sensitive to memory processes and to emotional factors on cognitive processes, e.g. face recognition. In addition, a frontal positive activity starting around 250 ms post stimulus has been described for emotional stimuli which were more pronounced when subjects were instructed to focus on the emotional connotation of the stimulus.

We identified ERPs as a tool to investigate memory processing in depressive patients with a special emphasis on electrophysiological correlates of the emotion/cognition-coupling. Therefore, we presented words on a video monitor with some words being repeated after a number of intervening items in a continuous word recognition paradigm. For every presentation of the words, the depressive patients or control subjects had to decide whether this word was presented for the first (first presentation) or the second time (repetition).

For the repeated words the event-related potentials have more positive potentials (deflection) of about 200 – 800 ms post stimulus, which is the result of a priming or repetition effect (cf. Figure 2). The presented words in our experiment were classified into three groups depicting different emotional content: negative words like "to die", positive words like "to kiss" or neutral words like "to go". These differentiations were not known by the subjects.

The question arises as to how depressive patients respond to the presentation of the words with different emotional content compared to healthy control subjects?

Figure 2 shows the average ERPs for the 3 different categories of words for 11 healthy control subjects for the midline electrode positions (from frontal to parietal). In particular, frontally, the negative and positive toned words (verbs) induced a greater difference between the first and second presentation compared to the neutral words. This difference is called old/new-effect ("new" for the first presentation and "old" for the second presentation of the words) or EM-effect (as episodic memory is mainly involved in the underlying processes (Friedman & Johnson 2000).

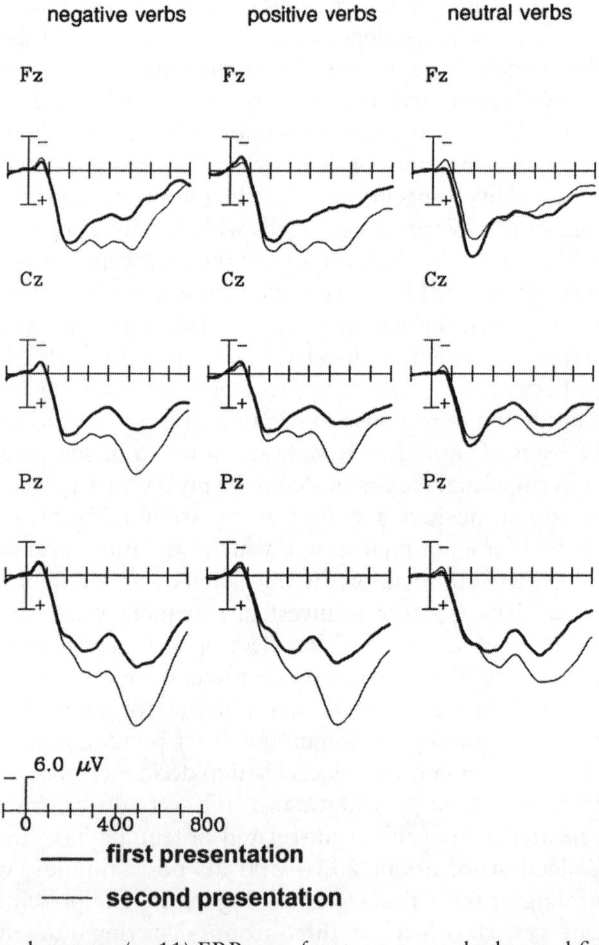

Figure 2: Grand average (n=11) ERP waveforms to correctly detected first (thick line) and second (thin line) presentations of the words (verbs) for the control subjects. The second presentations of words elicited a more positive waveform starting at about 200 ms after onset of the stimulus. This old/new-effect demonstrated here for the central electrodes (Fz, Cz, Pz) is more pronounced for the presentation of the "emotionally toned" negative and positive words.

In the depressive patients (cf. Figure 3) this difference is almost eliminated.

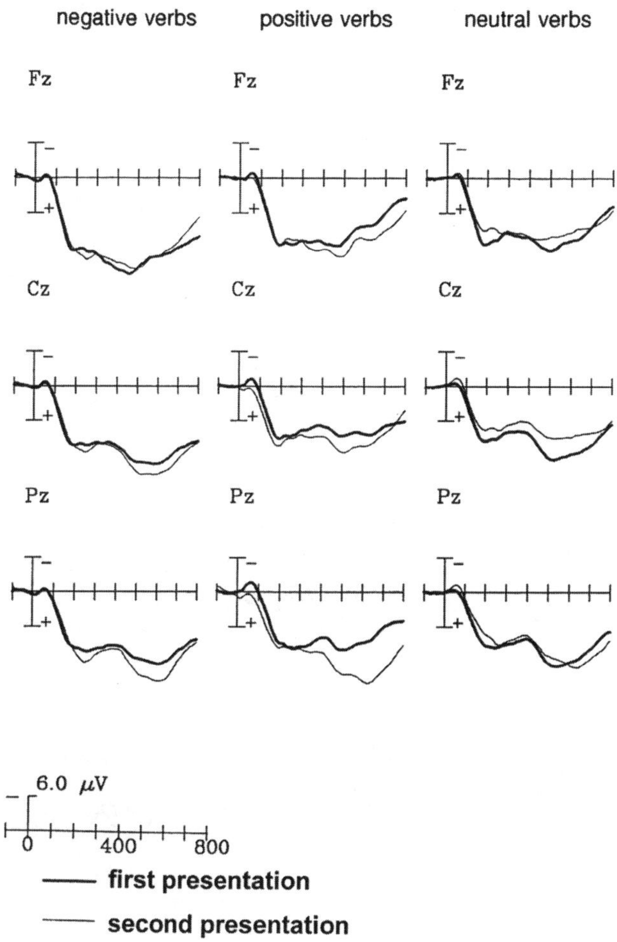

Figure 3: Grand average (n=9) ERP waveforms to correctly detected first (thick line) and second (thin line) presentations of the words (verbs) for the depressive patients. The old/new-effect is significantly reduced compared to the control subjects.

This may be understood by suggesting that the cognitive hippocampal memory system, including the frontal cortical structures, was influenced by the negative emotional memory system: it seems to be primed and influenced especially by negative cognitions and memories which lead to this massive reduction of the old/new-difference. The system appears to be influenced by negative cognitions. This may be clarified by demonstrating the ERPs for the first presentations only as shown in Figure 4.

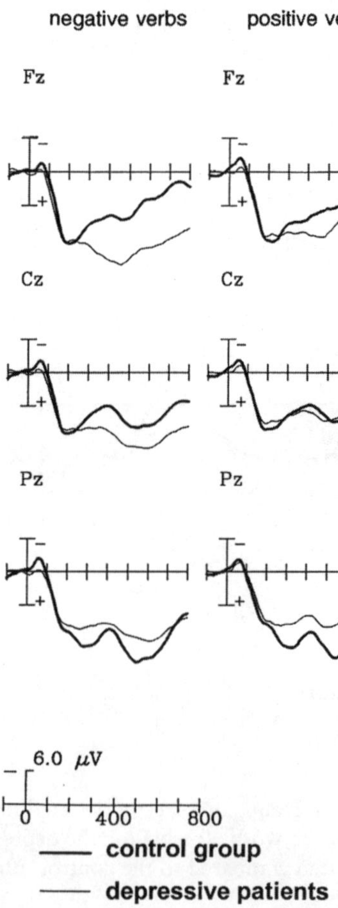

Figure 4: Grand average ERP´s to correctly detected first presentations of the words only for the control group (n=11; thick line) and for the depressive patients (n=9; thin line).

The depressive patients' event-related potentials for the first presentation are so pronounced, it is as if they had been presented before. This is congruent with the account of Theunissen, i.e. that depressive patients appear to be under massive pressure due to their negatively toned cognitions, their negatively charged memory system, and the dominance of time.

7. Psychotherapeutic Aspects: "Active" Forgetting

Following Theunissen's concept of "resistance to the dominance of time" (1992), we will now deal with a type of "active" disregard as a type of "forgetting process", namely disregard in the sense of forgetting as a creatively interpretative representation. What is involved here is a means of dealing with the past by using the imagination to gain access to the life-path that lies behind one while including all the options which were not chosen; also by using the imagination to bring to life subliminal "experiences" in the context of the "processes of choosing" which took place when travelling along this path. One might term this the "Proustian method". Theunissen describes it as follows:

> Proust is able to recall 'regained time' precisely by destroying it. Memory which functions as an organ of reconciliation is spontaneous in that it springs forth from the solid context of occurrences and opens itself to the unique in which the subject perceives the internal subjective world, this specific world which he has continually suppressed on the basis of what appeared to be external. In that it reveals the surface of memory. It is similar to Hegel's 're-collection' (Hegel 1973).

This type of active forgetting entails an imaginative time travel to the past and integrating the past into present life. Thereby it is possible to forget, and thus "solve" depression.

References:

Bar-On, D. 1988. "Did Holocaust perpetrators feel guilty in retrospect?" In: Bar-On, D., Beiner, F., Brusten, M. (eds.) *Der Holocaust – Familiale und gesellschaftliche Folgen.* Ergebnisse eines internationalen Forschungs-Kolloquiums an der Bergischen Universität, Wuppertal.

Cramer, F. 1993. *Der Zeitbaum. Grundlegung einer allgemeinen Zeittheorie.* Frankfurt: Insel Verlag.

Desimone, R., Miller, E.K., Chelazzi, L., Lueschow, A. 1995. "Multiple Memory Systems in the Visual Cortex", in: Gazzaniga, M. (ed.) *The Cognitive Neurosciences.* Cambridge, Massachusetts: MIT Press, 475-486.

Ehlers, J. 2003. "Concepts of Time in Physics: Insights Obtained and Open Questions", Lecture at the International Conference "On Time", Einstein Forum Potsdam.

Emrich, H.M. 1992. "Konstruktivismus: Imagination, Traum und Emotionen", in: Schmidt, S.J. (ed.) *Kognition und Gesellschaft. Der Diskurs des Radikalen Konstruktivismus*. Frankfurt: Suhrkamp, 76-96.
Emrich, H.M. 1998. "Synästhesie, Emotion und Illusion", in: Kunst- und Ausstellungshalle der Bundesrepublik Deutschland (ed.) *Der Sinn der Sinne*. Schriftenreihe Forum Band 8. Göttingen: Steidl, 126-139.
Friedman, D., Johnson R. Jr. 2000. "Event-related potential (ERP) studies of memory encoding and retrieval: a selective review". *Microscopy Research and Technique* 51: 6-28.
Gondek, H.-D. 1990. "Das Versprechen und seine Verbindlichkeit", in: Holz, K. (ed.) *Soziologie zwischen Moderne und Postmoderne. Untersuchungen zu Subjekt, Erkenntnis und Moral*. Gießen: Focus, 39-65.
Gray, J.A., Rawlins, J.N.P. 1986. "Comparator and buffer memory: an attempt to integrate two models of hippocampal functions", in: Isaacson, R.L., Pribram, K.H. (eds.) *The Hippocampus*. Plenum vol. 4, New York, 151-201.
Hegel, G.W.F. 1973. *Phänomenologie des Geistes*. Frankfurt a.M.: Suhrkamp.
Heisenberg, M. 1989. "Über Universalien der Wahrnehmung und ihre genetischen Grundlagen", in: *Mannheimer Forum 1989*. München: Piper.
Kohut, H. 1973. *Narzißmus*. Frankfurt a. M.: Suhrkamp,
Nietzsche, F. 1981. *Unzeitgemäße Betrachtungen*. Frankfurt a.M.: Insel.
Peitgen, H.-O. 1993. "Fraktale – gezähmtes Chaos". Lecture at XVI. Deutscher Kongress für Philosophie, Berlin 20.-24. Sept. 1993.
Pöppel, E. 1985. *Die Grenzen des Bewußtseins*. Stuttgart: DVA.
Proust, M. 1993. *Auf der Suche nach der verlorenen Zeit*. Frankfurt a.M.: Suhrkamp
Rugg, M.D. 1995. "ERP studies of memory", in: Rugg, M.D., Coles, M.G.H. (eds.) *Electrophysiology of mind, event-related brain potentials and cognition*; Oxford Psychology Series, No. 25. Oxford: Oxford University Press, 130-170.
Singer, W. 1990. "Search for coherence: a basic principle of cortical self-organization", *Concepts in Neuroscience*, 1: 1-26.
Theunissen, M. 1992. *Negative Theologie der Zeit*. Frankfurt a.M.: Suhrkamp.

Compulsion, Volitional Disorder, and Freedom of the Will

Rigidity: The Strange Preference for Compulsion

Martin Löw-Beer

This article aims to describe certain patterns of behaviour that are usually criticized as rigid. By "description" I do not mean to give mere examples nor do I wish to give a definition of rigidity. Rather my aim is normative. I wish to show what is wrong with rigidity.

Before I can go into the analysis of rigidity I would like to point out what I mean by this concept, what I mean with "normative critique" and why I think it is important in the case of rigidity.

What is "rigidity"?

To what classes of objects does "rigidity" apply? Persons, their relationship to themselves and also their behaviour can be rigid. "Rigidity", Shapiro says, is a "way of life", a system of reasoning, motivation and behaviour that persons do not choose in the sense of having an alternative. Nevertheless, it would be wrong to say that "rigidity" is a compulsive character trait, because rigid people usually identify with the way they behave and reason. However, rigidity is also compulsive: The rigid person typically needs pressure, emergencies, duties, pseudorationality in order to be motivated. He seems to search for situations or a description that force him to act. The pressure that forces him to act is not freely chosen but nevertheless self-created. Superficially, it is similar to willpower. The latter applies when a person chooses a task that is difficult for him and, therefore, has to concentrate and discipline himself to manage. Willpower is often necessary for being successful in those projects with which one identifies. But this is not the case with the rigid person; he is not involved in something which he values deeply. On the contrary, he needs pressure to find out what he should do.

I mentioned before that the rigid person identifies with the way he is reasoning. How can someone not value his projects and still be identified with what he is doing? The answer is that the rigid values reason and duty. He believes that he does what everybody in his situation should do and that he argues in a way that everybody should accept. The rigid person believes that he is doing his duty and that he follows rules that everybody who is in a similar situation should, according to him, accept. Often the rigid does not succeed in these endeavours. It is not surprising that he has difficulties to find binding maxims in situations of freedom of choice, where neither moral obligation, nor self-preservation, nor reasonable considerations do determine what one should do. That is when the rigid is afflicted with decision problems. He is suffering from freedom.

Why is a description of rigidity important?

Why is it interesting to find out what is wrong with the rigid? Because the usual criteria of autonomy apply in his case. He is a caricature of rationality and morality. In asking himself reflectively what to do and reverting to principles to answer this question, he seems to comply with the criteria of autonomy and rationality. Still, for the person who observes the rigid, he will be judged as heteronomous and irrational. Therefore the rigid case renders doubtful the standard model of autonomy. I will not argue for a revision of the model, but merely wish to point out that the rigid case makes us pay attention to presuppositions of the model. For instance, one has to be in touch with one's likes and dislikes to be able to reflect on what one should do.

Normative critique

In what sense is rigidity wrong? I will argue that it is irrational and objectively compulsive. The rigid is irrational in the sense that his style of living harms himself without compensating this disadvantage.

One can compare that with a driver who passes a red traffic light. By doing so purposely he is risking the lives of others as well as his own. Why does he do that? Perhaps he was elsewhere with his thoughts. To drive absent-mindedly is irrational in a weak sense of the word; one should be concentrating when behind the steering wheel. Otherwise there is a grave risk of causing an accident and harming somebody. Another supposition would imply that the driver has good reason to believe that passing the red light is a matter of life or death. Under these circumstances his act of risk could be justified. It could also be that the driver does it with purpose but without any reason, just because he has the urge to do it. This would be grossly irrational and is comparable with rigidity. The latter involves an action in which a person does harm to herself without having any sound reasons to do so.

This comparison is not accurate. It just gives a drastic hint. One significant difference is that the rigid usually has no choice. He has no alternative to the rigid way of orientation. This is what I mean with "objectively compulsive". Although most of the time the rigid has no alternative because he cannot articulate his subjective likes and dislikes, he does not feel forced into his rigid way of life. This is certainly true if feeling forced implies being aware of it in an articulate way. But one could argue that there is indirect knowledge: By failing in his disciplinarian exercises the rigid indirectly expresses his opposition. In some examples one gets the impression that the rigid has alternatives but that they are too painful to be even articulated. It is the hypothesis of this article that rigidity as a way of life has the function to escape suffering from painful experiences. In such cases rigidity does not seem to be a crazy choice but an understandable alienating mode of defence against adverse situations in life. By leaving the position of a participant and becoming an observer of oneself the rigid becomes less exposed to painful circumstances. But for this defence the rigid pays a high price: no strong satisfactions, no subjective orientation in life, in the sense of discovering what is important for oneself, no pursuing of projects in the mode of identification.[1] The danger is that rigidity becomes independent of this useful function and turns into a dominating mode of being.

---

1 It makes good sense to describe the genesis of the irrationality of rigidity by a defence story. If subjective orientation becomes too painful, one substitutes personal likes and dislikes by impersonal maxims. What was useful in defence situations becomes irrational as a mode of orientation that is independent of a defensive purpose. While it is certainly a relief to get rid of one's sufferings, it is ridiculous to install pressure with the aim of getting to know what one should do in situations where one would be otherwise free to do what one wants. The development of irrational modes of behaviour out of rational reactions in stressful situations is the normal fate of defence mechanisms.
Such descriptions derive from experiences and reflections in therapeutic encounters. Empirically these stories invite doubts especially if one gives in to the temptation to generalize and leave behind the retrospective perspective. When persons have to live through certain kinds of painful situations then they will act defensively in the mode of y and this will have the consequences x. Generalized or lawlike statements like this tend to be falsified by counterexamples. One will almost certainly find people who have experienced the same kind of sufferings and did not react in the same experience erasing way.
This is why it seems to me reasonable to understand the genetic story in a different way. If a person is unable to articulate subjective likes and dislikes, if his wants are boiled down to what is reasonable for everybody to want in most situations – self-preservation is an example – then there is something wrong with him. He represses subjective inclinations that are presuppositions that he can care about things and people. This is supported by the trivial anthropological hypothesis that persons have – besides insight in impersonal imperatives – the ability to have personal wants and engagements that are important for them, without being necessarily important for everybody. If this individualizing ability is missing, then something is wrong with the person. If interpretations and other interventions that derive from the genetic defence story are effective in generating subjectivity without using manipulative tools, then this supports this kind of genetic defence stories. Rigidity, if it is understood as developing out of repressions serving defensive purposes, does not seem to be the whole defence story that applies in cases of rigidity. There seem to be other examples of rigidity with a genesis where people aim to get rid of being a wanting, feeling and dependent animal. Rigidity develops when they change from a participant and performative position into the stance of an observer, who looks for prescriptions. They are unable to deal individually with the expectations of others and the society and just able to subjugate to roles and expectations in a passive way. Again we have a supporting anthropological thesis: The performative position cannot be given up totally but one can motivate the participant from an observer position or one can reduce the participant to a conformist.

Conscious alienation: Obsessive compulsive disorder

Before turning to examples of rigidity, I wish to explain the difference between objective and subjective compulsion.[2] Objective compulsion is the case in which a person arranges situations in a way which makes all alternatives but one unreasonable. Here he does not feel forced in an alienating way. The pressure that tells him what to do seems to correspond with his wants. He is unaware that he needs the self-installed pressure for orientation.

Quite the contrary, subjective compulsion is a felt force that the subject classifies as ego-dystonic. He feels forced to comply with certain thoughts through actions that seem to him irrational. This forced activity depends on behaving towards certain thoughts as if they were true, although the actor himself does not believe in them. This is what is meant by "ego-dystonic". Another classifying name for the same phenomena would be "conscious alienation" while rigidity could be called a form of "unconscious alienation". But can a person be forced to believe in what he does not believe? He cannot, but he may be forced to perform actions that usually presuppose beliefs that he does not accept. Usually compulsions are a reaction to obsessions that are disturbing and frightening for a person. Compulsions are understood as a means to get rid of frightening obsessions. That is why psychiatry speaks of obsessive-compulsive disorders that are subsumed under the broad category of anxiety disorders. Obsessions are frightening because of their content but

---

The participant stance in its individualized form presupposes that one is taken seriously in one's place in society and in one's utterances. If this acknowledgement of oneself is missing then people lose self-respect. They have no acknowledged place in society and even less a symmetric relationship to others. They try to relieve the resulting pain by retreating into an observing position from which they construct what everybody should want, who is in their situation. These are situations where people try to get rid of the participant role because they want to fend off painful meanings. In the last part of the paper I wish to describe this form of defence. Again, the therapeutic effect of applying this interpretation will support or weaken it. The therapeutic aim is to give people back their ability to react spontaneously to the expectations of others who take their reactions seriously. And again, this is a hypothesis that can be applied only retrospectively. Not everybody who is not taken seriously in his roles will retreat into the self-observing position. But probably nearly everybody who does it is suffering from failures of recognition and can perhaps be healed by relations in which he is taken seriously as a speaker and which enables him to exert influence on others by his utterances.

2 In an interesting discussion of mental and somatic illness, Schramme (2000) distinguishes between the lack of important functions as pathological and the subjective suffering that leads to the judgement: "I feel ill". While the standard of physiological functions is the normal ability to cope and to reproduce, the deficit of functions that are connected with feeling ill are not only associated with the former functions but also with important presuppositions of a good life, like the ability to have social contacts or to enjoy life.

even more important because of their penetrating and disturbing presence. The suffering person tries, without success, to eliminate them. Frightening obsessions force people to act as if certain doubts that the person judges as irrational were true. This can be illustrated by the following examples: A person loses a lot of time by checking that he has turned off the gas in the kitchen. The doubts that he has forgotten to do this are so tormenting that the person finally gives in to them. From this it does not follow that he believes in the doubts: his aim in checking again and again is to gain peace of mind. He is like the compulsive hand washer who is obsessed by the idea that his hands could be infected by dangerous bacteria. In empirical matters there is always the logical possibility of error. That is why orientating oneself in the empirical world by a standard that does not allow for the logical possibility of mistakes is self-defeating. But this knowledge does not help the compulsive person, because he cannot control the doubts that are based on the possibility that something terrible could happen. The similarity between rigidity and these cases is not limited to the trait of compulsiveness. Both have alienated motivational systems that are dysfunctional for orientation in the world and for living a good life. They are both irrational in the explained sense of Gert, meaning that these people do harm to themselves without adequate compensation (Gert & Culver 1982, pp. 27-31).

Until now we have given just an abstract description of rigidity. I would now like to introduce the phenomena by giving examples. Fortunately, there are two excellent books by David Shapiro that give detailed descriptions of the cluster of phenomena (Shapiro 1965, 1981).

Cases of rigidity

Let us start with an example that is typical of the inflexibility involved in rigidity:

> Two friends K and L are discussing the purchase of a house in which K is interested.
>
> K: So you think I shouldn't buy it?
>
> L: Never buy a house with a bad roof. It will cost you its price again in repairs before you're finished.
>
> K: But the builder I hired to survey it did say it was in good condition.
>
> L: The roof is only the beginning. First it's the roof and then comes the plumbing and then the heating and then the plaster.
>
> K: Still, those things seem to be all right.
>
> L: and after the plaster it will be the wiring.
>
> K: But the wiring is...
>
> L (interrupts with calm assurance): It will cost double the price before you are finished. (Shapiro 1965, p. 25)

L pays wilful inattention to the reasons that make his decision-rule doubtful. Knowing clearly what to do seems to him more important than an adequate account of the situation. The rule to which the rigid is clinging does not derive from a reflection on the situation, but is defended by closing his mind to relevant information that speaks against the "roof–theorem".

- Making decisions:

"(...) one patient maintained that he must avoid watching television since he might enjoy it, wish to watch more, become addicted and then do nothing else and, what would become of the book he was writing?" (ibid., p. 44)

The trivial wish to watch TV is interpreted as making him ill and unable to work. If one happens to be successful in describing alternatives in a contrasting way – life or death, culture or barbarism, relaxation as losing control and becoming crazy – then decisions become easy. The rigid person needs contrasting scenarios, in which all but one alternative are unreasonable to choose: this enables him to decide in the name of reason.

- Pressure makes decisions easier:

> One patient decided that he must have a better job by his next birthday or else he would have to regard himself as a failure. Of course he then felt greatly under pressure as the day approached, as anyone would given his assumption. With the passing of his birthday the deadline was shifted to the first of the year, and so on. (ibid., p. 33)

Weak normative expectations are interpreted as duties. "Thus such people feel that propriety requires them to dress neatly, duty obliges them to visit Aunt Tilly (...) mental health necessitates a number of hobbies and a certain degree of 'relaxation', culture a determinate amount of reading and music (...)" (ibid., p. 39)

- Trivial decisions are derived from principles:

The time-planning of the rigid is strange: "One such person carefully scheduled his Sundays with certain activities in order to produce 'maximum enjoyment'" (ibid., p. 32). These people do not find satisfaction as such in performing the activities but in the knowledge that they are spending their free time efficiently.

> When he is confronted by the necessity for a decision, even one which may be trivial from a normal standpoint, the obsessive compulsive person will typically attempt to reach a solution by invoking some rule, some principle, or external requirement

> which might with some degree of plausibility, provide a 'right' answer (...). Thus, if he can remember that it always makes more sense to go to the cheapest movie or 'logical' to go to the closest, or beneficial to go to the most educational, the problem resolves to a technical one, simply finding which is the most educational, the closest or such. In an effort to find such requirements and principles, he will invoke morality, 'logic', social custom, propriety (...). (ibid., pp. 46f.)

- The function of roles:

Roles tell rigid persons what to do, to wish and to feel and even more important, they inform the rigid persons who they are:

"A patient felt well only as long as he knew what role he was supposed to 'play' When at work he thought 'I am a worker' and this gave him the necessary security; when at home, 'Now I am the husband who comes home from work to his beloved family.'" (ibid., p. 38)

- Value judgements are derived from "objective" standards:

> One patient, for example, said of the girl he planned to marry, 'I must be in love with her – she has all the qualities I want in a wife (...) The same point is illustrated by the case of a lawyer who selected his clothes every morning with the aid of a colour wheel. He apparently did not experience the thought or feeling, 'this looks good' or 'this is nice,' but rather 'This fits-according to the rules, it must look good.' (ibid., p. 50)

These examples show that rigid persons prefer being dependent on pressure in the form of pseudonecessities or sanctions to self-determination. Nevertheless the will plays an important role in the life of the rigid:

> Wilful directedness has been distorted from its normal subjective significance as an extension and, so to speak, representative of one's needs to a position of precedence over needs, aimed even at directing them (...). Thus for these people impulse or wish is only a temptation which can corrupt their determination, interrupt their work, interfere with what they feel they 'should' wish to be doing (...). They are, therefore, cut off from the sources that normally give wilful effort its direction (...) (ibid., p. 37).

The rigid person wants to forget the problems that define what is subjectively meaningful for her and identify instead with perspectives that derive from principles that are reasonable. These principles should show her the way to a new life. They are made plausible for the rigid in a way that is more or less independent of the individual biography. Willpower should be the tool to fulfil these principles.

An example of the development of rigidity

The following example tells of a wish for such a new beginning, in which the person plans to become someone else, liberated from the dependencies that were caused by her emotions. The case is especially interesting because it describes a motivated transformation into rigidity that is prevented by the interventions of a therapist.

After an unhappy love affair a patient declares that she wants to move and make a new start. She complains that she cannot bring herself to fulfil this project of moving into surroundings where she would be alien. She criticizes herself of being weak-willed in the following dialogue with her therapist:

> Patient: What is the matter with me! I want to move, but I can't seem to get started! It's nothing but inertia, typical of me (...). That's the way I live my life, by inertia. Not doing what I really want to do.
> Therapist: Usually people don't have to overcome so much inertia to do what they really want to do. As matter of fact, when they are that eager, it's hard to hold them back.
> Patient: Well it's not exactly that I'm eager. But I know that's what I want in the long run.
> Therapist: Evidently the short run looks bad.
> Patient: But I know it would be good for me!
> Therapist: That's quite a different thing from wanting to do it.
> Patient: Whether I want to do it or I don't want to do it; I should do it! I have to learn to become independent! I have to go to some place where I can't call people all the time, where there's nobody to go to, where I have to take care of myself because I don't know a soul and I will either sink or swim!
> Therapist: I see why you are not rushing off to do it.
> Patient: It would be horrible. (She bursts into tears.) (Shapiro 1981, p. 72)

This patient has a rigid ideal and a rigid way of dealing with herself. She has the ideal of becoming independent of her wishes and emotions. Her wants, which she is not able to identify anymore, inhibit her not to move in this direction. She misidentifies them as inertia, weakness of the will. She believes in willpower as a mechanism that should bridge the gap between what she wishes and what she believes she should do.

The main lesson of the example seems to me that the person has given up her ability to orientate herself according to her wants, beliefs and experiences. Instead, she attempts to bring herself to believe what she should want and think. Her low sense of self-confidence and her wish to be rid of her problems motivate her to adopt an ego-ideal that she thinks she should believe in. Her will should help her to fulfil the task of coping with day to day life according to an alienated ideal that should fend off and substitute her painful self-interpretations.

Rigidity: A substitute for self-orientation?

In the following I wish to point out that rigidity is a symptom of disorientation. The rigid person is tormented by a decision problem and invents all kinds of devices that narrow his freedom of choice. This disorientation is a result of turning his back on his problems together with his wants and what is important for him. He has erased the context of his life and is now confronted with the task to orient himself by drawing on nothing but his place in society, conventions and impersonal principles. This explains the strange preference for the lack of freedom which the rigid person imposes upon himself. He gives the impression that he wishes to turn into a robot activated by decisions prescribed by a program. Remember that he feels more secure when he reminds himself in which role he happens to be – "a husband who comes home from work to his beloved family". Remember also the contrasting descriptions he constructs, that make only one option reasonable and also the pressure he puts upon himself by organizing deadlines. Even to get a clear notion about his emotional relationship to others he needs objective clues as if he were a disengaged observer who is guessing what a person whose situation he knows, might feel. Remember the rigid person who deduces from the objective qualities that he sees in a woman that he is in love with her. He is in need of objective reasons, because he does not know how he feels towards her. All this becomes comprehensible if one assumes that the rigid person needs these attributes to orientate himself, that by them he gets to know who he is and what to do. The rigid person is in the position of an observer who finds out his place in society and then asks himself what is best to do for any person in this position. He only subscribes to rational principles or conventions to answer this question. The thesis I wish to bring up is that the rigid person has lost his sense of self, i.e. that he has given up his role as a participant who finds things right or wrong, important, unimportant, attractive or repulsive. On the one hand, he overcomes his problems that were the problems of a participant, but, on the other hand, acquires instead the decision problems of an observer who knows just where he is located in society and what is considered reasonable for anyone. That is why he is faced with terrible difficulties in making trivial decisions like how to spend his free time or to which movie to go: because there are usually arbitrary principles that give answers to these questions. Only by taking the participant view can a person know who he is in the sense of knowing what is important for him, how he sees others, what his interests, desires, also his inhibitions are, and what sense of self-worth he has.

Observational and participant view

People need to coordinate the following abilities to orientate themselves. 1) A person needs to know which position he has in society. Where he is, which role he is performing. What the expectations of others are, what his possibilities are. Here the person is taking the view of an observer. 2) Participant view: how does the person feel in his roles, is he doing what he really wants? People experience relationships as agreeable, unsuitable, they fall in love, get annoyed by certain kinds of behaviour, are impressed by certain organisations and alarmed by others, have a sense of what is important for them, want to keep certain things private and make others public, feel inhibited in the presence of certain people, become interested in something, are absorbed by a book. "Participant" also means reacting to issues in communication as right or wrong, interesting, relevant, to speakers as being truthful etc. If there is any doubt about the "validity claims" in communication, reasons come into play. In the participant stance there should be room for spontaneity and reflection.

If statements are surprising or if one is impressed, attracted or repulsed by a situation and does not understand why this is so, one has reasons to reflect to get a clearer view on one's situation. Spontaneous reactions and intuitions provide a basis for the resource of reflection. Reflection is not just a reason-giving activity, it is also an activity that gives room for articulation and to the ability of imagination: How would I feel if I were in his situation? How would I wish the relationship to develop?

Sometimes we do not need to talk because we can already assess the expectations of others (second person perspective) and also what is generally expected from us (third person perspective). Many of our performances can be understood as reactions to these expectations.

Integrated in the participant stance is a biographical dimension. We cannot understand the importance that success has for a person, if we do not understand the difficulties that lie behind this person. One cannot comprehend why a person engages so much time in an activity, if one does not know about the hopes and desires and the memories connected with it.

I describe all these dimensions because they are missing or are transformed in rigidity: There is no spontaneity, because it is interpreted as a loss of control. Openness is missing, which is necessary for spontaneity as well as reflection. Shapiro tells the story of "the compulsive man, who examines each woman with a checklist in mind of certain qualifications for marriage (...). This is (...) an awareness that is not open and attentive to the world but is restricted and prejudiced by the necessity to satisfy pre-established requirements and fixed purposes." (Shapiro 1981, p. 75) In addition, the rigid person is negligent of the second-person-perspective because the application of dogmatically believed principles decides matters for him. For the rigid person, impersonal principles and rules are the passpartout for all circumstances.

On a more general level, the observational stance is taking part in a discourse about function. So it tells us about institutions and their function for the reproduction of society and it even tells us about the psychic states of individuals. There could be someone who registers that he feels hate towards somebody who has offended him. From an observational point of view, the person will recognize that the offence was the cause of the hatred and he will ask himself what to do with the negative emotion. Perhaps he remembers the hydraulic model, which states that emotions need to be expressed like steam under pressure, or he subscribes to a functional model, which states that retaliation leads to an endless unproductive chain that swallows valuable energy.

From the participant stance, the person will ask: how much pain does he feel; what were the reasons for the offence? Can he share them? Or are they irrational like e.g. a racist attack? Seen from the participant stance, history is understood by imaginatively participating in a praxis. This is helpful if one wants to understand the significance that activities have for many people. For instance, without reading books ourselves, we are unable to understand how this praxis can become something fascinating, or without engaging in love and intimacy we cannot understand the feeling of jealousy and how it hurts. On the other side, seen from the observational stance, the story will be all causal and functional.

It is an analytical fiction to think that the observational and the participant view are normally separated. Only as means of defence against painful interpretations it can happen that the participant stance, in which the person used to be, is given up with its wants, emotions and projects.

It is possible to give up self-orientation, but as long as one is conscious and acting, one remains in the participant perspective in the sense that a person must act and make decisions. The rigid person tries to feed the participant stance with stuff that is delivered from the observational perspective. He has to rely mainly on the observational and impersonal views in order to answer the questions who he is and what he is going to do. By thereby cutting himself off from the context in which activities make sense, he acts in a deeply confused way. Living a decontextualized life the rigid person is similar to the philosopher who is criticized by Wittgenstein in his *Philosophical Investigations*. Instead of taking into account the context that makes activities meaningful, the philosopher concentrates on the mental events that accompany statements, falsely identifying them with their meaning. Think again of the example of the transformation of the flexible competence to concentrate. So "these people not only concentrate, they seem always to be concentrating" (Shapiro 1964, p. 27). It is as if they have to decide between a life spent in concentration or living in an uncontrolled way. Being dissociated of the problems in which they were involved, the decision to concentrate has no particular object apart from one's whole life. To admonish oneself "to concentrate" makes sense, if one realizes that one is making mistakes in an activity like driving, but concentration without an apt object becomes an empty ritual. The same is true of effort: it makes sense in relation to certain tasks, but the mental experience of effort is nothing but a sign that one tries to achieve something. It is like the woman who complains how hard it is to stop smoking, who makes noises, e.g. sighs, in order to express her mental effort, while she is lighting a cigarette.

The rigid person is like somebody who lives in a society but merely in the position of an observer. He finds out where he is located and then scrutinizes what would be the best thing to do for anyone in such a situation, without even thinking what he cares about. He can draw only on abstract principles and directives that are prima facie plausible and can be formulated in imperatives: Do your duty! Don't harm yourself! Try to survive! Enjoy your free time! Work hard! Pay attention and concentrate! Find out what you really want and do it! Follow your obligations! Such imperatives are useful in a context where people are confronted with problems they have to deal with. But they are not self-sufficient in the sense that they alone can inform a person what is best to do. Now we can see why the rigid person has difficulties with decisions: because he is isolated from the problems of his life and interests, and has given up all effort to find out what is important to him. He ceases to take a participant perspective, but knows only how he is situated in society and that some principles are rational, while others have to be chosen arbitrarily. These impersonal principles serve the function to substitute his self-orientation based on being an individual in this world.

If this diagnosis is correct in principle, then it supports the intuition that rigid persons are not autonomous. They have renounced their self-orientation and are dependent on impersonal principles that cannot be reasonably applied, because the context and the wants and interests that would give them some meaning is missing.

Conclusion

Of course this analysis of rigidity is rather one-sided and the chosen aspect sometimes exaggerated. Perhaps there are no real cases where the release of one's problems and the transposition into an observational perspective is total.

Do persons have a choice to change over to the position of an observer? Can they choose to distance themselves from their problems and erase their sense of what is important to them? I am not sure, but I assume that it is a transformational process that does not happen suddenly but slowly, involving a combination of intentional and unintentional elements.

My excuse for disregarding other aspects of the phenomena is that for the purpose of gaining a clearer picture of a fundamental human ability, namely, contextually informed self-orientation, it was useful to concentrate on this one aspect. The loss of orientation by leaving the participant stance in rigidity is severe enough to support the view that one should refer to it as form of mental illness. We saw in the examples given above how difficult it is to cope without a participant perspective.

The transposition from the perspective of a participant to the perspective of an observer who chooses in a detached way what principles should be motivating for him, is the most impressive feature of rigidity. I have shown that there is some evidence to understand rigidity as the result of a defence mechanism that does not function in the usual way of repressing or transforming wishes but turns against the participant point of view in which persons develop likes and dislike and discover what is important for them. Being a participant has intersubjective presuppositions that I wish to mention in the end: others need to take one seriously, give one the chance to influence them, be open for cooperation and be valued as a human being, as a friend or as valuable member of society. The importance of others is obvious if one considers that they can exclude us, take away from us the right to be a participant. I guess that everybody has made the experience of being excluded in some contexts, be it as a member of a club, as a lover or friend or as being refused admission into a certain professional position. Reciprocally I have to take others seriously, value them. If I do not interpret others as valuable and do not understand them, there is no sense in participating with them.

References

Culver, C., Gert, B. 1982. *Philosophy in Medicine*, Oxford: Oxford U.P.
Schramme, T. 2000. *Patienten und Personen, Zum Begriff der psychischen Krankheit.* Frankfurt: Fischer.
Shapiro, D. 1965. *Neurotic Styles*. New York: Basic Books.
Shapiro, D. 1981. *Autonomy and Rigidity*. New York: Basic Books.

Towards a Psychiatric Anthropology of Addiction

Jann Schlimme

Psychiatric models of understanding often seem inappropriate as regards the inner perspective of the patient. When trying to comprehend the inner perspective of the afflicted person, these concepts lack insight into his everyday life, appear less vivid and even vague or seem burdened with controversial theoretical considerations. Initially, this problem of understanding appears merely to manifest the established difference of subjective and objective perspectives. As psychiatrists, we are forced to acknowledge that this problem extends far deeper, namely, that the "subjective" perspective is nothing else but the inner perspective of an individual. But is there an alternative perspective other than our own? Is the "objective" perspective the result and effect of a complicated process in which the people involved gain a "perspective out of nowhere"? It may well be assumed to be their own perspective but it is not acknowledged as "subjective" because of the complex process of "objectivation". This process of "objectivation" enforces a disregard for many aspects that are important for each individual perspective. This is not only a scientific predicament but also a theoretical problem of cognition.

It could be said that we face the problem of self-illusion, since everyone's self image and image of his own world is more or less an illusion from the viewpoint of others. This would appear to express the traditional difference of the individual and the social side of the single person. If we wish to understand the inner perspective, it is then necessary to take for granted these illusions as part of the inner perspective. All in all, do we not have any illusions about ourselves? Are self illusions as usual in the common "we-self" as in the individual "I-self"? If this is the case, then even we have to admit that these deceptions about oneself/ourselves can only be referred to as illusions, once they have been identified as such. As Feuerbach once expressed: Neither the individual nor the social self of a person is more fundamental or primary, however, they originate simultaneously (Feuerbach 1996). With regards this quotation, our theory of cognition appears to be quite different: we should forget the differentiation of "subjective" and "objective" and consider the synchronism of individuality and sociality.

According to this approach, a common perspective is explained as the result of a common process which incorporates many people. A common self – a "we-self" – evolves in this process so that the involved persons reach an understanding of themselves or their world (Rombach 1994). This explanation of scientific perspectives and scientific psychiatric models is similar to Ernst

Cassirer's theory, especially his distinction between symbol and object. Cassirer defines the human being as an "animal symbolicum". For him, terms, ideas and symbols are "primary" compared to the existent object. Objects correspond to these terms, ideas and symbols. Since the scientific process is one way of objectivation (like myths or religion) and understood as an approximation between scientific understanding and objects, "absolute objectivity" is an illusion comparable to "absolute subjectivity" (Cassirer 1990). Even if we claim the simultaneousness of symbol and object and hold on to this concept like Cassirer, namely, standing in the tension of "evolution" and "consolidation", the objectivated perspectives will still be "subjective" since we are unable to estimate ourselves completely by means of understanding or cognition. This understanding is anthropocentric, since our own perspective is all we have. It can be a social or a common perspective, or even an individual one.

Understanding of "Addiction" in the Age of Enlightenment

The Age of Enlightenment plays a focal role in the psychiatric anthropology of addiction. The changes in the understanding of regular or constant consumption of psychotropic substances (especially alcohol) at this time will be considered. In the Age of Enlightenment the knowledge of oneself as a human being was orientated at the individual self-enlightenment and the principal independence of situational aspects due to rational participation of the reason. The idea of freedom became equal with individual *autonomy* (Baruzzi 1993). This affords the distinction of "object" and "subject" and a definition of the subject as the individual person independent of a possible creator, of its world or society.

Historically, this distinction of "subjective" and "objective" was preformulated by René Descartes (1596-1650) in his concept of *res cogitans* and *res extensa* (Descartes 1994). However, for Descartes this distinction brought about reassurance as a free human being. Freedom was the new central point of being human in the New Ages, initially proposed as *dignity of man* (Mirandola 1990) in the Renaissance era. Since Descartes understood the *res cogitans* without primary contact with the *res extensa*, he, as a human being, was not subject to the mathematical or mechanical processes fundamentally structuring the *res extensa* in natural law. These processes were accepted as conditions of possibilities for the *res extensa*, but not the independent *res cogitans*. According to Galileo Galilei (1564-1642), these distinctive spheres could come into defined contact via experiments understood as the start of scientific research from our point of view (Galilei 1980, Rombach 1993).

This understanding of the human being changed radically in the Age of Enlightenment and especially with Immanuel Kant (1724-1804), however, the difference of subject and object was deepened even further and not overcome.

Kant argued that the inner perspective was preformed by conditions *a priori* always structuring the possibilities of perception and cognition. Therefore, it is impossible for a human being to know something about the *Ding an sich* (Descartes was of the opinion that humans knew something about the real thing for itself), since all knowledge is prestructured by unchangeable conditions of being human. Beginning with Kant, the world "rotated" around the subject comparable with the copernicanian change.

In connection with this self-understanding as rational and autonomous human beings, new and "sober ecstasies" like coffee, cocoa, tea or tobacco conquered the enlightened or civil classes. The societies were divided and polarized between sobriety and intoxication (Spode 1993). Problems of repeated or constant alcohol consumption were named (organic damages or apoplexy) and the question arose, how it was possible to overcome the vice or habit of drinking. Traditional understanding of repeated, constant and often excessive alcohol consumption as a Christian vice, referring to Augustine's concept of a "wrong will" (Flasch 1994) or as a customary and conscious decision (as formulated especially by the German physician Heinrich Stromer in 1531, Spode 1993), dominated culturally the common idea of chronic alcohol consumption. This can be seen in movements of moderation evident particularly in Europe and in the United States, which called for a more moderate consumption of alcohol. A transformation of this understanding was necessary for the enlightened individual. Following Kant in his *Grundlegung der Metaphysik der Sitten* (1785), chronic intoxication simply made a rational way of life impossible. The rational way of life was laid down as a basis for morality of the individual. Therefore, a drunkard was not a sinner, rather a more or less irrational person (Kant 1990).

Nevertheless, an important question still remained unanswered. Although the enlighteners and the sanitarians claimed that teetotalism would be advisable for a healthy and rational way of life, many people were reluctant to reduce their alcohol intake. If drunkenness was not considered a vice, then how could a lack of rationality be interpreted?

Parallel to enlightenment, another movement took place, namely, "*irrationalism*". It appeared as a counterpoint, emphasizing non-rational phenomena and the importance of emotions for being human. Non-rational phenomena – e.g. culminating in *magnetism* of Anton Mesmer (1734-1815) – demonstrated that a person was not only rational but always "irrational". According to this theory, each person possessed deeper structures that were always associated with the *ratio* and appeared as the other or dark side of himself. As Henry Ellenberger once claimed, this movement was important for the concept of unconsciousness and, therefore, the origin of the modern dynamic psychology and psychiatry (Ellenberger 1996). The understanding of the human being as always having subconscious or deeper structures besides his rational mind gained great significance for the increasing knowledge concerning addiction.

This holds especially true for *Brownianism*, important for a new and more rational understanding of addiction (Wiesemann 2000).

The Scottish physician and philosopher John Brown (1735-1788) developed an understanding of living organisms divided from inanimate matter, due to irritability and excitation, connecting vitalism and actual physiological insights. An equilibrium of environmental and bodily excitations and irritability of the organisms donated health. Pathologic processes – understood as an inequilibrium – were caused by over or underexcitation. Nowadays, Brownianism has been established as an "unspecific" model of disease because excitations influence organisms only indirectly and unspecifically, thus changing the relation between excitations and irritability. Therefore in Brownianism normal and pathologic processes are fundamentally comparable with each other (concerning the difference of "specific" and "unspecific" medical concepts of disease (Shyrock 1971, Wiesemann 2000). Furthermore, Brownianism was based on the concept of vitalism. Vitalism defined *vitality* as the central and unchangeable condition of life, as immaterial and animating inanimate matter (Putscher 1974). Concerning vitalism, a central question remained: how is it possible that the surroundings or, for instance, medicine are able to affect the organism and that the organism is still able to preserve its unity? Where does the connection lie between vitality and inanimate matter? This problem was solved by Brownianism, since excitations affected the organic irritability, thus changing the equilibrium, however, without vitality, all excitations would contribute nothing to an organism. For Brownianism, excitations do not cause specific diseases but are influenced in a more general way via changes of the equilibrium (Tsouyopoulos 1984).

Brownianism contributed to the success of an in-depth structured understanding of being human, later, understood as the division of consciousness and unconsciousness in the early 19th century (Wiesemann 2000). No less important was the medical discussion between followers of "unspecifism" and "specifism", developing the idea of a deceptive feeling of health, criticizing, in particular, the medical use of spirits in Brownianism. The knowledge of the effect of alcohol in Brownianism was determined in the file of excitation, overexcitation and indirect weakness in the sense of reduced irritability of the organism (*asthenie*).

In particular, Benjamin Rush (1745-1813), Thomas Trotter (1760-1832), Christoph Wilhelm Hufeland (1762-1836) and C. von Brühl-Cramer (unknown-1821) developed a concept of "dependence" as a possible understanding of addiction. Rush studied in Edinburgh, was a confessed "Brownianist" and later, a physician and politician in Philadelphia. He was engaged in movements of moderation, relying on the theses of the School of Edinburgh (Shyrock 1971). Hufeland, a famous sanitarian in Germany, known for his engagement in social medicine and his "*Makrobiotik oder die Kunst, das menschliche Leben zu verlängern*" (1796), personal physician to Goethe and Schiller and theoretically influenced by vitalism and more critically, by Brownianism (Busse 1982). In spirits, he recognized a "slow poison" which served to induce a kind of pathologic compulsion to consume more and more spirits (Hufeland 1802). More emphatic was Trotter who also studied in Edinburgh and was therefore strongly influenced by Brownianism. He wrote an important dissertation on drunkenness in 1785 ("De ebriate ejusque affectibus in corpus humanum"), published in English as "Essay on drunkenness", 1804, translated into German in 1821 (Trotter 1821). In this essay he described the chronic effects of alcohol consumption and, in this context, explicitly emphasized the increasing and willfully invincible compulsion for continued alcohol intoxication. As Trotter revealed, this held especially true for the "sober drunkard" who appeared to be sober, but drank alcohol in constant amounts regularly. He argued that this compulsion, comparable with other kinds of human urges, should be interpreted as the chemical effect of chronic alcohol consumption in the human body (Trotter 1821).

The Original Paradigm of "Dependency"

Besides Trotter, this existing new knowledge was mainly influenced by Brühl-Cramer with his book *"Über die Trunkenheit und eine rationelle Heilmethode derselben"* (1819). Little is known about his own life. He was a physician in Tomsk (Sibiria, Russia), in 1818 joined the "medical-physiologic society of Moskau" and died in 1821 (Kielhorn 1990). His work can be classified as a work of a follower of "specifism" and he was influenced partially by Hufeland who wrote the preface. With Brühl-Cramer's arguments and concepts, it was possible to define chronic alcohol consumption as a disease and no longer as a vice. Therefore, the chronic drunkard now stood in contrast with the rational and sober way of life of the enlightened citizens.

On defining his concept, we are confronted with two central ideas. Firstly, he states:

> durch den nur einige Zeit fortgesetzten mäßigen Gebrauch des Spirituosen wird der Genuss desselben zuletzt schon notwendig, welche Notwendigkeit sich in einem Verlangen, desselben zu genießen, und in einer unaussprechlichen Unbehaglichkeit, wenn dasselbe (...) nicht genossen wird, ausspricht. [through constant regular consumption of spirits over a short period of time, this consumption then becomes compulsive, shown in the necessity to drink spirits and the unspeakable discomfort if this is not possible.] (Brühl-Cramer 1819).

The origin of this urge is the spirit itself:

> Der Genuß des Branntweins gebieret das, was wir als nächste Ursache der Krankheit aufstellen, und dieses führt wiederum zum Genuß des Branntweins. [The excessive

intake of spirits leads to what we postulate as the greatest cause of this disease, resulting in further drinking of spirits.] (Brühl-Cramer 1819).

On the one hand, chronic drunkenness becomes partially a disease of the will: also those

> die mit dem festen Vorsätze wohl mehrer Male zu Werke gegangen sind, sich Zwang anzutun und sich des Trunkes zu enthalten. Es tritt der Zeitpunkt der Trunksucht ein, und siehe da, sie bitten flehentlich um ein wenig Branntwein, wenn man ihnen denselben gewaltsam vorenthält, und hernach versichern sie, daß es ein mächtiger unüberwindlicher Trieb, ein Drang sey, der sie zum Genuß des Branntweins führe, und äußerste Quaal, wenn er nicht befriediget würde [[Also those] who have tried many times with a firm purpose to quit drinking, there comes a time of dipsomania and again, they beg imploringly for a drop of spirits. On refusal, they are reminded that it is a strong and invincible urge, a drive, leading them to the consumption of spirits, or unbearable pain if this is not granted.] (Brühl-Cramer 1819).

On the other hand, this urge is a bodily phenomenon which cannot be influenced directly by the will of the afflicted. Furthermore, he differentiated a continuous and an episodic course of this disease and named feelings like anger, shame or insults as triggers of relapse. He also indicated that boredom or other intolerable states of mind could be interpreted as a disposition for chronic or episodic drunkenness. He claimed that education and enlightenment on this new and dangerous effect of alcohol would be the most effective cure, since he hoped, as an enlightener, that individuals would practice teetotalism armed rationally with the knowledge of this danger. Primary teetotalism would be the best solution because that way there would be no induction of alcohol urge or compulsion (Brühl-Cramer 1819).

Brühl-Cramer's concept of addiction or dependence shows two important "moments of structure": 1. The conscious and voluntary invincible dependence on an object; 2. The "dependence upon" is induced and provoked by this object itself (Schlimme 2000a). Brühl-Cramer recognized that this is not merely some kind of degeneration or inability to control an urge already present. It is important to realize that this is a new compulsion, installed inside the addicted person through chronic consumption and a specific urge. The focal point of this latest knowledge on alcohol, this "paradigm of dependency", is therefore the binding to a specific object that takes over the consciousness of the afflicted person and has direct contact with its unconsciousness or body.

As can be seen, this concept is only possible when the human being is recognized as a primary independent and a rational being. Every person can realistically retain this independence when following a rational way of living. The primary independence is only present as a possibility and can be undermined by an object such as alcohol or later, by other psychoactive drugs, thus leading to an irrational way of life and a pathologic dependence. This process uses a direct contact with the "dark side" of human nature that is demonstrated in the unconsciousness or the body. Therefore, it is also essential to accept that each individual also has an irrational dark side to his nature.

Tasks for a Psychiatric Anthropology of Addiction

If we wish to determine the inner perspective of the addicted, we have to ask ourselves the following question: What is it like to be addicted? This is also a philosophical question since the question "What is it like...?" asks how we see ourselves as human beings. A psychiatric anthropology is, therefore, based upon a philosophical anthropology. The focal point of the following psychiatric anthropology is the actual experience of the addicted individuals and refers to the philosophical anthropology of Heinrich Rombach (born 1923).

The central idea of his anthropology is no longer the anthropological constant factor known as the unchangeable condition of being a human being, but the fundamental "genetic" character of the human being in his world. "Genetic" stems from the Greek word *genesis* and means a creative growth and development. Rombach names this process of development *autogenesis*, which could be translated as *self-origination.*

For a better understanding, let us place ourselves in a certain situation. As humans we do not stand before or vis-a-vis a situation or the world in the sense of being on the outside. We cannot just walk away from our situation. The self-image of existing without any situation at all from this point of view is surely an illusion – whether or not somebody believes or experiences it. We are always *in* our situation, *in* our world, although situations can be varied and diverse. On the other hand, the respective situation always corresponds to the respective self and vice versa. This signifies "being in", which is the unbreakable structure separating itself into world and self. Heidegger named this unbreakable structure as *In-der-Welt-sein* [Being-in-the-world] (Heidegger 1993). This unbreakable structure can, however, be understood only as a process. We have to come to terms with ourselves and our situation as actual events corresponding to each other. Everything is revealed as the result of a creative process which involves, in due parts, ourselves and the world. Furthermore, we should accept ourselves as a multidimensional being with various and equivalent selves, since no one self can be seen as the core or the basis or the unchangeable and constant condition of the actual one. From this point of view, the self-image of a "core self" is also an illusion. The self-image representing one person or as many persons as desired as and when, is also an illusion, since you become what you are as a result of a process involving your situations. This process also requires the assimilation, integration, overcoming or fading out, disintegration, splitting off or annihilation of your own history, your other selves and situations and is only partially open for our own personal creative activity. This is why Rombach says: "*Wesensaufbau* und *Wesensverfall* macht den eigentlichen Inhalt des menschlichen Lebens sowohl im Individuum wie in der Gattung aus." (Rombach 1993, p. 15) ["The development of the essence and the decay of the essence contributes to the virtual content of a human life, in the individual as well as in species."].

Surely this kind of self-understanding poses questions about the origin of this *autogenesis*, since it is questionable how something can start from within itself, respectively on its own. Rombach recognizes this "ontological problem" and argues that a new *autogenesis* requires a breach (comparable to the concept of the "qualitative jump", Kierkegaard), in which the *autogenesis* starts, coming into existence suddenly in an undifferentiated manner.

The following, arising as a constant process of development, differentiates more clearly the structure and develops the corresponding self and situation which, in a retrospective view, appear as the result or product of this process. It must be pointed out that in this article this important question cannot be clarified in due fashion.

A psychiatric anthropology of addiction based upon this philosophical anthropology leads to the question "What is it like to be...?", since the self-illusions of the addicted can be accepted as aspects of the inner perspective and understood as necessary conditions in the experience of addiction. This philosophical anthropology does not require everybody to understand himself in the same way, but offers an understanding of the inner perspective as a central point and basis. The aim is to comprehend the addicted person from his own perspective and describe him as an addicted self (or selves) in terms of "moments of structure". These "moments of structure" are also constituted moments. The arising of an addicted self in an addicted world, therefore, is known as an *autogenesis*.

There are two important themes for a psychiatric anthropology of addiction: firstly, it is essential to understand the process of addiction as a continuous process; secondly, the understanding must demonstrate the possibility of becoming totally "hooked" by a psychotropic substance, a compulsion that cannot be controlled by the will or by the consciousness of the addicted. The first point is significant since most psychiatric models of understanding addiction or dependence argue that there comes a certain point in time during consumption when a sudden change takes place, a transition from abuse to dependence. This point is often associated with a bodily transformation from a quenchable positive pleasure to an inquenchable negative pleasure i.e. withdrawal symptoms. From a philosophical point of view, this is often referred to as a bodily transformation (e.g. Giulia Sissa 1999). The second point is of significance because if such an overwhelming compulsion would not arise, then the addiction would be put down to a "problem of consciousness or of the will", which, apparently, is not the case. It is essential in our psychiatric anthropology to be aware of the whole scope of addiction e.g. taking drugs or gambling which was certainly not the case before the time of Hufeland, Trotter or Brühl-Cramer.

The following solution would appear feasible: the dynamics of the process of addiction, respectively, the arising of an addicted self, develops a sufficient compulsion which the afflicted person experiences as "dependence" in specific phases of this process. These phases of insight evolve from this process in such a way that control of the addiction consciously fail and, thus, lead to e.g. further consumption or gambling. Options of cessation are possible, however, are not open to self-conscious control. These considerations focus on the central problem of a psychiatric anthropology of addiction in that insight into the addiction or dependence is not totally sufficient but still deemed necessary in order to stay clean. In terms of Rombach's philosophical anthropology: insight is no breach but possibly a necessary disclosure to an arising non-addicted self.

What Is It Like to Be Addicted?

In order to understand the inner perspective of the addicted person, we can refer to a number of authors who wrote about their own addiction. They offer us the chance to observe addiction through their own eyes and to find an answer to understand more clearly our question: What it is like to be addicted?

William S. Burroughs (1914-1997) is an example of such a person. Burroughs was an opiate addict and had great success with his confessional book, *Junky*, published in 1953. He was immensely influential amongst Beat writers, working with cut-up techniques and combining his stories with citations and borrowed ideas from all cultural areas. Besides other aspects, he succeeded in relating the most extraordinary descriptions of the inner perspective of the addict. This inner perspective was also used as a metaphor for life in general in the modern societies. In the following, I wish to present citations from his book, *Naked Lunch*, published in 1959.

Junk is quantitative and accurately measurable. The more junk you use the less you have and the more you have the more you use. (Burroughs 1993, p. 8).

> Junk yields a basic formula of 'evil' virus: T*he Algebra of Need*. The face of 'evil' is always the face of total need. A dope fiend is a man in total need of dope. Beyond a certain frequency need knows absolutely no limit or control. In the words of total need: '*Wouldn't you?*' Yes, you would. You would lie, cheat, inform on your friends, steal, do *anything* to satisfy total need. Because you would be in a state of total sickness, total possession, and not in a position to act in any other way. (Ibid., p. 8).
>
> I found this vaccine at the end of the junk line. I lived in one room in the native quarter of Tangiers. I had not taken a bath in a year or changed my clothes or

> removed them except to stick a needle every hour in the fibrous grey wooden flesh of terminal addiction. I never cleaned or dusted the room. Empty ampoule boxes and garbage piled up to the ceiling. Light and water had been long since turned off for non-payment. I did absolutely nothing. I could look at the end of my shoes for eight hours. I was only aroused to action when the hourglass of junk ran out. If a friend came to visit – and they rarely did since who or what was left to visit – I sat there not caring that he had entered my field of vision – a grey screen always blanker and fainter – and not caring when he walked out of it. If he had died on the spot I would have sat there looking at my shoes waiting to go through his pockets. Wouldn't you? Because I never had enough junk – no one ever does. (Ibid., pp. 9f.).
>
> 'What are you *thinking*?' says the squirming American tourist. To which I reply: 'Morphone has depressed my hypothalamus, seat of libido and emotion and since the front brain acts only at second hand with back-brain titillation, being a vicarious type citizen can only get his kicks from behind, I must report virtual absence of cerebral event. I am aware of your presence, but since it has for me no affective connotation, my affects having been disconnect by the junk man for the non-payment, I am not innarested in your doings (...). Go or come, shit or fuck yourself with a rasp or an asp – 'tis well done and fitting for a queen – but The Dead and The Junky don't care (...).' They are *Inscrutable*. (Ibid., p. 181).

Let us go over the focal moments of this particular experience Burroughs is describing. Firstly, we are confronted with his unquenchable need for "junk". But "junk" only serves to make normal life possible and no longer induces any blissful pleasure. Furthermore, we find a rhythm of life orientated solely at the consumption and procurement of "junk". Burroughs refers to this as the "hourglass of junk". Thirdly, he describes an inscrutability and indifference for everything else apart from "junk" or aspects of life connected with consumption or procurement of "junk". This indifference is the outcome of total orientation of his life towards the phenomenon "junk". The rhythm of life through the consumption of opiates (the "hourglass of junk") not only orientates everything towards opiate consumption, but also renders everything else insignificant. For Burroughs it seems that the answer lies in this indifference. The important aspect of this indifference is that everything else beside the phenomenon of "junk" becomes unimportant and only a side-issue of his life. His life is totally orientated towards the availability of "junk", whereas other aspects and issues of his life have little significance only.

Psychiatric Anthropology of Addiction

To our knowledge, we could say that the difference between addictive and non-addictive behaviour can be directed to the moment that this behaviour becomes absolute. As Burroughs says: the algebra of addiction is total need. This process of becoming absolute can only be understood as the arising of a self and a world determined by the "hourglass of junk", totally orientated at the phenomenon of "junk" and concerned only with the availability of "junk" that makes this self and its world indifferent towards everything else, indifferent to other and former identities. Therefore, the arising of the addicted self can be interpreted as the "development of the essence" of this being. But this addicted self was once a part of the ordinary and former selves which have disappeared and become indifferent.

There are three structural moments: firstly, the "availability of" something, secondly, the "orientation of" self and situation at this availability and, thirdly, the "lifting off" of this self from all other selves or identities. For Burroughs "junk" was displacing him from other situations, rendering him indifferent for everything and everyone else including his own past. But this displacement is only possible so long as adequate special agent e.g. "junk" is available, affording total orientation of this self at the availability of the special aspect. Former identities, maybe even of central importance for the person or his experience, are eliminated and concealed. The addicted and displaced ("lifted off") self gradually becomes more aware of the conviction that he stands above everything, since the central point of his new life – e.g. the "junk" – is in conscious availability. This disappearing of former selves corresponds to the "decay of the essence" – as can be seen by other people, respectively, non-addicts – and is a parallel process in the arising of the addicted self.

The hidden aspects are, therefore, of central importance for the addicted self, however, only if they are not present. They must remain hidden which affords constant "lifting off". The addict is still involved in these former selves and their situations but is under the conviction that he stands above them. This would appear to other people as an illusion of independence as the addict can experience during withdraw or by consuming moderate amounts only (e.g. insufficient intoxication). These former identities will then return to mind, they are no longer hidden – the position of standing above everything else other than the aim of total need is a fragile and insecure position, always depending on the availability and total orientation towards this substance or the behaviour to guarantee this displacement. However, being in this position, one is in the inner perspective of an addicted self and everything else is totally insignificant and indifferent compared to the substance or the behaviour to guarantee the position of standing above.

With this knowledge of addiction, there is no specific point of transformation or qualitative jump *inside* the consuming and now addicted self, but a *qualitative difference in the transparence* of this self for other identities (Schlimme 2000a). The dynamics of this self correspond to the growing disappearance of the former and other selves and the seclusion of a single self until this displacement and hiding is more or less complete. If this arising of self takes place, a compulsion for further consumption in the perspective of this self increases in order to remain superior to the other and therefore "hidden" identities. The shame evolving from his own impotence to change or bear the situations of those selves, respectively, the experience of those selves, corresponds to the impossibility of controlling this behaviour of addiction by will or consciousness.

The compulsion is then best understood as an estrangement. In the view of the addicted self, whose self-image is that of the independent, rational and conscious human being ("lifted off"), he becomes a stranger to himself. The strange aspect is his own invincible compulsion, his addiction. This reflects the concealment of deeper dimensions, becoming gradually more and more estranged and, therefore, developing a more and more invincible compulsion while raising the actual self above everything else. This would clarify the point that insight into ones own addiction reveals that options of cessation are possible, however, are not open to self-conscious control.

References

Baruzzi, A. 1993. *Die Zukunft der Freiheit*. Darmstadt: Wissenschaftliche Buchgesellschaft.

von Brühl-Cramer, C. 1819. *Ueber die Trunkenheit und eine rationelle Heilmethode derselben*. Berlin.

Burroughs, W.S. 1993. *Naked Lunch*. London: Flamingo.

Busse, H. 1982. *Christoph Wilhelm Hufeland. Der berühmte Arzt der Goethezeit*. St. Michael: Bläschke.

Cassirer, E. 1990. *Versuch über den Menschen*. Frankfurt/Main: Fischer.

Descartes, R. 1994. *Meditationen über die Grundlagen der Philosophie*. Hamburg: Meiner.

Ellenberger, H.F. 1996. *Die Entdeckung des Unbewussten*. Diogenes.

Feuerbach, L. 1996. "Grundsätze der Philosophie der Zukunft", in: Jaeschke, W., Schuffenhauer, W. (eds.) *Entwürfe zu einer neuen Philosophie*. Hamburg: Meiner, 25-99.

Flasch, K. 1994. *Augustin. Einführung in sein Denken*. Stuttgart: Reclam.

Galilei, G. 1980. *Sidereus nuncius*. Frankfurt/Main: Suhrkamp.

Heidegger, M. 1993. *Sein und Zeit*. Tübingen: Niemeyer.

Hufeland, C.W. 1802. *Ueber die Vergiftung durch Branntwein*. Berlin.

Kant, I. 1990. *Metaphysik der Sitten*. Stuttgart: Reclam.

Kielhorn, F.-W. 1990. "Die Trunksucht als Krankheit, v Brühl-Cramer", C. *Nervenarzt*, 61: 431-434.

de Mirandola, G.P. 1990. *Über die Würde des Menschen*. Hamburg: Meiner.

Putscher, M. 1974. *Pneuma, Spiritus, Geist. Vorstellungen vom Lebensantrieb in ihren geschichtlichen Wandlungen*. Wiesbaden: Steiner.

Rombach, H. 1993. *Strukturanthropologie. "Der menschliche Mensch"*. Freiburg: Alber.

Rombach, H. 1994. *Phänomenologie des sozialen Lebens. Grundzüge einer phänomenologischen Soziologie*. Freiburg: Alber.

Schlimme, J. 2000a. *Sucht. Zur philosophischen Anthropologie eines "misslingenden" Selbst*. Würzburg: Königshausen & Neumann.

Schlimme, J. 2000b. "Zur Philosophie der Sucht. Giulia Sissa", *Handlung Kultur Interpretation*, 9: 179-188.

Shyrock, R.H. 1971. "The Medical Reputation of Benjamin Rush. Contrasts over Two Centuries", *Bulletin of the History of Medicine*, 45: 507-552.
Sissa, G. 1999. *Die Lust und das böse Verlangen*. Stuttgart: Klett-Cotta.
Spode, H. 1993. *Die Macht der Trunkenheit. Kultur- und Sozialgeschichte des Alkohols in Deutschland*. Opladen: Leske + Budrich.
Tsouyopoulos, N. 1984. "German Philosophy and the Rise of Modern Clinical Medicine", *Theoretical Medicine*, 5: 345-357.
Wiesemann, C. 2000. *Die heimliche Krankheit. Eine Geschichte des Suchtbegriffs*. Stuttgart: Frommann-holzboog.

Neurophilosophical Perspectives on Conservative Compatibilism[1]

Henrik Walter

Introduction

More than 30 years ago, Harry Frankfurt introduced examples into the debate of free will and responsibility, now referred to as Frankfurt-type examples (Frankfurt 1969). They were designed to argue for the compatibility of moral responsibility and determinism. According to Frankfurt, moral responsibility does not require a person to have genuine alternative possibilities. Imagine the following scenario.

Sally is driving a car. She wishes to make a right turn. As a result of her intention to turn right, she signals, turns the steering wheel and carefully guides the car to the right. It is perfectly sensible to say that she was controlling the car by her own will. Thus, she herself is responsible for turning right. Traditional philosophers of free will, i.e. libertarians, would insist, however, that she is responsible because she could have done otherwise, i.e. she could have also turned to the left. In other words, what makes her responsible is that there were genuine alternative possibilities open to her. Frankfurt denies this. To argue for his view, he changes the scenario as follows. Imagine the same situation. Everything happens as before and Sally turns to the right by her own will. However, unbeknownst to her, the car she drives is an "driver instruction" automobile with dual controls. In the car a hidden instructor is present. The instructor is quite happy to allow Sally to steer the car to the right. That is what she did. However, *if* Sally *had* shown any inclination to steer the car in some other direction, the instructor would have intervened and steered the car to the right (as actually happened). Now, does this different scenario change our judgement that Sally was controlling the car by her own will? Does it change our holding her responsible for turning right? Frankfurt says no. He says, if we assign responsibility in the first case, we should also assign it in the second case because the situation remains the same, except that there were no alternative possibilities. If this is so, you agree that there can be responsibility without there being alternate possibilities.

---

1 Reprinted (with minor changes), with kind permission, from: Walter H., "Neurophilosophical perspectives on conservative compatibilism" in: Kanzian C., Quitterer J., Rungaldier E. (eds.) *Persons. An Interdisciplinary Approach*. Proceedings of the 25th International Wittgenstein Symposium. öbv-hpt, Wien 2003, pp. 299-308.

The aim of this paper is to analyse recent compatibilist theories of moral responsibility using neurophilosophical means based on these examples. But before I do so, I would like to give a short sketch of my own neurophilosophical account of free will. However, firstly, I feel the irresistable urge to also say a little about what neurophilosophy is. The reason being that neurophilosophy appears to have a poor reputation in most philosophical communities.

On Neurophilosophy

To begin with, I think it is important to say what neurophilosophy is not, at least neurophilosophy Walterian style, that is. Neurophilosophy is not identical with scientism, namely, that science is the best method for solving any human problem. There are many problem domains in which science is of no great help whatsoever. Secondly, neurophilosophy, from my point of view, is not identical with eliminative materialism, i.e. the view that all mental terms will and should be eliminated in favour of neuroscientific terms. However, what holds true to me is that neuroscience has a strong revisionary impetus. Thirdly, neurophilosophy is not possible without making some metaphysical assumptions or without having some unproven premises. However, this is a feature that neurophilosophy shares with every empirical and philosophical theory and I do not consider this general point as any form of a self-refutation argument against neurophilosophy.

So what exactly is neurophilosophy? The main concern of neurophilosophy is to question and understand very general ideas about mental phenomena with the help of neuroscience, i.e. ideas that are used daily by all of us without thinking. Neurophilosophy can be practiced in two ways. Either you study philosophical problems arising in the neurosciences themselves. This is philosophy of neuroscience. Or you start with a philosophical problem, e.g. the problem of free will, and use neurobiological knowledge in order to solve, dissolve, redefine or, at least, advance the solution of this problem. Neurophilosophy, as I understand it, is thus nothing more than reflection and (re)construction of philosophical theses and theories in the light of our knowledge of the brain.

As mentioned above, neurophilosophy – as any other theoretical approach – is not possible without any presupposition. Instead of leaving the task of finding out what I presuppose to the reader, I will state them explicitly, although, due to space, this will be more in a confessional style (but cf. Walter 2001). First of all, I do presuppose that substance dualism is wrong and that the most promising approach is revisionary monism. What do I mean by that? I mean that empirical discoveries will lead to some – perhaps even major – revisions in our folk psychological conceptions of the mental, as has always been the case. For example, I believe that no reasonably informed person still holds the once upon a time widely shared beliefs that people with epilepsy are possessed by demons, that there is a *elan vital* or that it is feasible to hold people directly responsible for the weather. At least, I strongly hope so. Why is this the case? Because we are more knowledgeable about how the world really is. So why will neurophilosophy change folk psychology?

Until very recently, folk psychology only had three sources of information. First person information (from personal experience), third person experience (observing the behaviour of others) and tradition (theories about persons). Now we have another perspective, namely, a third person perspective on the mechanisms of the first person perspective. Call this the fourth person perspective. The fourth person perspective was not available to us until just recently. Basic knowledge about the brain is already beginning to become part of folk psychology and this will alter our view of ourselves and infiltrate folk psychology, like it or not.

Secondly, I assume that there is supervenience of the mental on the neural plus x. This leads to two things. Theories of mind cannot be correct if they contradict neuroscientific knowledge. This follows from the asymmetric nature of the supervenience relation. The plus x is important here because I believe that, at least, for some kinds of mental properties, the neural is not a sufficient subvenient base. For example, I do believe that intentional content is dependent on the past of the system having intentional properties.

Thirdly, I do not suggest searching for neural correlates but for neural mechanisms of the mental. Why? The search for neural correlates is severely contaminated with an implicit Cartesian dualism stance. I do confess that the talk of mechanisms has strong monistic implications. But as monism is true, as I believe, this is better than using a manner of speech which has strong dualistic implications.

Neurophilosophy of Free Will

Recently, I argued that the concept of a strong, libertarian free will is inconsistent, in other words, that there is no strong form of free will (Walter 2001). I claim there are three central components or intuitions about free will to which the arguments in the debate appeal. By *alternativism* I refer to the idea that free will entails the ability to do otherwise. By *intelligibility*, I refer to the claim that free will entails rational choice or acting for reasons. By *agency* I refer to the important idea that we are the true sources of our free volitional acts, i.e. that they originate in *us* and are our own.

Theories on free will can be reconstructed by giving these general components strong, weak or moderate interpretations. The traditional libertarian view can be reconstructed by the claim that free will means that we can do otherwise under exactly the same circumstances, that we nonetheless act intelligibly in a strong sense and that we are the real originators of our doings, namely, that we start a new causal chain.

I am deeply convinced that this is not a coherent position and I have argued extensively against such a concept of free will. Nonetheless, there is something we possess, a kind of autonomy, which is relevant for issues of moral responsibility. In order to find out what this autonomy consists of, one should adopt a neurophilosophical stance. In the first place, this means to see free will not as a moral problem but as a problem of natural philosophy. How does that work?

First, presuppose supervenience as a starting point (no change in mental properties without changes in physical properties). Then, go on to study if the different interpretations of the three components (alternativism, intelligibility and agency) are compatible with brain science. If not, ask yourself how much we have to give up in order to be compatible with the principles of brain science. You will finally end with a brain compatible concept of autonomy. We may then look at the (descriptive) results and only then consider their (normative) consequences. I will not go into more detail here because the theme of this paper is based on moral responsibility. I only wish to stress that I firmly believe that natural autonomy is not the same as libertarian free will. Rather, we have to give up some of our most cherished illusions in our ideas in the way we are in control of ourselves.

Unfortunately, others now often call me a compatibilist. However, I do not like to be regarded as such, at least, not as a traditional compatibilist. Why not? Because traditional compatibilists claim that determinism is also compatible with our traditional concept of moral responsibility. Let's call this conservative compatibilism. I do not believe in conservative compatibilism. Rather, I believe not only our idea of free will has to be revised but also our concept of moral responsibility.

However, I cannot present you with such a revised theory of moral responsibility at this stage, the reason being is that I have not yet worked out such a theory. So what I will do here is to analyse one of the most ambitious theories of conservative compatibilism I know of, confront it with some neurobiological case studies and thereby call conservative compatibilism into question.

A Compatibilist Theory of Moral Responsibility

In their book "Responsibility and control", Fischer and Ravizza (1998) promote what I refer to as *conservative compatibilism*: "We shall be trying to articulate the inchoate, shared view about moral responsibility in (roughly speaking) a modern, Western democratic society" (p. 10). In other words, they are of the opinion that the prevailing account of moral responsibility is not in need of revision, rather only the concepts on which it is founded. Most importantly, they claim that the component of alternativism plays no role in moral responsibility.

The central idea of their theory is that responsibility is associated with control. They contend that there are two distinct kinds of control: Guidance control and regulative control. Whereas regulative control involves the ability to do otherwise, guidance control does not. Guidance control should be understood in terms of two elements: the agent's ownership of the mechanism that actually issues in the relevant behaviour, and the reason-responsiveness of those mechanisms. A person, according to the theory of guidance control, is morally responsible if the mechanisms which have brought about his actions are his own and are responsive to reasons. The reference to mechanisms makes this theory highly attractive for a neurophilosophical approach.

Fischer and Ravizza depart from Frankfurt-style-examples. Consider again Sally, steering the car. The mechanisms which bring about the turn to the right are mechanisms which guide the behaviour of Sally. In virtue of these mechanisms it would be appropriate to say that Sally has a certain degree of control over the car. This kind of control is guidance control. What Sally, however, does not have, is regulative control. That is, she has no real alternative possibility, e.g. turning left, because if she showed an inclination to do so, the instructor would force her to make a right turn. But although there are no real alternative possibilities, there is a genuine sense in which she controls the car. Fischer and Ravizza say that the mechanisms which bring about Sally's behaviour are responsive to reason. Remember that there was the intention to take a right turn. The intention, i.e. a reason, plays an indispensable role in the steering of the car.

The second part of their theory is that the mechanisms accountable for bringing about the actions for which a person is responsible must be the person's own mechanisms. They contend that individuals make certain kinds of mechanisms their own by taking responsibility for them. In order to carry out this version of agency, they construct moral responsibility as a historical notion. A person makes mechanisms, e.g. practical reasoning, nonreflective habits and so on, her own, when she acquires certain views of herself as an agent, when she sees that the world depends on her choices and bodily movements and believes she is a fair target of certain reactive attitudes. This process comes about as a result of moral education.

The historical twist explains why we sometimes hold people responsible even if their actual action is *not* under guidance control. If a person has taken responsibility for certain mechanisms, then a person may be responsible for an action A even if the person has no guidance control over action A, if the mechanisms which bring about action A are the results of some other actions B which had been under guidance control or for which the person has taken responsibility in the past. Moreover, the historical approach helps to explain why an external manipulation in the past can render a person non-responsible for an action which is reason-responsive but brought about by mechanisms which are not the agent's own.

Neurophilosophy of Moral Responsibility

So much for the sketch of Fischer and Ravizza. I will grant that their theory does indeed explain our actual practice of holding people responsible without making any reference to the idea of alternativism. It is conservative in the sense that they are trying to save our traditional practices by giving them a different theoretical underpinning. However, I do believe there is something wrong with this theory. So let us put the theory to test by demonstrating some limiting cases. If I were primarily a philosopher of mind, I would think about a decisive- thought experiment. As I am a neurophilosopher, however, I will discuss instead real cases. Let me briefly explain my argumentative strategy.

- Lesions of the Ventromedial Prefrontal Cortex

Let us start with the well-known case of Phineas Gage. Gage was employed by an American company responsible for building railroads in the last century. He suffered an accident in which an explosion caused an iron piece to penetrate his brain, including the ventromedial part of his prefrontal cortex, i.e. the part of the brain lying right above the eyes. The most fascinating thing was that he survived at a time when antibiotics or neurosurgery did not yet exist. The second most fascinating thing was that he was not impaired in language or intelligence. However, being a formerly reliable worker and responsible husband, he became an irresponsible, disorderly and unsociable person, who was unable to lead a normal life, made personal decisions that were not in his own long-term interest and became unemployed and then divorced. Today such behaviour would be called "acquired sociopathy".

Antonio Damasio and his group have studied patients with similar lesions of the ventromedial prefrontal cortex, in short, VM-patients (Damasio 1994, Bechara et al. 2000). VM-patients show deficits similar to Phineas Cage: In cognitive tasks they perform well and their intelligence is surprisingly good and unimpaired. They are also unimpaired concerning theoretical reasoning, e.g. when they are tested on moral tasks in which they have to decide if certain actions are morally wrong or right. However, in real life, they behave similarly to Gage and show sociopathic behaviour. Why is this? Damasio and other groups examined these patients more carefully and discovered the reason. Very roughly summarized, the reason is that the sociopathic behaviour is a result of an impairment of emotional information processing leading to an inability to reason practically and a lack of concern for the future.

Given this, how do we judge the responsibility of VM-patients? Although they are responsive to reasons we think it justified not to hold them responsible if we know that their sociopathic behaviour stems from a brain lesion. Thus, VM-patients seem to contradict the theory of guidance control.

One can naturally modify the theory to handle these case studies. First of all, it can be argued that it is not the theoretical reasons one should be responsive to, but the practical reasons. A theory along this line has been proposed by R. Jay Wallace (Wallace 1998). In his theory, moral responsibility is justified if people are responsive to normative, i.e. practical reasons. Notice, however, that in this theory moral sentiments, that is, emotional processes, are important. Secondly, Fischer and Ravizza could argue that the mechanisms causing VM-patients' lack of responsiveness to moral reasons are not their own, because they are not the results of historical guidance control, but the results of surgery or a disease. So far, a modified theory can be saved. Let's proceed to less obvious cases.

- Psychopathy (Antisocial Personality Disorder)

We all have a rough idea of what psychopaths are like, at least, if we have seen the movie "The Silence of the Lambs". In psychiatry, psychopaths are diagnosed as patients with antisocial personality disorder (APD) when they fulfil certain diagnostic criteria which are very similar to those Phineas Gage and ventromedial patients fulfil. However, not only certain criteria have to be met, but there is also a negative criterion, namely, that a brain lesion or dysfunction has to be excluded (Diagnostic and Statistical Manual of Mental Disorders, 4th edition). It is often said that APD-patients tend to be offenders. And indeed, there is a very high incidence of APD-patients in jail. However, there are probably other social groups which also fulfil most of the APD-criteria, namely, in positions in which the characteristics of APD are of advantage, namely adventurers, politicians and certain types of entrepreneurs. However, these people are difficult to study scientifically, so the following refers mostly to people who are offenders.

Thus, the question arises, are APD-patients morally responsible? The common penal law says in general "yes", except for certain extreme conditions (Herpertz and Sass 2000). Actually, the penal code has taken great care to formulate its conditions of not being responsible in the face of the law in such a way that psychopaths are excluded by diagnosis. If, however, a person were diagnosed falsely as an APD-patient and discovered to have a brain lesion, he would not be held responsible in the majority of scenarios. So what would happen if APD itself were to be caused by a more subtle brain lesion or brain dysfunction in the VM-cortex? Evidence has accumulated over the last years making this point plausible. There have been psychophysiological studies, neuropsychological studies, as well as structural and functional neuroimaging studies that have shown this to be the case (Hare and Quinn 1971, Lapierre et al. 1995, Dinn and Harris 2000, Raine et al. 2000, Schneider et al. 2000, Kiehl et al. 2001, Diekmann et al. 2000, Soderstrom et al. 2002).

For the sake of argument, I will assume that these studies are valid in the sense that there is ample evidence that there are functional, perhaps even structural abnormalities in the brains of patients with APD to explain their defective behaviour. What is then the outcome? Guidance control theorists would argue that the mere fact of an actual brain dysfunction in APD, compelling as it is, does not *per se* threaten their theory. What really matters is how this brain function came about. Admittedly, this is a very crucial question which is not answered by these studies. However, there is some evidence from two case studies that a fully fledged clinical picture of psychopathy after a brain lesion will only develop as a result of early damage of the VM cortex (Anderson et al. 1999). An intact VM-cortex, so the authors argue, is necessary to learn moral practice.

Although there is no proof as yet, whether or not APD is the result of early VM-brain dysfunction, if this would be the case, then it would stand true that APD behaviour would not arise from guidance controlled behaviour in the past. Thus, Fischer and Ravizza would have to conclude that these persons are not morally responsible. Would this threaten the theory of guidance control in general? Not necessarily. It would only follow that certain people would have to be excluded from being morally responsible in a full fledged manner. But for the majority of people it could still well hold true. So let us turn to this majority in non-psychiatric populations.

- Murderers, Personality and Temperament

The first example I wish to consider is a study by Raine et al. (1998). He studied murderers pleading not guilty with the technique of PET, i.e. he studied the glucose metabolism of their brains. He found that murderers showed reduced prefrontal metabolism. Moreover, he detected differences between two groups. He distinguished the two groups by the history of the offenders. One group included murderers with a typical broken home situation incorporating violence, i.e. a psychosocial situation explaining partly their own behaviour and a situation which sometimes leads to diminished responsibility in a juridical sense. The other group had a normal family history. How did these two groups differ in terms of brain metabolism? Most surprisingly, the group which showed the most significant reduction in brain metabolism, especially in the medial PFC, was the group which had a standard history, i.e. which had not experienced a broken-home situation. Raine concludes from this that a physiological brain dysfunction does explain violent offences especially if there are no standard psychosocial explanations.

But what about normal, healthy persons who are not murderers? There is some evidence that sociopathic behaviour not corresponding to the diagnostic criteria of APD is associated with VM-brain dysfunction in children of school age (Blair et al. 2001). Furthermore, there are twin studies showing evidence that antisocial behaviour is genetically transmitted (Kaplan and Sadock 1998, p. 859). This does not necessarily threaten the theory of guidance control. It only implies that a greater number of people have to be excluded from the category of morally responsible persons.

So what about us "normal" people, people with no psychiatric diagnosis, who are not murderers, who do not show sociopathic tendencies? At this point I would like to remind you that because of the findings in VM-patients, we have now changed our reason-responsiveness theory to include responsiveness to moral reasons which are based on emotional information processes or moral sentiments. But how are our moral sentiments, our emotional information-processing mechanisms determined? In traditional terms: How is our temperament determined?

There are several influential theories of temperament which do give neurobiological explanations for the dimensions from which our temperament is formed. One influential theory is the one formulated by Cloninger (1993). He distinguishes several personality dimensions like novelty seeking, reward dependence, harm avoidance, or persistence. Furthermore, he postulates a close link between the kind of temperament we have and the receptor profile of our brains.

Now, what does that imply in terms of moral responsibility? Probably Fischer and Ravizza may say that it depends whether the receptor profile we have is a result of processes which were under guidance control. But what if our receptor profile is given to us by our genes or, at least, in early childhood where there is no guidance control? There is indeed a great deal of evidence that our emotional character is more or less fixed in early childhood as a result of endogenous dispositions, as shown by transcultural studies (McCrae et al. 2000), and early childhood experience, as shown by developmental psychology and animal experiments (Braun et al. 2002). What then if our emotional information processing mechanisms are crucial for practical reasons and moral behaviour? Are we responsible for our emotions? If not, what does that mean? Why is it that people in very similar circumstances react differently to drastic influences like war, deprivation, trauma or stress? Why do some of them suffer from subsequent serious mental disorders? Why do others stay stable and healthy? One good explanation for that is the concept of *susceptibility*. By this psychiatrists mean that the specific composition of the human brain determines how they will react to external influences. How much sense does it then make to appeal to guidance control? I think all of these questions call a conservative theory of moral compatibilism very much into question. At the very least, I have shown that conservative compatibilism a la Fischer and

Ravizza will present problems if some facts turn out to be true, pertaining to the period in which the biological mechanisms of our emotional information processing mechanisms are formed.

Fortunately, I am writing this paper as a neurophilosopher and not as a scientist and so I can make it a virtue to wind up with questions rather than with answers. Nevertheless, let me draw some preliminary conclusions.

Conclusions

I wish to draw three conclusions. Firstly, I do believe that one reason for the failure of conservative compatibilism is that it declares alternativism to be irrelevant for responsibility. I consider this a mistake. To be sure, I do agree that regulative control or strong alternativism is not at stake. However, there are weaker versions of alternativism appealing to the potential flexibility of our actions, e.g. to the fact that we are able to act otherwise under similar circumstances (Walter 2001). If we discover persons to be totally rigid and inflexible, we do not treat them as morally equivalent to non-rigid, flexible persons, at least, so I claim. Also, the old deterministic intuition that the possibility of influencing one's behaviour, i.e. a forward-looking approach to responsibility, should play a role in an empirically adequate theory of responsibility.

This leads to my second conclusion. Whatever holds for free will holds also for moral responsibility. If there is no strong form of free will, then there is also no strong form of moral responsibility. Our concept of moral responsibility has to change and this change will be influenced by facts concerning the brain. One important point is to figure out exactly what role emotions and moral sentiments play in the real brain and in what way they are or can be under guidance control and how they can be influenced. There are now ways to study this experimentally in healthy human subjects (for a review compare Greene and Haidt 2002).

My third conclusion is somewhat vague and more of a hypothesis or a provisional idea. Moral responsibility, in my view, is characterized by two features. First of all: Moral responsibility is not a property of a person but a practice we live by on the basis of certain properties of persons, like e.g. normative competence, moral sentiments, reflective judgement, etc. Put into other terms: Moral responsibility is in itself a normative principle because it includes an evaluative component on the basis of which we decide to include persons in the range of moral agents or not. The implication that certain properties and abilities justify the attribution of responsibility leads to a problem. As Dennett (1984) stated: We do not search endlessly for the reasons why a person is responsible, rather we just hold him responsible because time is limited and decisions have to be made. I agree. However, it has to be acknowledged that this is an act of evaluation. This leads to the conflict of two normative principles, namely, between justice and equality. If we wish to be just, we would have to figure out in each individual case to what degree a person is responsible. Moreover, we would have to adjust our retributive measures according to the degree of responsibility. However, this has the implication that people are not equal in moral terms. It also has the implication that people are not equal in the face of the law. This conflict between two moral principles is, I think, the reason why a libertarian view, which regards free will and ultimate responsibility as all-or-none-properties, is such an appealing, but, as I hope to have shown, nonetheless an illusionary idea.

References

Anderson, S.W. et al. 1999. "Impairment of social and moral behavior related to early damage in human prefrontal cortex", *Nature Neuroscience*, 2: 1032-1037.

Bechara, A. et al. 2000. "Emotion, Decision Making and the Orbitofrontal Cortex", *Cerebral Cortex*, 10: 295-307.

Blair, R.J.R. et al., 2001. "Somatic Markers and Response Reversal: Is There Orbitofrontal Cortex Dysfunction in Boys with Psychopathic Tendencies?", *Journal of Abnormal Child Psychology*, 29: 499-511.

Braun, A.K. et al. 2002. "Frühe emotionale Erfahrungen und ihre Relevanz für die Entstehung und Therapie psychischer Erkrankungen", in B. Strauß, A. Buchheim, H. Kächele: *Klinische Bindungsforschung*, Stuttgart: Schattauer, 121-128.

Cloninger, T.R., Svrakic, D.M., Przybeck, T.R. 1993. "A psychobiological model of temperament and character", *Archives of General Psychiatry*, 50: 975-990.

Damasio, A. 1994. *Descartes' Error*. New York: Grossett/Putnam.

Dennett, D.C. 1984. *Elbow Room*. The Varieties of Free Will Worth Wanting. Cambridge: MIT Press.

Dikmann, Z.V., Allen, J.J.B. 2000. "Error monitoring during reward and avoidance learning in high- and low-socialized individuals", *Psychophysiology*, 37: 43-54.

Dinn, W.M., Harris, C.L. 2000. "Neurocognitive function in antisocial personality disorder", *Psychiatry Research*, 97: 173-190.

Fischer, J.M., Ravizza, M. 1998. *Responsibility and Control. A Theory of Moral Responsibility*. Cambridge: Cambridge University Press.

Frankfurt, H.G. 1969. "Alternate possibilities and moral responsibility", *Journal of Philosophy*, 66, reprinted in: H. Frankfurt 1988. *The Importance of What We Care About*. New York: Cambridge University Press, 1-10.

Greene, J., Haidt, J. 2002. "How (and where) does moral judgement work?", *Trends in Cognitive Sciences*, 6: 517-523.

Hare, R.D., Quinn, M.J. 1971. "Psychopathy and Autonomic Conditioning", *Journal of Abnormal Psychology*, 3: 223-235.

Herpertz, S.C., Sass, H. 2000. "Emotional Deficiency and Psychopathy", *Behavioral Sciences and the Law*, 18: 567-580.

Kaplan, H.I., Sadock, B.J. 1998. *Synopsis of Psychiatry*, 8th edition. Baltimore: Williams & Wilkins.

Kiehl et al. 2001. "Limbic Abnormalities in Affective Processing by Criminal Psychopaths as Revealed by Functional Magnetic Resonance Imaging", *Biological Psychiatry*, 50: 677-684.

Lapierre, D. et al. 1995. "Ventral Frontal Deficits in Psychopathy: Neuropsychological Test Findings", 33, 139-151.
McCrae, R.R. et al. 2000. "Nature over Nurture: Temperament, Personality, and Life Span Development", *Journal of Personality and Social Psychology*, 78: 173-186.
Raine, A. et al. 1998. "Prefrontal Gluccose Deficits in Murderers Lacking Psychosocial Deprivation", *Neuropsychiatry, Neuropsychology, and Behavioral Neurology*, 11: 1-7.
Raine, A. et al. 2000. "Reduced Prefrontal Gray Matter Volume and Reduced Autonomic Activity in Antisocial Personaliy Disorder", *Archives of General Psychiatry*, 57: 119-127.
Schneider, F. et al. 2000. "Functional Imaging of Conditioned Aversive Emotional Responses in Antisocial Personality Disorder", *Neuropsychobiology*, 42: 192-2001.
Soderstrom, H. et al. 2002. "Reduced frontotemporal perfusion in psychopathic personality", *Psychiatry Research Neuroimaging*, 114: 81-94.
Wallace, R.J. *Responsibility and the Moral Sentiments*. Cambridge: Harvard University Press.
Walter, H. 2001. *Neurophilosophy of Free Will. From libertarian Illusions to a Concept of Natural Autonomy*. Cambridge: MIT Press, publ. in German as: H. Walter 1999. *Neurophilosophie der Willensfreiheit*. Paderborn: mentis.

Freedom of Will, Freedom of Action and Psychiatry: Concerning the relationship of empirical to intelligible character and so-called freedom of choice in the view of forensic psychiatry

Rainer Luthe and Michael Rösler

Seen historically, psychiatry is the junior partner in a triangular relationship with philosophy and law where the former has little association with either of the latter two subjects. Conversely, the question of what a psychiatrist can expect from the latter two is rarely conveyed in daily psychiatric practice. This was not always the case. During the romantic era of psychiatry, the natural philosophy of Schelling (Orth 1914, Boenke 1995) had a great influence on psychiatric thinking (Feuchtersleben 1841, Carus 1846) and one could understand the course of the still relatively new science as a tributary of the great river of philosophy.

Since this psychiatric thinking was holistic, body and soul were considered as subject to natural law, as a unity and as indivisible. The in itself strained term of mental illness was not only concerned with illness but also with the mind. But in a scientific sense the mind was hard to grasp so the ways parted. True to the traditional division of the university into the arts and sciences, the psychiatrist now considers himself a man of medicine and medicine an applied science (Friedreich 1835, Griesinger 1843). For some time psychopathology played a unique mediating role in this environment but under the influence of psychopharmacology its importance waned. Meanwhile psychiatrists have learnt to diagnose and treat mental illness as a brain disorder with huge success. Although the term "psychiatric drug" in its wording still contains a reference to something psychic, it seems to involve an understandable thoughtlessness only, since the word stem also appears in the occupational description, "psychiatrist". The development of new diagnostic methods, especially the picture rendering process (magnetic resonance scanning), and the further development of electroencephalography have now resulted in sensational discoveries and made man, so to speak, transparent. Formerly, it was the exclusive privilege of God to see through man, now man, left to his own devices, manages even to conjure this trick. In doing so, instead of a mind, the finest neurobiological processes are depicted.

Now that the "vagaries of the mind" can be visualized in three dimensions and many colours, the old discussion about the essence of mental illness seems definitely to have been brought to an end (Müller and Hajak 2003). Since acquiring optical proof of the surprising neuronal plasticity of the limbic system, psychiatry can no longer be defined as dealing with the "pathology of freedom" as it was by Henri Ey (Ey 1975, Witter and Luthe 1977) in the last century, but rather with the "pathology of the limbic system". It is assumed that the complicated decision-making processes take place in this central region of the brain (Singer 2002), which are mistakenly experienced by many as being "free". Beyond this, important representatives of neurobiology, with incomplete knowledge of the current stance in philosophical discussion, assume that now, due to the knowledge gained through their experiments, there is proof to finally allow a definite judgement pertaining to that old metaphysical problem of free will. The verdict is: *Man is determined!* His belief in freedom was an illusion (Roth 1997).

The consequences that result from this for general psychiatry seem at first glance to be relatively small. Whether a case of schizophrenia or depression is regarded as "pathology of freedom" or "pathology of the limbic system" does not affect the choice of psychiatric drugs specifically used to combat it. The situation is quite different in forensic psychiatry which must, as its name implies, bridge the gap to law (Rösler 1987). In the interest of reliable communication, one must ask where its foundations lie (Grasnick 1987, 1991). Freedom plays a fundamentally vital role in the dynamics of the triangular relationship of law, philosophy and psychiatry. There is, however, not only in the field of psychiatry, disagreement concerning the question of whether man is free to act as he chooses, or whether he cannot avoid acting as he does. A clear doctrine on this subject first gained acceptance during the revolutionary atmosphere of the Council of Carthage [418 A.D.] (Wermelinger 1975). It was the position of Augustine that determined the course and had drastic practical consequences. Very much later Luther was one of the most active among those who considered man to be determined. Modern criminal law has, for the most part, indeed freed the idea of guilt from its ethical implications (Luthe 1981), but it has not fundamentally escaped the question of freedom despite the emancipation of morality and conscience. The perpetration of a criminal offence explicitly presupposes, apart from the act and the unlawfulness, that the perpetrator was capable of guilt at the time of the crime. The assumption of criminal responsibility, on the other hand, presupposes that man can "freely" choose his actions (Lenckner 1972). The attempt, supported by noted forensic psychiatrists (Haddenbrock 1992, Witter 1970), to turn this into a socially functional term of law (Schild 1990), met with serious doubts.

In the practice of law one does not check in individual cases whether the assumption of criminal responsibility is justified or not. Rather, it is still generally taken for granted in the case of a member of society who is sane and of age. Only in exceptional cases must courts decide whether this assumption is justified, namely, to what extent there are well-founded doubts relating to a special case (Luthe 1996). Grounds for such doubts can be the lack of a mature personality, its illness or disturbances of consciousness. In this case the court consults psychiatric experts from whom it expects, as regarding criminal responsibility, that they are able to inform the court about the mental condition of the perpetrator at the time of the crime. In order to be able to do this, psychiatric experts, whether they want to or not, will have to concern themselves with the question of whether human actions can be freely chosen or whether the acting person could not avoid acting as he did. Furthermore, the special authority of psychiatric experts is based on evidence – not questionable by human systems of law and shared by every reasonable person – that the mentally disturbed person cannot be held legally responsible.

Therefore, one must ask what distinguishes the mentally disturbed perpetrator, who therein resembles the child (Luthe 1977), from the perpetrator in the case that this evidence does not emerge from the start. Consequently, it becomes immediately understandable, why Ey (1975) could ever succumb to the idea of defining psychiatry as grounded in the *pathology of freedom*. Illness is forced upon man. Responsibility presupposes the absence of constraint. The freedom referred to here, remarkably lacking in the child as well as the mentally disturbed person, is the freedom of self-determination (Luthe 1985). The child lacks this freedom because, due to its stage of development, it has not yet reached a certain level of understanding and reason. The adult lacks this freedom if he is in want of understanding and/or reason due to illness or as a consequence of a developmental disturbance. For children the language uses the personal pronoun "it". "It", as a neuter noun, is a designation for that which has yet to be defined. What five o'clock is, is not explained, only It. What "it" is, as far as the child is concerned, is also not explained. However, what is meant is not what has already been defined from a child's view, but rather something specifically childlike: That, which will in all probability develop out of the temporary situation, the definite man or the definite woman. Thus, It will turn into a more or less definite evening, but perhaps also another indefinite one, such as the light at the beginning of the story of creation, that fits so poorly to the dark It (id) of the subconscious, of which it is said that it shall become "I" (ego) (Groddeck 1978/79).

Words are always words for something. In his time, Duns Scotus (Luthe 1993) received the honorary title of *Doctor subtilis* for this clarification. "It" is a word that specifically means only the "word ", whose material supposition – in analogy to the method of so-called Negative Theology (Heiser 1989) – consists of its determinability which presupposes that which is not yet defined. So we are not dealing with the sex specific endowment of chromosomes, which the child shares with the adult, but rather with the question of why the child is neither man nor woman. To that extent the child is everything possible, it is also determinable, but at the moment not determined. Its indefiniteness, however, should not be confused with freedom. What the child lacks in this regard is what distinguishes an arbitrary act from an act of will. For a fired bullet to hit the target direction must be added to the dynamics of the process. Whether the child can prove itself depends on the direction, which is determined by its developing a balance between analytic understanding and synthetic reasoning. Only in this way can the antinomy of freedom be clearly illustrated, not however, by attempting to escape the certainty of the word "it" by thinking positively of a supposed meaning and continually fragmenting it in a categorizing manner. According to Dath (2003) the attempt ends up on a heap of rubble.

During the transition from natural evidence of illness-conditioned irresponsibility, in the sense of a lack of understanding or reason, to a comprehensible scientific explanation, the search for psychiatric orientation found it very accommodating that a similar duality has always been postulated in the system of law. When dealing with the term, criminal liability, one differentiates between the cognitive and voluntary elements and speaks of the ability of reason and control (Schreiber, 2000). Finally, from the psychological viewpoint, we have Jean Piaget (1965), whose book about the wisdom and illusions of philosophy, though having already appeared in 1965, is still well worth reading. He also describes the normal development of the personality as dual, namely, as a consequence of equilibrations, by which a continuum of movement is controlled through the balance of two functional principles (Piaget 1967). Although Piaget did not speak of understanding and reason in this context (rather about accommodation and assimilation) and also not specifically about free will, he did expressly refer to the dynamic principle of subjective spontaneity, which is based on Kant's idea of synthetic judgement a priori (Kant 1983, Kaulbach 1991). This idea is fundamental for the dissolution of the antinomy of empirical and intelligible character realized by man. Its importance goes far beyond the forensic psychiatric practice since it follows that the question of freedom can, in accordance with its nature, never be decided with empirical means, even if they are so highly developed as those of modern neurobiology (Frank and Zanetti 1996).

To the extent that man, in regard to his empirical character, can only be understood as fully determined and forced to exist, progress in modern neurobiology has perhaps vastly extended the boundaries of empirical knowledge. This does not, however, affect the relationship of empirical character to intelligible character as such, upon which the judgement concerning so-called free will solely rests. Moreover, the importance of thinking in terms of synthetic judgements a priori, can be seen therein, that in regard to spontaneity, the *discontinuity* of the (as "appearance") empirically ascertained, *on the one hand*, is confronted with the dynamics of movement as *continuity, on the other hand* [Nicholas of

Cusa's *Quellgrund* is alluded to here, where, by using source as a metaphor, he tries to explain the continuous activity of its origin, apparently *ex nihilo*] (Bormann 1975). By means of synthetic reasoning a priori, the essence of man does not only consist of its being bound to the temporal/spatial existence of discontinuous bodies. Rather, man is also part of that principle called *arche* (Cherniss 1970), which in the continuity of movement, is always carried on through him. While everything that is completed is always subject to principles in its certainty of time and space (and therefore cannot be free), the principle as such is not subject to this limitation. Kant speaks in this sense of the "thing in itself" (Cohen 1917).

The course of this discussion, which has been pursued in a lively manner since Augustine, should interest the forensic psychiatrist from a professional standpoint. No later than Hobbes (1988), an action is termed "free" if its execution is not hindered by internal or external resistance. The following makes reference to the treatise concerning the freedom of will by Schopenhauer (1977). It was written in the year 1839. In it one is warned not to equate the freedom of being able to act with the freedom of wanting to act (volition). After completing a day's work, I can decide to visit the club or a movie theatre. I could, however, just as well hail a taxi, let myself be taken to the airport and fly to Patagonia. I do nothing of the sort, but instead drive home to my wife, as I do every day, convinced that this is my free will. *You're mistaken, my dear friend, says* Schopenhauer, *you're confusing the freedom to act with the freedom of wanting to act* (volition). The next day the same thing happens. Well not quite, since Schopenhauer is lurking behind me wondering what I'll do next. To prove to him that I can indeed decide freely, I opt this time for the movie theatre, although the film does not interest me in the least. Schopenhauer laughs in his sleeve, *Patagonia appears to be too lavish for you.*

Here is an additional example taken from court life: The defence attorney of a heroin dealer requests acquittal and maintains, the compulsion of his client to procure drugs was so strong at the time of the crime that he could act in no other way than as accused. Due to his craving for drugs he was not able to control himself. The attorney mistook the freedom of being able to act as one wants (which in this case actually was impaired) with the freedom to want. According to legal guidelines, the expert is only called upon in questions of controllability, not in questions of freedom of action. That is why he could ignore how the latter's situation, with regard to the constrained position due to drug craving, compared with the truth. To explain the difference that exists, relating to this, between criminal liability and its respective use, the expert did something else. He compared the situation of the addict with that of a person who is being threatened with a pistol and asked to put up his hands. If such a predicament of the most extreme kind really suspended the ability to control in the threatened person, then one could expect that what he does after that – having become uncontrollable – is in a very dangerous way dependent on chance. He might not be able eventually to recognize the position as being one of constraint or if he did recognize it correctly, interpret it incorrectly by considering himself invulnerable, for example. Thirdly, he could also do the only reasonable thing, namely, raise his hands. In the event of loss of control, this would depend completely on chance.

It would be another matter, if in prevailing criminal law one proceeded from a gear-like automatic mechanism of action rather than from the ability to control action. In the former case, the sight of the pistol would have triggered the raising of hands virtually mechanically, similar to a puppet. Apparently, this is what the defence attorney was actually thinking of, since he pointed out to the court that in 99.9 % of the cases the hands are indeed raised. The fact would prove that in such cases of constraint, free will is ruled out, so it would follow that criminal liability was absent in the case at hand. The court went along with the expert rather than the defence attorney. It explained in reference to the high rate of 99.9 %, that at best, only in the case of one of a thousand test persons could the absence of self-control be assumed. Only in the case of the one person, who did not act as the other 999, could it be presumed, that he was "crazy". All the others would have done what was for them the most obvious under the given circumstances.

So the court realized that the man who is capable of self-control makes use of it as he wishes and that is usually as he considers right under the given circumstances. The high percentage of those who react similarly in a given situation only proves their lack of ambiguity. It does not prove *eo ipso* the absence of the ability to form autonomous, i.e. under normal circumstances, rational judgements. (In the case of heroin addiction it is not put into question that the circumstances are not normal. That *behaviour* in such a case is not voluntary means that in making use of one's will, one has only few choices in this case.) – Regarding the so-called freedom of will, it does not follow from what has been established so far, however, that it exists or not. The preceding examples only serve to stress the difference to be made, according to prevailing criminal law, between ability and its use. This is of utmost importance for the work of the expert. It signifies, methodically and economically, an enormous simplification for him, as regarding criminal liability, to be able to ignore the search for and assessment of motives. And as for the verifiability of his conclusion, this constitutes a colossal increase of confidence for both himself and the court. In order to serve the interests of legal certainty and legal equality, the boundary between the authority of the court and that of the specialist can be maintained only in this way and the court be put in the position to make its own judgement.

The difference between the freedom to act and criminal liability is easy to see, but nevertheless both are continually confused in the courtroom. The confusion, however, does not just occur in the courtroom; the commonly held view of the interested public that the will is obviously free is also based on this confusion. Being able to move the right or left hand, however I want, only implies the freedom of the respective action from any external or internal constraints – paralysis or handcuffs, for example – but no more. What is decisively important for our problem is the additional remark: *However I want*. The question of whether the will is free or not also remains open in regard to this experience (Schopenhauer 1839). In addition to the experience that I can move my hand when and how I want, there is another basic human experience that is not reflected upon but rather felt. Accordingly, I am the executor of my acts and naturally responsible for them. It is an experience of the moral kind (Kant 1983). The question of how this experience, which can normally appear in any healthy and reasonably mature person, can be explained or rather whether it can be explained at all, leads to the actual problem of so-called will. Its significance goes way beyond the forensic application, for example, in regard to the political and religious relevance of fatalistic attitudes towards life and theological doctrine of mercy (Flasch 1988).

The basic experience that one is the doer of his deeds and naturally responsible for them usually manifests itself, when pertaining to criminal law, as remorse and a guilty conscience in the form of guilt, shame and similar emotions. The fact that one recognizes oneself as guilty can support the notion that man knows in his innermost being that he is *free*, because that is the way he is. But it is also possible that this feeling is an externally induced result (Witter 1962). This standpoint has been especially supported in the context of sexual morality. Since the phenomenon of a guilty conscience will not be taken into consideration as an argument here, it is only mentioned in passing that in this respect the Christian moral codex certainly does not have the great significance to whom it is prescribed. There were already at least traces of such a sexual morality in pre-Christian antiquity, which was not especially prudish; otherwise one could not understand why in depictions of the divine Venus, she holds her pudenda covered with her left hand (Papaioannou 1977). Whether the feeling of a fundamental morality of man is based on an original or on an acquired condition, a proof that leads to certainty will only be handed to that person, who, with Schopenhauer (and Kant) is already sure concerning his subject. It points to the road upon which a clarification beyond canonized moral ideas and educational programmes is eventually possible. This road is spoken of when the Socrates of the Platonic dialogues (Platon 1925) maintains that *no one voluntarily does bad things*. Therewith Socrates does not say that the committing of crimes or sins already *eo ipso* proves the absence of free will, whether it be in regard to the internal state of mind or the external one (to which the bodily condition also belongs, including that of the brain). Rather, he says that the wrongdoer or the sinner considers the "bad" of his deed to have been "good" at the time of the deed and therefore wanted to do it. In other words: The voluntariness of an action may be objectively bad in its outcome, but for the acting person it is considered good at the time of the action. Man acts freely as long as he is capable of doing good. *Goodies* owe their name to the fact that children consider them good. If the child gets a toothache later or becomes overweight, its preferences usually change. Children who consider pickles rather than sweets to be good are a great exception; but such children exist too. This fact shows that the "good" is not objectively a characteristic of the intended object but rather a changeable expression of subjective estimation (Luthe 1993).

Those who – empirically – reject a concept of man that is based on self-determination, usually use one of two methods of argument in which they refer to the human cognitive capacity (Singer 2002, Roth 1997). They say if there were a will, then the will, being the internal prerequisite for cognition, would not be able to recognize itself. They aptly conclude from this that it does not exist, since whatever exists, must also be able to be recognized scientifically. What is called "will" outside of science is in their eyes, only the – as such unknown – epiphenomenon of chemical-physical processes at certain synapses which, in the course of research, have always become easier to identify. If recently such processes in the living brain can be made three-dimensionally visible by means of contrast methods even in their temporal sequence, then this only shows, however, as is objected to here, what was already generally presupposed, i.e. that certain psychological processes with certain somatic correspondences occur together. That, in principle, is not different from the bending of an arm and its electromyographically objectified parameters. The second chain of argument refers to the proof of the nervous system's unbroken unity in a hierarchy of stimulus and response curves without it requiring the implementation of a special instance of will at any point. According to this argumentation, what seems to intervene really is a reservoir of energy understood as a reinforcing agent that always acts when the triggering stimulus is of the nature that it – in consideration of internal linguistic and other filtering systems – corresponds to an already set response pattern similar to a key which fits the lock. Reduced to the essential, it is a matter of man being morphologically and physiologically programmed in a way so that he is able to react to situations in such a way that he recognizes them by virtue of his endowments. Following the passage of the stimulus through the cerebral filtering station and its organic executive to the resulting constellation of promoting and restraining factors, an individual must indeed react in a certain way and cannot do otherwise (Singer 2002, Roth 1997).

This, by the way, is also how Schopenhauer (1839) essentially judges free will in the above mentioned text. All further expectations of the human cognitive capacity would exceed the borders that this capacity is naturally bounded by, in that the cognitive capacity is directed outwards in accordance with its origins of sensory activity, i.e., away from the will as the innermost centre of man, centrifugally. The direction of the human cognitive capacity is generally not recognized as a defect, since the inner self is usually accepted without reflection as being simply given. To be able to recognize the *will as such* was for the longest time in the history of mankind not an urgent task. It was vital then and is vital now that it exists *de facto*. And so the additional fact that at least since the days of Augustine (Flasch 1989) it is a desideratum of the arts to recognize the will as such should also not upset the scientist who considers himself to be a scientifically minded psychiatrist or psychologist (Carneri 1876) and still believes he must apologize when he happens to speak of the will in the old phenomenological sense of the word. The centrifugal character of cognition thereby corresponds to the view that the properties by which we recognize things must obviously be objective – as objective as the things themselves and in this sense man is a being that reacts, according to Aristotle (1995).

That the "good" is not a special property of a preferred object, but rather, as in the case of the child that loves pickles in a capricious manner, a changeable expression of subjective estimation, seems to be unusual. This makes it advisable to investigate the characteristic features of the "good", which, as it seems, constitutes a task of moral philosophy (Frank and Zanetti 1996). The crucial setting of the course regarding the solution of this task took place in the third century B.C. At that time the ways of Plato and Aristotle parted. In the so-called *Oldest Metaphysics* (Book 12.7) Aristotle states: "*for the thinking is the starting-point. And thought is moved by the object of thought.*" Plato doesn't say so anywhere expressly but he thinks that *the starting point is knowledge*. Ideas are not thought. In complete accordance with the saying, *Let there be light,* ideas as original knowledge consequently lead to thinking. In the "idea of the good", as Plato expressly points out, even *being* is surpassed, to which thinking of being belongs (Chomsky 1973). According to Aristotle, it is the commonly held opinion that we strive for something because it is desirable. Plato maintains, incidentally: Something becomes desirable because we pursue it. That is also the interpretation of Spinoza (Ethics III, sentence 9, cf. Luthe 1993), who equates free will with the term "God", and Hobbes (1988) in the *First principles*. We do not like something because it is beautiful, but rather something becomes beautiful because we love it. That is the quintessence of the lesson that Diotima gives the young Socrates in the Platonic *Symposium*. In modern times, offshoots of this concept can be found, for example, in McDougall 1961, von Bertalanffy 1924 or Köhler 1968. Gödel (cf. Dawson 1999, Piaget 1968) produced a mathematical version.

The empirical outwardly directed character of man is not everything; he needs an intelligible counterpart to prove himself worthwhile. In reference to this Schopenhauer justifies – a priori – the moral consciousness of freedom which corresponds to our intuition that we are doers of our deeds and responsible for that what we do. He justifies it as being *transcendental*. That means that we cannot recognize the circumstances but we can imagine them. The reason why we can imagine them is that we *are* them. Schopenhauer says accordingly: *Freedom is not a result of our actions, but rather of our being* – an old scholastic position (operari sequitur esse). The contention however, is only unproblematic in regard to the scholastic distinction between existence and essence [Dasein and Sosein] (Flasch 1989), but highly problematic if this distinction is dropped. For if our being as such were really free, then it could not be simultaneously determined or formed in any way at all. It is determined by our existence in time and space. Hence, by justifying the freedom of will on Schopenhauer's account, we arrive at a super-temporal and super-spatial dimension of existence and it goes without saying that science does not want to and cannot follow such an argument (Stegmüller 1978).

In the roughly 150 pages of his essay, Schopenhauer (1839) continually presupposes that what "will" is, is known (a dark natural force in our interior that lends the cause the ability to effect). And in complete accordance with Aristotle (1995) it is generally agreed that the relationship between the interior and the exterior is one of a reacting person to the reagent, i.e. objective. To illustrate this thesis Schopenhauer refers to, among others, the example of the tree. The seed reacts upon the conditional makeup of earth, water, light and heat, from which it germinates, and thus, strictly causative as stimulus, brings about the tree. Nowhere does a tree develop out of earth, water, light and heat without the seed. The seed as the cause of the tree reacts to the outside conditions fulfilled on the spot by growing into a tree in order to, at a given time, produce further seeds. Reading this, it amazes us not so much the morphological range of the development curve endowed in the seed for other seeds, the constantly transitory existence, as regards the phenotypic development of the genotypic constitution, but rather the thought of a dynamic that can uninterruptedly push this process forward through time or let it rest.

Where and based upon which existential coordinates should the natural force be imagined that, according to Schopenhauer, provides the ability to work in the seed as the will of the cause? Can we seriously imagine that it – in its being valid specifically for this tree – originates in a reservoir inside the seed that must be imagined to be virtually inexhaustible in regard to the following generations? It can also not be present in the existence of the tree, since its nature must first mature. If the last resort is taken, i.e. the force is localized externally – for example as solar or food energy – nothing of a will remains. Additionally, this assumption also contradicts the further prerequisite of human reaction to the external stimulus as the object of thought, which triggers movement according to Aristotle. The reacting must already be latently, from within itself, dynamically prepared, as the roundness and the elasticity in the form of the hit ball. It does not react by calling it. So it is a matter of the already chemically preformed responsiveness to light in the photosynthesis of reacting plants, and the composition of the drive bound to certain smells etc. in humans and animals that a cherry tree and not a buttercup actually develops from the seed. It must always proceed from a specific relationship.

Schopenhauer (1839) bases his argument on Kant (1983) and the a priori. He does this in different places in his essay, but always merely in an analytical sense. For this reason it remains unknown from the beginning how the will as a natural force can empower the cause to achieve its effect. The analysis in the sense of the analytical a priori can never lead to something new, or all-encompassing, but always to something that is already there, something already enclosed in the cause and therefore small and elementary. This can discover, cause and set it free, but cannot create something beyond itself, not even in the imagination. Thus the ability of the cause to have an effect does not really need any will at all, as Aristotle (1995) already noted. It rather needs the externally initiated, suitable and circumstantially directed inducement to action, i.e. the physical shove, the physiological stimulus or the psychological motive whose result is the respective action. There is just as little room for the will being a natural force as for it being a manifestation of the mind. In God everything there is is already determined in a teleological manner from the beginning. What happens must and can only happen in the way that it happens. The way to Hell, to which the "bad" is headed, is its predetermined way. The eo ipso good cause justifies every means for the chosen one and if we still feel responsible in our innermost being, then we are poorly advised or have not thought about it properly.

The actual, the synthetic meaning of the a priori can be recognized in the fact that it does not lead to something increasingly smaller, to the element, but rather to surplus value (Cohen 1917). It does not occur in Schopenhauer's prize essay concerning the freedom of the will, which is taken paradigmatically as the basis for the deterministic standpoint as a whole here. Schopenhauer repeats *from nothing comes nothing* and determinists keep repeating it with an abundance of expressions. The intelligible character of Kant, however, can therefore only logically become a moral authority because it is based on the Platonic idea of spontaneity, i.e. the effect "by itself". That nothing comes from nothing *(nothing exists that does not exist)* is then only a cheap and worthless phrase if "nothing", as linguistic invention, is the self-imposed limit of recognition, comparable to the linguistic mystification of being only as being. In "Sprache" [Xenien and Votivtafeln] Goethe (1998) maintains: Does the soul *speak*, so alas! The soul speaks no more. The reason for speech cannot be expressed through speech. Banal and subtle. Spontaneity is just as difficult to determine or "something" as the reason for being. In regard to its spontaneity the subject does not react to an outside world to which not only its ideas but also its brain and the rest of its body belong; rather it constructs the outside world using the seed, piece for piece according to the stipulation of what is "good" in proving itself in the inter-subjective sphere of action. That is the constructivist definition of the border term "subject".

The will that is expressed in this spontaneity can be compared to growing and can only be "free" because that is the definition of spontaneity. *It happens by itself*. That is why it is tautological to speak of "free will". If will exists in this way, then it is the epitome of that freedom which is systematically prevented from being arbitrary by its opposing forms of foreign activities and thus has the chance to prove itself inter-subjectively in the community. Plato (1950) uses a graphic expression for this dialectic: *gigantomachy*. It is the ingenious formulation of the old pre-Socratic picture of the sawing giants. This will differs from arbitrariness therein that it is, according to Socrates, principally directed at the good, since no one voluntarily does bad. The good that each individual wants its his own survival. To survive, each must prove itself in what it achieves, with regard to the community. That is how we create the world. It is this criterion of truth of probation that Plato refers to when he speaks of the idea of the good and says, as is repeated here, that it even surpasses being. The recognition of the fact that the existence and essence of man have a partially fictitious character is directly relevant to the solution of the problem of free will.

If we again cast a glance at general psychiatry at the end of this essay, then upon closer inspection it turns out that it is wrong to assume that the consequences that arise from the concept of man based on it – free or determined – are small. If man is determined, then Jaspers's (1913) prognosis is confirmed, according to which psychiatry must be unsystematic and can only describe what is given in its boundless variety and get to the heart of it as a target symptom. If, on the other hand, we are dealing, in the case of the development of human personality, on the basis of a synthesis a priori, with a forward-oriented, open equilibration process, then the two-sided nature of this equilibrium gives us the opportunity to see such a similar ordering structure at work in a system of psychopathology (Luthe 1982). And this is the basic idea through which general psychiatry, in the sense of structural psychopathology, could give itself a systematic character.

References

Aristotle 1995. *Philosophische Schriften*. 6 Bd. Darmstadt: Wissenschaftliche Buchgesellschaft.

Boenke, M. 1995. *Schelling*. München: Diederichs.

Bormann, K. 1975. "Die Koordinierung der Erkenntnisstufen (Descensus und Ascensus) bei Nikolaus von Kues", in: Haubst, R. (ed.) *Mitteilungen und Forschungsbeiträge der Cusanus-Gesellschaft*, Mainz: Grünewald.

Carneri, B. 1876. *Gefühl, Bewusstsein, Wille*. Wien: Braumüller.
Carus, C.G. 1846. *Psyche. Zur Entwicklungsgeschichte der Seele*. Reprint in: Kröner Taschenausgabe, Bd. 95. Leipzig: Kröner
Cherniss, H.F. 1970. "The Characteristics and Effects of Presocratic Philosophy", in: Furley, D.J., Allen, R.E. (ed) *Studies in Presocratic Philosophy*, vol. 1, London: Routledge and Kegan
Chomsky, N. 1973. *Über Erkenntnis und Freiheit*. Frankfurt: Suhrkamp.
Cohen, H. 1917. *Kommentar zu Immanuel Kants Kritik der reinen Vernunft*. Leipzig: Meiner.
Dath, D. 2003. "Wie aus sprachphilosophischer Entrüstung der Ansatz zu einem neuen Verständnis der Welt entsprungen ist. Die mathematische Kategorienlehre lehrt das Machen, nicht die Sachen", *Frankfurter Allgemeine Zeitung*, 272: 41.
Ey, H. 1975. *Des idées de Jackson à un modèle organo-dynamique en psychiatrie*. Toulouse: Rhadamanthe-Privat.
Feuchtersleben, E. von 1841. *Zur Diätetik der Seele*. Leipzig: Fock.
Flasch, K. 1988. *Das philosophische Denken im Mittelalter. Von Augustin zu Machiavelli*. Stuttgart: Reclam.
Frank, M., Zanetti, V. (eds.) 1996. *Kant – Kritik der Urteilskraft. Kants Schriften zur Ästhetik und Naturphilosophie – kritisch geprüfte Texte mit umfassender Kommentierung*. Frankfurt: Verlag Deutscher Klassiker.
Friedreich, J.B. 1835. *Systematisches Handbuch der gerichtlichen Psychiatrie*. Leipzig: Wigand.
Dawson, jr. J.W. 1999. *Kurt Gödel: Leben und Werk*. Wien: Springer.
Goethe, J.W. von 1998. *Werke. Dig. Biblioth*. Berlin: Directmedia.
Grasnick, W. 1987. "Wille und Willensbenehmen", in: Witter, H. (ed.) *Der psychiatrische Sachverständige im Strafrecht*. Berlin: Springer.
Grasnick, W. 1991. "Freiheit, die wir meinen", *JR*, 364.
Griesinger, W. 1843. *Pathologie und Therapie der psychischen Krankheiten*. Stuttgart.
Groddeck, G. 1978/79. *Ça et moi*. 2 Bd. Paris: Champ Libre.
Haddenbrock, S. 1992. *Soziale oder forensische Schuldfähigkeit (Zurechnungsfähigkeit)*. Berlin: de Gruyter.
Heiser, J.H. 1989. "Struktur. Augustine and neg. theology", *New Scholast*, 63: 66-80.
Hobbes, T. 1988. Court Traité des premiers principes. *Le Short Tract on first principles de 1630-1631*. La naissance de Thomas Hobbes à la pensée moderne. Texte, Traduction et Commentaire par Jean Bernardt. PUF Paris
Jaspers, K. 1913. *Allgemeine Psychopathologie*. Berlin Springer.
Kaufmann, A. 1976. "Schuldprinzip und Verhältnismäßigkeitsgrundsatz", in: *Festschrift für Richard Lange zum 70. Geburtstag*. Berlin: de Gruyter.
Kaulbach, F. 1991. "Der Übergang vom Bestimmt-Bestimmenden zum freien Schema in Kants Kritik der Urteilskraft", *Revue internationale de philosophie*, 176: 76.
Köhler, W. 1968. *Werte und Tatsachen*. Berlin: Springer.
Lange, R. 1985. "Hirnforschung und Kriminologie", *ZStW*, 97: 1
Lenckner, T. 1972. "Strafe, Schuld und Schuldfähigkeit", in: Göppinger, H., Witter, H. (eds.) *Handbuch der forensischen Psychiatrie*. 2 Bd. Berlin: Springer.
Luthe, R. 1977. "Aktuelle Positionen in der forensischen Psychiatrie", *Fortschr. Neurol. Psychiat*, 45: 635-648.
Luthe, R. 1981. *Verantwortlichkeit, Persönlichkeit und Erleben*. Berlin: Springer.
Luthe, R. 1982. *Das strukturale System der Psychopathologie*. Berlin: Springer.
Luthe, R. 1985. *Die strukturale Psychopathologie in der Praxis der Gerichtspsychiatrie*. Berlin: Springer.

Luthe, R. 1993. *Der fingierte Mensch. Wie die Seele den Leib bewegt*. Frankfurt: Lang.
Luthe, R. 1996. *Die zweifelhafte Schuldfähigkeit*. Frankfurt: Lang.
McDougall, W. 1961. *Psychologie*. 2.A. Bern: Francke.
Mohr, H. 1987. *Natur und Moral: Ethik in der Biologie*. Darmstadt: Wiss. Buchgesellschaft.
Müller, J., Hajak, G. 2003. *Über das Dürfen und Müssen der Forschung mit forensischen Patienten*. Aachen: Shaker.
Orth, J. 1914. *Der psychologische Begriff des Unbewussten in der Schelling'schen Schule*. Inaugural-Dissertation, Heidelberg.
Papaioannou, K. 1977. *Griechische Kunst*. 3. Aufl. Freiburg: Herder.
Piaget, J. 1965. *Sagesse et illusions de la philosophie*. PUF Paris
Piaget, J. (ed.) 1967. *Logique et connaissance scientifique*. Gallimard Paris
Piaget, J. 1968 *Le structuralisme*. PUF Paris
Plato 1925. *Staat*. Übs. Von K. Preisendanz. Jena: Diederichs.
Plato 1950. *Oeuvres complètes*. 2 Bd. Paris: Gallimard.
Rösler, M. 1987. "Wo liegt die Zukunft der forensischen Psychiatrie?" In: Witter, H. (ed.) *Der psychiatrische Sachverständige im Strafrecht*. Berlin: Springer.
Roth, G. 1997. *Das Gehirn und seine Wirklichkeit. Kognitive Neurophilosophie und ihre philosophischen Konsequenzen*. Frankfurt: Suhrkamp.
Schild, W. 1990. *Der freiheitliche Straftatbegriff*. München: Luchterhand.
Schneider, K. 1932. "Zur Psychologie und Psychopathologie der Trieb- und Willenserlebnisse", *Zentralbl Gesamt Neurol Psychiat*, 141: 351.
Schopenhauer, A. 1977. "Über die Freiheit des menschlichen Willens, gekrönt von der Königl. Norwegischen Sozietät der Wissenschaften zu Drontheim, am 26. Januar 1839", in: *Die beiden Grundprobleme der Ethik*. Zürich: Diogenes.
Schreiber, H.L. 2000. "Rechtliche Grundlagen der psychiatrischen Begutachtung", in: Venzlaff, U. Foerster, K. (eds.) *Psychiatrische Begutachtung*. München: Urban und Fischer.
Singer, W. 2002. *Der Beobachter im Gehirn*. Frankfurt: Suhrkamp.
Stegmüller, W. (ed.) 1978. *Das Universalienproblem*. Darmstadt: Wissenschaftliche Buchgesellschaft.
Wermelinger, O. 1975. "Rom und Pelagius", quoted from Ritter, J., Gründer, K. 1989. *Hist Wörterbuch der Philosophie*, Bd 7, Darmstadt: Wissenschaftliche Buchgesellschaft.
Witter, H. 1962. "Psychopathologie, Krankheitsbegriff und Freiheitsfrage", in: Kranz, H. (ed.) *Psychopathologie heute*. Stuttgart: Thieme.
Witter, H. 1987. "Zur gegenwärtigen Lage der forensischen Psychiatrie", in: Witter, H. (ed.) *Der psychiatrische Sachverständige im Strafrecht*. Berlin: Springer.
Witter, H. 1990. *Unterschiedliche Perspektiven der allgemeinen und der forensischen Psychiatrie*. Berlin: Springer.
Witter, H., Luthe, R. 1977. "La conception organo-dynamique dans la psychiatrie légale en Allemagne occidentale", *Evolut. Psychiatr.*, XLII: 701-708.

Personal Identity

Why Are Identity Disorders Interesting for Philosophers?

Thomas Metzinger

1. Identity Disorders and their Relevance for the Philosophy of Mind

"Identity disorders" constitute a large class of psychiatric disturbances that, due to deviant forms of self-modelling, result in dramatic changes in the patients' phenomenal experience of their own personal identity. The phenomenal experience of selfhood and transtemporal identity can vary along an extremely large number of dimensions: There are simple losses of content (for example, complete losses of proprioception, resulting in a "bodiless" state of self-consciousness, see Cole 1995, Gallagher and Cole 1995, Sacks 1998). There are also various typologies of phenomenal disintegration as in schizophrenia, in depersonalization disorders and in *Dissociative Identity Disorder* (DID), sometimes accompanied by multiplications of the phenomenal self within one and the same physical system. It is important to not only analyse these state-classes in terms of functional deficits or phenomenology alone, but as *self-representational* content as well. For instance, in the second type of cases just mentioned, we confront major redistributions of the phenomenal property of "mineness" in representational space, of what is sometimes also called the "sense of ownership". Finally, there are at least four different delusions of misidentification (DM[1]; namely Capgras syndrome, Frégoli syndrome, intermetamorphosis, reverse intermetamorphosis and reduplicative paramnesia). Being a philosopher, I will discuss two particular types of identity disorder in this contribution – disorders, which are of direct philosophical relevance: A specific form of DM, and the Cotard delusion. Why should philosophers do this? And why should psychiatrists care?

If we are seriously interested in a conceptually coherent and empirically plausible theory of the self-conscious mind, then it is important to test our conceptual tools at least against some examples of the enormous phenomenological richness of our target phenomenon. Generally, the relevance of

1 In using the abbreviation "DM" instead of "DMS" (for "delusional misidentification *syndromes*") I follow a recent terminological modification introduced by Nora Breen and colleagues in order to avoid the inaccuracy of assuming a whole cluster of symptoms as defining characteristics for the different categories. Cf. Breen, Caine, Coltheart, Hendy and Roberts 2000, p. 75, n. 1.

case-studies from cognitive neuropsychiatry consists in the fact that they allow for "reverse engineering": If we can develop an empirically plausible representationalist and functional analysis of identity disorders, we will automatically arrive at a better understanding of what precisely it means to consciously *be someone* in standard situations. Second, it is important to have an effective cure for what Daniel Dennett importantly has identified as "Philosopher's Syndrome" – mistaking a failure of imagination for an insight into necessity (Dennett 1991, p. 401). But there is much more to be learned.

The first thing psychiatrists have to learn from philosophers is that an identity is not something you can simply have, like a bicycle or the color of your hair. From a purely logical point of view identity is not a thing or a property, but a *relation*: Identity is the most *subtle* of all relations, the relation in which every thing stands to itself. On the neurophenomenological level of description, however, we only see how this relation is *represented*, how it is portrayed on the level of an individual brain and on the level of the individual person's conscious self-experience. And in psychiatric disorders we frequently witness how this self-representational process can be damaged in various ways. But even here there is no mysterious thing or property – "a" personal identity – that is damaged or lost. What is changed are certain representational and functional properties in the central nervous system. Of course, we could decide on purely theoretical grounds that a human being with a certain kind of damage to such properties – say, a patient who has irreversibly lost all autobiographical memory and all access to rational modes of cognition – does not fulfil the conditions of personhood anymore. But this would not directly change the patient's phenomenology. "Personal identity" can be either a complex theoretical concept or a concrete form of subjective experience, a conscious content – but it never is a thing, neither in the brain nor anywhere else. To put the point differently: Psychiatrists must stop being naïve realists about personal identity.

The first thing philosophers have to learn from psychiatrists, is that "personal identity" is not only the topic of a traditional *theoretical* field of research, which is centred around questions like, "What are the conditions determining the *sameness of persons*, synchronously as well as diachronously?" The identity of persons is something that is also *phenomenally* represented, by the human brain, prereflexively and pretheoretically, on the level of conscious experience itself. Philosophers have to understand that there is not only an analytical problem of personal identity, but a neurophenomenological one as well – and both are linked in an interesting way. Why is this so? The conscious self, constituted by the content of an organism's *phenomenal self-model* (PSM; for details see Metzinger 2003a), constitutes a concrete kind of standing-in-a-relation-to-oneself, sometimes even *by* representing identity for an organism. But what precisely is it that is being represented? What – given an appropriate cultural context – are the necessary and sufficient conditions for us to first experience ourselves as being *persons,* identical through time? Put very briefly, possessing a globally available and integrated self-representation enables an information-processing system to stand in new kinds of relations to itself (in functionally accessing different kinds of system-related information *as* system-related information), and if a certain portion of this information is highly invariant, the phenomenal experience of *transtemporal* identity can emerge. However, we have to be careful at this point: Conceptually, indiscriminability is certainly not equivalent to identity. Identity is a transitive relation, while indiscriminability is not. Indiscriminability in the self-model may just cause certain functional invariances – for example on the level of body image, background emotions, or autobiographical memory. However, a transparent representation[2] of such functional invariances can result in the *phenomenology* of being identical through time, of transtemporal sameness. And this phenomenology is what, first, functionally *enables* us to refer to ourselves as persons and, second, constitutes the roots of our theoretical discourse on personal identity. Without this phenomenology I could not write an article like this, and you could neither read nor understand it. Conceptual self-representation is anchored in phenomenal self-representation; personal-level properties are to a considerable degree determined by subpersonal properties in the brain. The first lesson philosophers have to learn, then, is how vulnerable and how fragile human beings actually are on the level of those subpersonal properties. More specifically, they have to take notice of the fact that there are strong neurophenomenological conditions of possibility for personhood, that there is no part of human self-consciousness which is immune to epistemic disturbances resulting from subpersonal disintegration, and that; therefore, empirical constraints are relevant and indispensable for anybody who is seriously interested in the philosophy of self-consciousness.

Philosophy and psychiatry share many common epistemic targets. The most central of them may lie in achieving some more substantial progress, a growth of knowledge with regard to human *self-consciousness.* What we need is a conceptually coherent theory of the self-conscious mind, which is phenomenologically and empirically plausible at the same time. Therefore, one important first step is to analyse unusual neurophenomenological configurations of self-consciousness from two directions at the same time: From the point of view of theoretical psychiatry and from the metatheoretical perspective developed by analytical philosophy of mind.

2 A transparent representation is one that cannot be experienced as such. (For more on the notion of "transparency", see Metzinger 2003a, section 3.2.7 and 6.4.2; Metzinger 2003b, section 2.)

2. Example 1: Delusional Misidentification

Let us begin with *reverse intermetamorphosis,* usually defined as "the belief that there has been a physical and psychological change of oneself into another person" (Breen et al. 2000, p. 75). I will argue that this kind of disorder rests on a deviant form of phenomenal self-modelling, and that in principle it could also occur in a non-linguistic/non-cognitive creature not able to form anything like "beliefs" in the more narrow philosophical sense. Here is a brief excerpt from a recent case study on a patient Roslyn Z, conducted by Nora Breen and colleagues:

> RZ, a 40-year-old woman, had the delusional belief that she was a man. This had been a stable delusion for two months prior to our assessment with RZ. During most of these two months she believed that she was her father, but occasionally she would state that she was her grandfather. At the time we saw RZ, she had taken on the persona of her father. She would only respond to her father's name, and she signed his name when asked to sign any forms. She consistently gave her father's history when questioned about her personal history. For example, she said she was in her 60s. (...) The following excerpts are from an interview with RZ. Throughout the interview RZ's mother, Lil, was sitting beside her.
> Examiner: Could you tell me your name?
> RZ: Douglas.
> Examiner: And your surname?
> RZ: B_____.
> Examiner: And how old are you?
> RZ: I don't remember.
> Examiner: Roughly how old are you?
> RZ: Sixty-something.
> Examiner: Sixty-something. And are you married?
> RZ: No.
> Examiner: No. Have you been married?
> RZ: Yes.
> Examiner: What was your partner's name?
> RZ: I don't remember. Lil.
> Examiner: Lil. And you have children?
> RZ: Four.
> Examiner: And what are their names?
> RZ: Roslyn, Beverly, Sharon, Greg.
> (...)
> *RZ standing in front of a mirror looking at her own reflection.*
> Examiner: When you look in the mirror there, who do you see?
> RZ: Dougie B_____ (*her father's name*)
> Examiner: What does the reflection look like?
> RZ: His hair is a mess, he has a beard and a moustache and his eyes are all droopy.
> Examiner: So is that a man or a woman?

RZ: A man.
Examiner: How old is Dougie?
RZ: Sixty-something.
Examiner: And does that reflection you are looking at now look like a sixty-something person?
RZ: Yes.
Examiner: It looks that old does it?
RZ: Yes.
Examiner: Do you think that a sixty-something year old man would have grey hair?
RZ: Well, I haven't worried a lot over the years so my hair didn't go grey.
Examiner: So it's not grey?
RZ: No. It's brown.
(Breen et al. 2000, p. 94p/98p)

Reverse intermetamorphosis is of philosophical relevance because it challenges the Wittgenstein/Shoemaker-principle of immunity to error through misidentification (Wittgenstein 1953, p. 67, Shoemaker 1968). Very obviously there are cases of phenomenal self-representation, of the phenomenal representation of one's own *personal identity* in particular, which are misrepresentations. What philosophers have to see is that there are subsymbolic, non-criterial, and phenomenally transparent forms of self-representation, which are fundamentally fallible and can lead to an obvious error through misidentification on the level of linguistic, personal-level self-reference. I will briefly come back to this point in section 4.

Delusional misidentification is a symptom rather than a syndrome comprising a stable collection of symptoms, and the particular variety of self-misidentification is closely associated with severe psychotic states (Förstl et al. 1991, p. 908p). I now want to shift my reader's attention to a full-blown syndrome, which, again, is of great relevance for the philosophy of mind.

3. Example 2: Cotard Syndrome

Let us briefly look at a second type of identity disorder, which once again is of particular theoretical relevance. This disorder is what I would like to call *existence denial.* In the year 1880 French psychiatrist Jules Cotard introduced the term *délire de négation* to refer to a specific kind of "nihilistic" delusion, the central defining characteristic of which consists in the fact that patients deny their own existence, and frequently even that of the external world (see Cotard 1880, for a more detailed account see Cotard 1882). From 1879 onwards this condition was referred to as the "Cotard Syndrome" in the scientific literature (Séglas 1879; for a concise review of the literature see Enoch and Trethowan 1991, p. 163pp). Although there still is considerable discussion about the notion of a delusion as such (see, e.g., Young 1999) and about the conceptual status of "pathological" belief systems (see Coltheart and Davies 2000, Marshall and Halligan 1996) in general, most researchers tend to agree that the Cotard syndrome is likely a distinct theoretical entity.[3] I will here simply treat it as a neurophenomenological state-class characterized by a specific form of deviant self-modelling, without entering into any further empirical speculations.

As a delusion, the Cotard syndrome certainly is quite dramatic – for instance, it violates the global logical coherence of the patients "web of belief" (see Young 1999, p. 582p) and simply *ends* biographical coherence, while exhibiting a more or less modularized damage to the cognitive model of reality to which the patient has conscious access. The Cotard syndrome is a *monothematic* disorder (Davies et al. 2002). As in many delusions, it is the rather isolated nature of a specific belief content that initially raises serious doubts about his status as a rational subject. However, as a closer look at the data will reveal, a Cotard patient may actually count as a rational subject, because he develops the only possible conclusion from a dramatic shift in his subcognitive PSM. A promising attempt towards a testable and conceptually convincing hypothesis may therefore start from the assumption that the Cotard disorder is simply a modularized, cognitive-level reaction to very uncommon perceptual experience (Young and Leafhead 1996). It must be clearly noted, though, that the phenomenology of firmly believing in one's own non-existence may also turn out to be too intricate and complex to be tractable under classical belief-desire-approaches – for instance, because it decisively involves pathology in *nonpropositional* levels of phenomenal self-representation.

Obviously, any good future philosophical theory of mind should be able to incorporate the "existence denial" exhibited by Cotard subjects as an important phenomenological constraint, one to be satisfied by its own conceptual proposals. There exists a whole range of neurological disorders characterized by an unawareness of specific deficits following brain injuries, all of them falsifying the Cartesian notion of epistemic transparency for phenomenal self-consciousness, i.e. the idea that one cannot be wrong about the contents of one's own mind, that unnoticed errors are impossible because the light of knowledge shines through and through the inner space opened by the conscious self. In pure and extreme versions of the Cotard delusion we are confronted with a

---

3 Young and Leafhead (1996, p. 154) argue that there is no specific symptom shown by every one of Cotard's pure cases, whereas Berrios and Luque (1995) offer a statistical analysis of historical clinical usage of the term, concluding that a pure Cotard syndrome (represented by "Cotard type 1" patients) does exist, and that its nosological origin *"is in the delusional and not in the affective disorders;..."* (ibid., p. 187) I will not take a position on this issue here.

particularly interesting example of this type of representational configuration: Patients may explicitly state not only that they are dead, but also that they don't *exist* at all. In other words, something that seems an *a priori* impossibility on logical grounds – a conscious subject truthfully denying its own existence – turns out to be a phenomenological reality. And phenomenology has to be taken serious. In this case the first lesson to be drawn is this: You can be fully conscious and still truthfully describe the content of your own phenomenal self-experience as "non-existence". In other words, there are actual, nomologically possible representational configurations in the human brain, which lead truthful subjects into logically incoherent autophenomenological reports. What is needed is a representationalist analysis of this target phenomenon, which can lay the conceptual foundations for a truly explanatory account on functional and neuroscientific levels of description.

Elsewhere (Metzinger 2003a, section 6.4.4; 2003b), when discussing cognitive subjectivity as a challenge to naturalism, I offered a representationalist analysis of the Cartesian thought:

- **[I am certain, that I* exist.]**[4]

In extreme forms of the Cotard delusion, we are faced with a delusional belief that can be expressed as follows:

- **[I am certain, that I* do not exist.]**

Weaker forms are delusional beliefs that can be expressed as follows:

- **[I am certain, that I* am dead.]**

What is the phenomenological landscape of the Cotard delusion? A recent analysis of 100 cases (Berrios and Luque 1995, see Fig. 2, p. 186) points out that severe depression was reported in 89% of the subjects, with the most frequent forms of "nihilistic delusion" concerning the body (86%) and existence as such (69%). Other very common features of the reported content of the PSM in Cotard patients are anxiety (65%), guilt (63%), hypochondriacal delusions (58%) and, even more surprising, delusions of immortality (55%; see cf. Berrios and Luque 1995, p. 187). In many cases, certain elements of the bodily self-model seem to have disappeared, or at least to be attentionally unavailable. For instance, one 59-year-old patient would say, "I have no blood" (Enoch and Trethowan 1991, case 5, p. 172), or another one would say, "I used to have a heart. I have something which beats in its place" (ibid., p. 173) while a further case study (Ahleid 1968, quoted after Enoch and Trethowan 1991, p. 165) reports a patient asking "to be buried because he said he was 'a corpse which already stinks'. A month later he said that he had no flesh and no legs or trunk. These ideas were unshakeable, so that the clinical picture

4 The asterisk is here used following the common notation introduced by Hector Neri Castañeda 1966.

remained unchanged for months". Such early stages will frequently proceed to states in which the body as a whole is denied, and the patient feels like a "living corpse", e.g., when saying "I am no longer alive"; "I am dead" (Enoch and Trethowan 1991, case 1, p. 168) or stating "I have no body, I am dead" (Enoch and Trethowan 1991, case 2, p. 168) or, like Young and Leafhead's patient WI (Young and Leafhead 1996, p. 154), simply being convinced that he was dead for some months after a motorcycle accident (involving contusions in the right hemisphere temporo-parietal areas and bilateral frontal damage), with this belief then gradually resolving over time.

Interestingly, there are a number of other phenomenological state-classes, in which a person may experience herself as bodiless or disembodied – ranging from cases like Christina (Sacks 1998) or Ian Waterman (Cole 1995) to certain types of OBEs and lucid dreams (see Metzinger 2003a, sections 7.2.3.2 and 7.2.5) What seems unique about the Cotard delusion is the additional belief that one is dead. The Cotard patient, on the level of his *cognitive* self-model acquires a new, consciously available content – and this content is specific in being highly irrational and functionally immune to rational revision. I would propose that the difference in the phenomenal content in the transparent and *subcognitive* layers of his self-model can be aptly described by employing a traditional conceptual distinction, which is only available in the German language, but not in Greek (e.g., Homer only uses "soma" as referring to corpses), Latin (with *corpus* only referring to the body-as-thing, being the etymological root of the English term "corpse") and other important languages like Italian, French, Spanish or English: The Cotard patient only has a bodily self-model as a *Körper*, but not as a *Leib* (see also Alheid 1968, and Enoch an Trethowan 1991, p. 179p). What is the difference? A *Leib* is a *lived body,* one that is connected to a soul, or, in more modern parlance, the body *as subject,* as locus of an individual first-person perspective. The body *as inanimate object,* on the other hand, is what the PSM in the Cotard configuration depicts. The Cotard-patient only has access to a *Körper*-model, but not a *Leib*-model.

It is interesting to note how one can arrive at a better understanding of the underlying neurophenomenological state-class by simply following the traditional line of thought. What kind of loss could make a *Leib*-model a representation of something inanimate, of something that is no longer tied to the inner logic of life (see Damasio 1994, 1999)? If the logic of survival is made globally available by conscious emotions, then a complete loss of the *emotional* self-model should have precisely this effect. Philosophically speaking this would mean that what the Cotard patient claiming to be a dead corpse is truthfully referring to is the transparent content of his self-model, predominantly concerning the spatial, proprioceptive and emotional layers. This content portrays a moving *res extensa,* from the inside, closely resembling a living human person, but, as a matter of phenomenal fact, not tied to the logic of survival any more. In traditional philosophical terminology, the patient has a new belief *de se*. Since the first-order, non-conceptual self-representational content grounding this belief, in the most literal sense possible, simply no longer *contains* the information that actual elementary bioregulation is still going on, and as technically speaking there is no subjective representation of the current degree of satisfaction of the adaptivity-constraint (Metzinger 2003a, section 3.2.11) any more, and as emotions are completely flattened out, the patient forms a hypothesis. This hypothesis, given his current internal sources of information, is absolutely coherent: He must be a dead object resembling a human being. The existence of this object, although experienced as the origin of an internal perspective, does not affectively *matter* to the patient in any way. An important author in the field, Philip Gerrans (Gerrans 2000, p. 112), writes: "The Cotard delusion, in its extreme form, is a rationalization of a feeling of disembodiment based on global suppression of affect resulting from extreme depression." Many Cotard patients make utterances like "I have no feelings" (Enoch and Trethowan 1991, case 4, p. 171) or, like Young and Leafhead's patient KH (Young and Leafhead 1996, p. 160), state that they are dead as a result of "feeling nothing inside". If it is the conscious self-model, which, as I would claim, mediates embodiment not only on the phenomenal, but also on the functional level, then these patients suffer from functional deficits, because they are, due a severe impairment in their PSM, emotionally disembodied. Computationally speaking it is a specific subset of system-related information, which can no longer be made globally available. This fact then triggers further changes on the cognitive level of self-modelling.

As Gerrans (1999, p. 590) has pointed out, on the level of representational content the Cotard delusion may be miscategorized if described as a DM. At least in weaker forms, the Cotard patient truthfully reports about the content of a very unusual PSM. This unusual PSM results from a globalized loss of affect, Gerrans hypothesizes, mirroring the *global* distribution of the neurochemical substrate that causes the actual deficit, which in turn is then cognitively interpreted. The issue is to first explain how such a PSM could actually come about. Classical belief-desire-psychology and a traditional philosophical analysis in terms of propositional attitudes may, however, not be very helpful in bridging the necessary levels of description in order to arrive at a fuller understanding of the target phenomenon. For instance, it seems plausible that a non-linguistic creature like a monkey could suffer from most of the Cotard phenomenology, without being able to utter incoherent autophenomenological reports. An animal could *feel* dead and emotionally disembodied, without possessing the capacity to self-ascribe this very fact to itself, linguistically or on the level of cognitive self-reference. What is special about the human case is that an isolated, and functionally rigid new element on the level of the cognitive self-model is formed. As soon as we arrive at a convincing representational and functional analysis of the human Cotard patient's self-model, we can proceed to the philosophical issue of whether it is possible to exhibit strong first-person phenomena in Lynne Baker's (1998; see also Metzinger 2003a,b) sense, while simultaneously entertaining the belief that one actually doesn't exist at all. I will return to this issue below.

The Cotard delusion may be analysed as a combination of loss of a whole layer of non-conceptual, transparent content and a corresponding appearance of new, quasi-conceptual and opaque content in the patient's PSM. Is there a more specific way of describing the causal role of the information now not available on the level of the patient's phenomenal model of reality anymore? What *triggers* the massive restructurization of his "web of belief"? A second, and more specific hypothesis may be the "emotional disembodiment"-conjecture: The PSM of the Cotard patient is emptied of all emotional content, making it, in particular, impossible to consciously experience *familiarity* with himself. What the Cotard patient loses may be precisely the phenomenal quality of "prereflexive self-intimacy", the experience of always being in an unshakeable, maximally direct contact with himself. The Cotard patient is not infinitely close to herself, but infinitely distant. If, in addition, it is true that emotional content, generally speaking, represents the logic of survival to an organism, then *self-representational* emotional content, in particular, will represent the internal logic of autonomic self-regulation, of its *own* life-process to this organism. For the Cotard patient, the logic of survival has been suspended: His life-process – although functionally unfolding as still continuously realized in the physical body – is not *owned* anymore, by being represented under a PSM. His life-process is not only not his own anymore, it may no longer even be part of his phenomenal *reality* – depending on the severity of the degree of psychotic depression. The fact that autonomous self-regulation, a continuous bodily process aiming at self-preservation is going on is not a globally available fact anymore; thereby this fact is no longer a part of the patient's reality. It is not appropriated under the PSM. It is important to note that the dynamic process of self-modelling does not generate static forms of mental content, that it is a process of *self-containing*. A Cotard patient may therefore be described as a living, self-representing system that cannot self-contain the fact that it actually is a *living* system anymore.

However, there is more to the Cotard delusion than emotional disembodiment, leading to a persistent false belief via the principle of phenomenal self-reference (i.e., *all* cognitive self-reference ultimately can only refer to the content of the currently conscious self-model, Metzinger 2003a, p. 436). Claiming to be dead – in terms of a dead *body* – is not the same as claiming to be *non-existent*. As Enoch and Trethowan write:

> Subsequently the subject may proceed to deny her very existence, even dispensing altogether with the use of the personal pronoun 'I'. One patient even called herself 'Madam Zero' in order to emphasize her non-existence. One of Anderson's patients

> said, referring to herself, 'It's no use. Wrap it up and throw "it" in the dustbin' [referring to Anderson 1968; TM]. (...)
> If the delusion becomes completely *encapsulated,* the subject may even be able to assume a jovial mood and to engage in a philosophical discussion about her own existence or non-existence. (Enoch and Trethowan 1991, p. 173; 175)

To my knowledge there is only one other phenomenal state-class in which speakers sometimes consistently refer to themselves without using the pronoun "I", namely during prolonged mystical and/or spiritual experiences. What seems to be common to both classes is that the phenomenal property of selfhood is not instantiated any more, while a coherent model of reality as such is still in existence. However, a Cotard patient may express his dramatic and generalized emotional experience of unfamiliarity by even denying the existence of reality as a whole. The phenomenon of explicit existence denial can not be ignored, because on the level of explicitly negated content, it is the second most common representational feature of the Cotard delusion, to be found in 69% of the cases (Berrios and Luque 1995, p. 187). Therefore, the pivotal question is: What kind of neurophenomenological configuration could lead a human being into a) denying his or her own existence, and b) stop using the personal pronoun "I" (or "I*" for that matter, see Metzinger 2003a, section 6.4.4; 2003b)?

Let us begin by considering the first issue. The conscious representation of existence is coded via phenomenal transparency (Metzinger 2003a, section 3.2.7). Phenomenally, we are beings experiencing the content of a certain active representations as *real,* if and only if, earlier processing stages of this representation are attentionally unavailable to us. This leads to the prediction that if a human being's self-model became fully opaque, then this person would experience herself as non-existent – the phenomenal property of selfhood would not be instantiated anymore. The subject-component of such a being's PMIR[5], the self-component in its consciously experienced first-person perspective, would be fully opaque, and only continue to function as the origin its first-person perspective for *functional* reasons, due to the ongoing source of continuous input making it the *functional* centre of its representational space. As there would no longer be a phenomenal *self as subject,* such a system would not have a PSM in the true sense of the term, and its PMIR, strictly speaking, would only instantiate a functional, but not a *phenomenal* first-person perspective. I take this to be the natural explanation for the pro-

5 A PMIR is a *phenomenal model of the intentionality relation*, i.e. a conscious representation of the subject as currently related to a specific object or as interacting with another subject, for instance the conscious experience of a "self in the act of knowing". A PMIR is a consciously experienced first-person perspective. See Metzinger 2003a, section 6.5 for details.

longed spiritual and mystical experiences mentioned above, but will not pursue this line of thought any further here. The second logical possibility is that in extreme Cotard configurations existence is denied because there is no PSM at all in existence. This is empirically implausible, because Cotard patients certainly exhibit a high degree of sensorimotor integration, of coherent speech, etc. – they certainly are not comatose or in deep sleep.

The third possibility, then, is that a transparent, conscious self-model is in place, but it is not a *subject*-model, only an *object*-model. Something still exists, something that looks like the model of a person, but something that is utterly unfamiliar, not alive, and not a phenomenal self in the act of living, perceiving, attending and thinking. The PSM has lost the emotional layer. The consciously experienced first-person perspective in such a case would not be a model of a subject-object-relation, but only one of an object-object-relation. It would not constitute a phenomenal *first-person*-perspective, but rather a *first-object*-perspective. The "first object", for purely functional reasons persists as the invariant centre of reality, because it is tied to an invariant source of internally generated input. Phenomenally, this functional centre is the place at which things happen, but all of them – as well as the centre itself – are not *owned*. The phenomenal property of "mineness" has disappeared from the patient's reality. As Philip Gerrans puts it:

> In this type of case the patient conceives of herself as nothing more than a locus, not of experience – because, due to the complete suppression of affect, her perceptions and cognitions are not annexed to her body – but of the registration of the passage of events. (Gerrans 2000, p. 118)

Let us now proceed to the second issue: Why would such a system stop using the pronoun "I" when referring to itself? The answer to this question would have to explain the phenomenon for two different phenomenal state-classes: Spiritual experiences and the Cotard delusion. In both cases, the system still operates under a functionally centred model of reality. Motor control, attentional processing and cognitive availability are in place, and in principle well integrated. Sensorimotor integration is successfully achieved. In both cases, the subject-component of the PMIR is not a *subject*-component any more on the level of phenomenal experience. Phenomenologically, both state-classes are constituted by *subjectless* models of reality. On the representational level of analysis we find that there is no globally available representation of a *self as subject*. We currently know very little about the minimally sufficient neural correlates for both types of states, but it is plausible to assume that the aetiologies are highly different: In one state-class it is a considerable elevation in the degree of attentional availability for earlier stages of processing contributing to the system-model, in the second state-class it is a loss of a particular layer, namely the emotional layer, which transforms a subject-model into an object-model, turning a first-person state into a "first-object" state. If my short analysis points into the right direction, we can give a new answer to the old philosophical question of what the personal pronoun "refers" to. "I*" inevitably refers to a specific form of phenomenal mental content: to the transparent, *subcognitive* partition of the currently active PSM depicting the speaker *as subject*. If this partition is lost or becomes opaque, then speakers will stop using "I*".

4. Conclusion

Of course, my brief philosophical interpretation of the empirical material may be false or utterly misguided. But I hope it has served to demonstrate the *relevance* of identity disorders to the philosophy of mind. Identity disorders, while being diagnosed on the *personal* level of description, result from subpersonal disintegration (see Gerrans 1999, see also Dennett 1998). Especially when operating from a genetic perspective, when investigating the causal history of such dramatic "personality shifts", subpersonal levels of explanation have to be taken into account. The concept of a PSM forms the logical link between subpersonal and personal levels of description: As a neurobiological, functional, and representational entity it is subpersonal, but by satisfying the transparency-constraint (see Metzinger 2003a, sections 3.2.7 and 6.2.6) it generates personal-level properties like phenomenal selfhood for the system as a whole, enabling "strong" first-person phenomena, social cognition and intersubjectivity. Classical, egologic, theories of mind simply fail by not being able to provide any satisfactory account when confronted with phenomenological material like the one presented. But certain standard assumptions underlying modern analytical philosophy of mind create major difficulties in developing a conceptually clear analysis as well.

Example 1, delusional misidentification clearly challenges the Wittgenstein/Shoemaker-principle of immunity to error through misidentification (Wittgenstein 1953, p. 67, Shoemaker 1968). Why? Very obviously there are cases of phenomenal self-representation, of the phenomenal representation of one's own *personal identity* in particular, which are misrepresentations. One can be entirely mistaken about which person one is, not only in a weak sense of being disoriented about one's own personal identity or of temporarily not knowing *who* one is, but in the strong sense of consistently experiencing oneself as *another* person. And this can happen without a chance to gain higher-order insight into this very fact, under the condition of epistemic opacity. What philosophers have to see is, first, that there are subsymbolic, non-criterial, and phenomenally transparent forms of self-representation and self-identification. Second, these non-linguistic and obviously internal (i.e., locally supervening) forms of self-identification are fundamentally fallible and can therefore lead to an obvious error through misidentification on the level of linguistic, personal-level self-reference. This error would then not be an error based on an object-use of the first-person pronoun "I", but on a subject-use *based on the content of a subpersonal misrepresentation, namely a delusional and phenomenally transparent PSM of oneself as another person.*

I have discussed the philosophical implications of Example 2 at greater length in the previous section. I can therefore be brief in pointing out its metatheoretical relevance: Existence denial is important for *theories of rationality,* because they show how an obviously false belief can be highly modularized, immune to revision, and embedded into a complex network of cognitive self-representation that remains largely coherent. It is also important, because phenomena like the Cotard delusion provide us with a valuable possibility to investigate, first, the relationship between phenomenally transparent and phenomenally opaque mental content in the constitution of human self- consciousness. Second, they permit for a closer description of the relationship between the emotional and the cognitive self, between the prereflexive and the reflexive layers in the human PSM. For reasons of space, I cannot penetrate deeper into these issues here (see Metzinger 2003a for a more detailed account). I nevertheless hope that my short comments could serve to establish the general conclusion that philosophy has a lot to learn from psychiatry.

One last question remains to be answered: Why should psychiatrists care about all of this? Here the answer can be even more simple and short: Theoretical progress is one of the most important factors in the alleviation of human suffering.

References

Ahleid, A. 1968. "Considerazioni sull'esperienza nichilistica e sulla syndrome die Cotard nelle psicosi organiche e sintomatiche", *Il Lavoro neuropsichiatrico,* 43: 927-945.

Anderson, E.W. 1964. *Psychiatry*, 1st edition. London, Baillière: Tindall & Cox.

Baker, L.R. 1998. "The first-person perspective: A test for naturalism", *Amer Phil Quart,* 35: 327-46.

Bermúdez, J.L., Marcel, A., Eilan, N. (eds.). 1995. *The Body and the Self*, Cambridge, MA: MIT Press.

Berrios, G.E., Luque, R. 1995. "Cotard's syndrome: analysis of 100 cases", *Acta Psychiatr Scand*, 91: 185-188.

Breen, N., Caine, D., Coltheart, M., Hendy, J., Roberts, C. 2000. "Towards an understanding of delusions of misidentification: Four case studies", in: Coltheart and Davies 2000.

Cole, J. 1995. *Pride and a Daily Marathon*. Cambridge, MA: MIT Press.

Cole, J., Paillard, J. 1995. "Living without touch and peripheral information about body position and movement: Studies with deafferented subjects", in: Bermúdez, Marcel, and Eilan 1995.

Coltheart, M. Davies, M. (eds.). 2000. *Pathologies of Belief*. Oxford and Malden, MA: Blackwell.

Cotard, J. 1880. "Du délire hypocondriaque dans une form grave de la mélancolie anxieuse", *Annales Médico-Psychologiques*, 38: 168-170.
Cotard, J. 1882. "Du délire des négations", *Archives de Neurologie*, 4: 152-170/282-295.
Damasio, A.R. 1994. *Descartes' Error*. New York: Putnam/Grosset.
Damasio, A.R. 1999. *The Feeling of What Happens: Body and Emotion in the Making of Consciousness*. New York, NY: Harcourt Brace & Company.
Davies, M., Coltheart, M., Langdon, R., Breen, N. 2002. "Monothematic delusions: Towards a two-factor account", *Phil Psychiat Psych* (special issue 'On Understanding and Explaining Schizophrenia', (ed.). Hoerl, C.) 8 (2/3, June/September 2001), 133-58.
Dennett, D.C. 1991. *Consciousness Explained*. Boston-Toronto-London: Little, Brown and Company.
Dennett, D.C. 1998. Postscript, in: Dennett, D.C. (ed.). *Brainchildren – Essays on designing minds*. Cambridge MA: MIT Press.
Enoch, M.D., Trethowan, W.H. 1991. *Uncommon Psychiatric Syndromes*. Oxford: Butterworth-Heinemann.
Förstl, H., Almeida, O.P., Owen, A., Burns, A., Howard, R. 1991. "Psychiatric, neurological and medical aspects of misidentifications syndromes: a review of 260 cases", *Psychol Med*, 21: 905-910.
Gallagher, S., Cole, J 1995. "Body schema and body image in a deafferented subject", *J Mind Behav*, 16: 369-390.
Gerrans, P. 2000. "Refining the explanation of Cotard's delusion", in: Coltheart, M. Davies, M. (eds.). *Pathologies of Belief*. Oxford and Malden, MA: Blackwell.
Metzinger, T. 2003a. *Being No One. The Self-Model Theory of Subjectivity*. Cambridge, MA: MIT Press.
Metzinger, T. 2003b. "Phenomenal transparency and cognitive self-reference", *Phenomenology and the Cognitive Sciences*, 2: 353-393. doi: 10.1023/B:PHEN.0000007366.42918.eb. German version: "Phänomenale Transparenz und kognitive Selbstbezugnahme", in: Haas-Spohn, U. (ed.). *Intentionalität zwischen Subjektivität und Weltbezug*. Paderborn: mentis.
Séglas, J. 1897. *Le Délire des Négations: Séméiologie et Diagnostic*. Paris: Masson, Gauthier-Villars.
Shoemaker, S. 1968. "Self-reference and self-awareness", *J Phil*, 65: 555-567. Reprinted in: Shoemaker, S. 1996. *The First-Person Perspective and Other Essays*. Cambridge: Cambridge University Press.
Wittgenstein, L. 1953. *Philosophical Investigations*, trans. G.E.M. Anscombe. London: Macmillan.
Young, A.W., Leafhead, K.M. 1996. "Betwixt of life and death: Case studies of the Cotard delusion", in: Halligan, P.W., Marshall, J.C. (eds.). *Method in Madness: Case studies in cognitive neuropsychiatry*. Hove, UK: Psychology Press.
Young, A.W. 1999. "Delusions", *Monist*, 82: 571-590.
Young, A.W., Robertson, I.H., Hellawell, D.J., de Pauw, K.W., Pentland, B. 1992. "Cotard delusion after brain injury", *Psychol Med*, 22: 799-804.

The Influence of Brain Implants on Personal Identity and Personality – a Combined Theoretical and Empirical Investigation in 'Neuroethics'

Georg Northoff

Introduction

The intimate connection between our brain and our behaviour, as well as the peculiar relation between our brain and our selves, generates questions that beg for the interplay between anthropological, ethical and neuroscientific issues. Accordingly, there is a need for the development of a "neuroethics" (Roskies 2002) or an "ethics of the brain" (Northoff 2001) which, however, have neither been defined nor delineated so far in full detail.

Recent results from neuroscience reveal the close linkage between brain function, personal identity and the personality (Northoff 2001, 2003). In addition to neuroscientific problems, the close linkage raises both anthropological and ethical questions (Birnbacher 1995, 1998, 2002, Northoff 1995, 1996, 2001, 2003). The anthropological issues concern predominantly the definition of 'personal identity' and 'personality', potential modes of their relation and general criteria for the differentiation between 'preservation' and 'alteration' in both cases.

The ethical questions concern the border between 'restitution' and 'manipulation' of 'personal identity' and 'personality' in therapeutic interventions in the brain and their consequences on the 'competence' to give informed consent. Do brain implants change and thus manipulate persons in order to be therapeutically effective? Can brain implants enhance or suppress certain traits of the personality or even the identity in healthy persons? Are the patients more 'competent' to give informed consent after surgery? Will certain medical and technological therapies therefore change who we are and what we are doing?

These issues remain difficult to investigate since the terms 'brain', 'personal identity' and 'personality' cover different domains which require different methodological approaches. 'Personal identity' is discussed as a theoretical-conceptual term in philosophical contexts where it describes predominantly the numerical i.e. diachronic aspect of the identity of persons (see Northoff 1996 and 2001). The term 'personality', in contrast, is rather an empirical term which describes the character and individuality and thus the synchronic aspects of a person which are closely related with psychological functions. Finally, the term 'brain' is an empirical term which is not primarily associated with psychological functions but rather with physiological processes.

All three terms require consequentially different methods of investigation. 'Personal identity' can be revealed in theoretical-philosophical reflections, 'personality' presupposes empirical-psychological investigation while the 'brain' renders an empirical-physiological approach necessary. In order to elucidate the relation between 'brain', 'personal identity' and 'personality', all three methods should therefore be combined and linked with each other.

In the first part, we therefore refer to the philosophical discussion about personal identity by relying predominantly on the theories as put forward by Thomas Nagel and Derek Parfit. We focus predominantly on their assumptions about the relation between brain and personal identity from which criteria for personal identity are inferred. In the second part, these criteria are operationalized, transformed and empirically investigated by relying on a semistructured interview and a visual analog scale. In addition to these instruments, a standardized scale for the assessment of the personality is included. All three, semistructured interview, visual analog scale and standardized personality scale, are investigated in patients with Parkinson's disease who underwent either fetal brain tissue transplantation or electrode implantation. Based on both theoretical-philosophical reflections and empirical-psychological results, anthropological criteria for the ethical evaluation of 'personal identity' and 'personality' in brain surgery are developed in the third part (see Figure 1).

Theoretical-Philosophical Account of the Linkage between Personal Identity and the Brain

In the philosophical discussion about necessary and sufficient ontological criteria for personal identity, the role of the brain still remains unclear. Either the brain is regarded as a necessary and sufficient criterion for personal identity as it is, for example, suggested by Thomas Nagel. Or the brain is neither regarded as a necessary nor sufficient criterion for personal identity as it is, for example, reflected in the account by Derek Parfit. In addition to these positions, there are various intermediate positions (for example, Shoemaker, Williams, etc. see Northoff 2001 for an overview) which relate personal identity with the brain, though not exclusively. However, in order to reveal the relation between personal identity in a paradigmatic way, the positions from Nagel and Parfit shall be illustrated briefly in the following whereas the intermediate positions will be disregarded for the time being.

• "I am my brain": Nagel

Nagel (1986, pp. 37ff.) considers the brain as both necessary and sufficient criterion for personal identity which results in the statement "I am my brain". Both terms "I" and "brain" as well as their relation shall be defined in further detail in the following.

The "I" is defined by the First-Person Perspective which accounts for the "What is it like" as determined by phenomenal-qualitative experience i.e. so-called qualia (Nagel 1979). Due to the First-Person Perspective, there is a point of view from which the respective person experiences the world. Accordingly, the First-Person Perspective provides a "centre" i.e. "centralization" for the person by means of which it is anchored and embedded within the world (see also Metzinger 1993, pp. 236-7). Interestingly, as pointed out by Metzinger (1993, pp. 231-2) and Northoff (2001, p. 59), this "centralization" may be altered and dissoluted in ego-disturbances in schizophrenia and drug-induced psychotic states. In addition to the First-Person Perspective and the "centralization", the "I" may be characterized by a so-called "relation of mineness". The "I" can distinguish itself i.e. its own person from the "I" of other persons. For example, I can relate the phenomenal-qualitative states which I experience with my own person while I cannot relate those phenomenal-qualitative states which I do not experience by myself with my own person. Subsequently, the phenomenal-qualitative states which I experience are 'my' phenomenal-qualitative states so that one can speak of a "relation of mineness" (Metzinger 1993, pp. 177, 204, 237, 265-7; Northoff 2001, pp. 156-7). The same remains true with the body. I experience a particular body which I consecutively characterize as "my body" – there is a "relation of mineness" between my "I and this particular body". Whereas there is no such "relation of mineness" between other bodies and my "I".

Nagel (1986, pp. 35, 37f.) considers the term "identity" as a definitive and non-conventional term. The term is definitive in the sense that it necessarily implies a Yes-No i.e. All-or-Nothing decision with regard to the identity of persons. Either a person is identical or non-identical. There are no intermediaries. The term is non-conventional in the sense that it does not imply its own necessary and sufficient conditions. Since the term does not imply its own necessary and sufficient conditions, it contains a "blank space" which must be filled by a "further feature" (Nagel 1986, p. 39). He compares the term 'identity' with the term 'gold'. Before the chemical formula for 'gold' was detected, the term 'gold' contained a "blank space" which later was filled by a "further feature" i.e. the chemical formula. Analogous to the situation before the detection of the chemical formula of "gold", we currently have no idea about the "further feature" which might potentially fill the "empty position" in the term 'identity'.

According to Nagel (1986, p. 40), the "further feature" in the case of the term 'identity' must bridge the gap between the subjective experience of the person i.e. its First-Person Perspective and its "I" on the one hand, and the objective necessary structures i.e. its body of its existence on the other. Since the brain might bridge this gap between subjective experience and objective structures, it may be considered as a suitable candidate to fill the "blank space" as a "further feature" in the case of the term "identity". On the one hand, the brain must be considered as the necessary foundation for the possibility of subjective experience since without a brain we are unable to make experiences in First-Person Perspective. On the other hand, the brain is the carrier of psychophysiological processes which are essential for regulation and maintenance of the body. In contrast to other organs, like the liver or kidney, the loss of the brain is accompanied by loss of personal identity. The brain must subsequently be regarded as a necessary and sufficient condition for personal identity. However, due to our current lack of empirical knowledge, this assumption must be considered as a preliminary hypothesis which may be either verified or falsified in both regards empirically and ontologically (see also Northoff 2003a).

If the brain is the foundation of subjective experience, it cannot be considered as a purely physical organ since mental states and thus subjective experience cannot be reduced to physical properties (Nagel 1986, pp. 29, 40). In addition to physical properties, the brain must be subsequently characterized by mental properties. Nagel (1986, 1987) assumes an intimate relationship between mental states and their physical conditions. Due to these mental properties, the brain shows a special kind of "insideness" which accounts for its foundational character for subjective experience: "It [the brain] can be dissected, but it also has the kind of inside that can't be exposed to dissection. There's something it's like from the inside to taste chocolate because there's something it's like from the inside to have your brain in that condition that is produced when you eat a chocolate bar" (Nagel 1987, pp. 34-5). The brain can subsequently be described mentally and physically which both may be traced back to a common foundation i.e. a "fundamental essence" (Nagel 1979, p. 199). This "fundamental essence" can be defined by complex forms of organization and combination ("unusual chemical and physiological structure") of matter which therefore shows both proto-physical and proto-mental properties (Nagel 1979, p. 201). However, the exact definition of and relation between both kinds of properties remains yet unclear.

- "I am not my brain": Parfit

Parfit (1989) challenges Nagel's definition of personal identity by the brain. He claims that the brain is neither a necessary condition for personal identity nor a sufficient one.

According to Parfit, there is no "I" which as a separate entity reflects and remains essential for personal identity. Instead, there is only the "Relation

R" which he defines by "psychological connectedness" and "psychological continuity" (Parfit 1989, p. 206). "Psychological connectedness" points out direct psychological connections ("particular direct psychological connections") as, for example, those between the memories in the sense of Locke. In contrast, "psychological continuity" is defined by "overlapping chains of direct connectedness". If there are no direct connections i.e. "psychological connectedness", as in the case of amnesia, "psychological continuity" can nevertheless still be maintained.

Due to the fact that the "Relation R" replaces the "I", the term "identity" is replaced by the term "survival". According to Parfit (1989, pp. 476-7), "what matters" is not "personal identity" but "survival" of the person ("identity is not what matters"). Unlike the term "identity", the term "survival" neither implies a one-to-one relationship nor an All-or-Nothing relationship. In the case of fission in hemispherectomy, the "Relation R" may be preserved so that the person "survives". However, the person cannot be considered as identical since in this case there is a one-to-two and more-or-less relationship. "What matters" for the person itself in this case is therefore rather "survival" than "identity".

In addition to rejection of an "I", Parfit challenges Nagel's assumption of "identity" as a non-conventional term. If the term "identity" can be replaced by the term "survival", the question for characterization of the latter has to be raised. Persons can survive without reference to something else so that the term "survival" can neither be characterized by a "blank space" nor a "further feature", as suggested by Nagel (see above). He illustrates his point by an analogous example, the one of nations. Although nations neither refer to a separate existing entity nor to other objects, properties, entities, etc. (governments, territorium, etc.), they nevertheless "survive". Analogous to nations, the term "survival" refers exclusively to itself. In contrast to Nagel, the assumption of a "further feature" is therefore not necessary (Parfit 1989, pp. 471-2). The brain is subsequently no longer needed to fill the "blank space" within the term "survival" since there is no such "blank space".

However, even if the brain is neither needed as a "further feature" nor as a sufficient condition, it may nevertheless be regarded as a cause i.e. necessary condition for the possibility of the "Relation R" and thus for "survival". Parfit concedes that the brain is the "normal" cause of the "Relation R" which, however, does not necessarily imply that it is the necessary cause. Following Parfit (1989, pp. 207-8), there may also be other causes i.e. "wide" and "widest" causes which refer to "any reliable cause" ("wide causes") and "any cause" ("widest causes") respectively. For example, a computer which reliably simulates the activity of the brain may be considered as a "wide cause" for the "Relation R". The brain can therefore no longer be considered as the necessary cause for the "Relation R" so that "survival" and brain are not necessarily related with each other ("Relation R is not its brain").

Even different kinds of accentuation in the definition of the brain do not pose a challenge to Parfit's assumption. Parfit concedes that Nagel's definition of the brain carries a certain ambivalence. On the one hand, Nagel (1986, p. 41) speaks about "a brain"/"intact brain" and on the other, about "a brain in certain (mental) states". Only the second meaning of the term "brain" i.e. the "brain in certain states" may be regarded as the "normal cause" for the "Relation R". The first meaning, namely, the "brain", focuses rather on anatomical structures than functional states and may not be linked with the "Relation R". In the first case, the brain cannot be linked with the "Relation R" at all while in the second case the "brain" can be replaced by "any cause". Accordingly, there is no necessary relation between brain and "Relation R".

Finally, the emphasis of Parfit on "psychological continuity/connectedness" suggests that "physiological or physical continuity" may be considered as a necessary condition for the "Relation R" and thus for "survival". Parfit (1989, pp. 474-6) rejects this argument of "physical continuity" by comparing two different kinds of surgical procedures in the brain. In the first procedure, 100 brain cells are exchanged sequentially in 100 steps while in the second procedure the same 100 brain cells are exchanged simultaneously in one step. According to Parfit, the results of both surgical interventions remain the same and can only be distinguished in their procedures. Moreover, both surgical interventions differ with regard to "physical continuity" which is preserved only in the first i.e. the sequential case but not in the second one. If "physical continuity" is considered as essential for "Relation R" and thus for "survival", the person should "survive" only the first procedure but not the second one. This, however, is absurd since both procedures lead to the same results. Accordingly, neither the brain nor the "physical continuity" of the brain can be considered as a necessary condition for the "Relation R" and thus for "survival". Moreover, the example underlines "what matters". In the first procedure, the identity of the person would be preserved, however, this would no longer be the case in the second procedure where the person would only "survive" but, due to lack of "physical continuity", no longer be identical. Since the person "survives" both surgical procedures, any additional differentiation between "identity" and "survival" remains meaningless and therefore no longer significant for the person itself.

Empirical-Psychological Investigation of Personal Identity and Personality in Brain Surgery

- Methods

Patients: Five patients with severe Parkinson's disease were investigated. All patients showed only motor symptoms (akinetic-rigid type) since any kind of psychological symptoms (depression, dementia) were not present (i.e. patients with those symptoms were excluded). Consequently, they received only medication for their motor symptoms but no psychotropic drug in order to ensure reliability of reports, self-observation and judgement. Two of these patients received fetal brain tissue transplantation (transplantation of fetal cells into the basal ganglia (i.e. striatum) as a subcortical structure) and three patients received electrode implantation into the basal ganglia (i.e. internal globus pallidum) (see Brundin et al. 2000 for exact details about both patient selection and surgical procedures). All five patients were investigated with a standardized interview (see Appendix 1), a semi-quantitative visual analog scale (see Appendix 2) and a personality scale (see below) before (t1) and six months after (t3) implantative surgery. In addition, we investigated five age- and sex-matched Parkinson patients at the same time points (t1) and 6 months after (t3), who received only pharmacological treatment (drug-treated), and five healthy controls with the personality scale.

Personal identity: The different items in both the standardized interview (see Appendix 1) and the visual analog scale (see Appendix 2) focused on the various kinds of kinds of criteria for personal identity as raised by Nagel and Parfit in particular.

Firstly, as derived from Nagel, subjective experience of the own "I", the First-Person Perspective i.e. "What is it like", the "centralization" i.e. point of view and the "relation of mineness" is asked for with regard to the mental states and the body. These questions focus on the conscious awareness and integration of material to be implanted into their brains.

Secondly, the subjective experience, perception, role and relation to the own brain and the importance of the brain for personal identity, as compared to other organs of the body, is requested so that the direct relation between brain and personal identity can be explored. Thirdly, after the implantative surgery, the influence of the surgery on personal identity/personality/individuality, brain/relation to own brain, mental states and subjective experience and body and environment is asked for. This allows for exploration of the direct relation between changes in the brain and personal identity.

The qualitative interviews were analysed according to a qualitative analysis of content with a consecutive phenomenological analysis (see Mayring 1990, pp. 46-80 for details and Northoff 2001, pp. 435-466 for the interviews i.e. the results). The lines of the different items in the semi-structured visual analog scales were divided into centimeters and the respective answers were measured (see Appendix 2).

Personality: In order to investigate the personality, we applied the German version of the Minnesota Multiphasic Personality Inventory (MMPI) which includes various dimensions of the personality like hypochondriasis, depression, conversion hysteria, psychopathic deviate, masculinity/feminity, paranoia, psychasthenia, schizophrenia, hypomania and social introversion. Statistically, comparisons between groups (surgically-treated patients versus drug-treated patients versus healthy controls) at the different time points (ANOVA with post-hoc t-tests), as well as between time points (before-after) within the surgical group (paired t-tests) were calculated. Moreover, we compared the differences between the different time points between the groups using analysis of variance (ANOVA) (see Table 1).

- Results

Personal identity: Firstly, no patient experienced a change in the "I", the First-Person Perspective and her/his point of view by implantation of either fetal cells or an electrode. The electrode is regarded as a "purely technical device". However, it nevertheless becomes individualized so that, for example, one patient spoke of "my electrode" – one may characterize this relation as a "relation of mineness" with regard to the electrode. Moreover, patients reported that the function of the electrode may be influenced by psychological factors including the own emotional status and attitude towards it. The fetal cells are regarded as "substitutes for dopamine" (i.e. the lacking transmitter) and are thus experienced as "natural and physiological"substitutes. However, the fetal cells may be influenced by psychological factors. For example, one patient performed meditation before and after surgery in order to "create a good and beneficial mental-moral environment for the growth of the cells". Another patient asked whether he would speak Swedish after the implantation (the surgery was performed in Sweden with fetal cells derived from Swedish women).

Secondly, some patients say that during the course of their illness they "became much more aware of their brain". One patient reported that "she would feel her brain during the on and off switching of her electrode" and all patients had the feeling that they were able to influence the function of the brain by means of their mental and psychological states. Moreover, all patients attribute a "special role" to the brain as compared to other organs. Although implantation of cells and electrodes in the brain does not lead to changes in personal identity, it nevertheless cannot be compared with other organs like the heart because the "brain constitutes psychological and mental functions". Accordingly, patients experience a principal difference between brain surgery and surgery in other organs with regard to personal identity and personality.

Thirdly, neither the disease itself nor the implantative therapy was related with any felt changes in personal identity and personality. Some patients spoke about a "greater freedom and individuality" in their movements after surgery. The fetal cells were regarded as a "natural and physiological substitute" for the dopamine deficiency in their own brain, whereas the electrode was considered as "technical device" "which enables the brain function in the correct way".

In summary, surgically-treated patients did not experience changes in their personal identity since they were well able to psychologically integrate the implant within their experience in First-Person Perspective.

Personality: Surgically-treated patients differed in several different subscales regarding dimensions of the personality from drug-treated patients and healthy controls at either time point i.e. t1 and t3 (see Table 1). While, in contrast, only the dimensions of 'schizophrenia' and 'social introversion' showed significant differences between t1 and t3 within the surgically-treated group, which was neither the case in drug-treated patients nor in healthy controls. This is supported by the fact that the difference between t1 and t3 (t1-3) was significantly higher in surgically-treated patients than in the other groups (see Table 1).

In summary, surgically-treated patients showed changes in their personality after surgery especially in the dimensions of 'social introversion' and 'schizophrenia'.

Anthropological Criteria for Ethical Evaluation of the Impact of Brain Surgery on Personal Identity and Personality

Based on theoretical-philosophical reflections and empirical-psychological results, we aim to develop anthropological criteria for the impact of brain surgery on personality and personal identity. These anthropological criteria may serve for the distinction between preservation and alteration of personal identity and personality in the case of brain surgery which, in turn, may be presupposed for evaluation of ethical problems like, for example, informed consent (see Figure 1 as well as Birnbacher 1995, 1998, 2002, Northoff 2001).

Firstly, our empirical results suggest dissociation between personality and personal identity after implantative brain surgery. While the own personal identity was not experienced as different, several dimensions of the personality showed changes after surgery (see above and Table 1). This further underlines the importance of the distinction between both terms 'personal identity' and 'personality' (see above and Birnbacher 1995). Both must therefore be distinguished in terms of context, being either theoretical-philosophical or empirical-psychological, and content, focusing either on numerical i.e. diachronic or characterological i.e. synchronic aspects of the person.

Due to these differences in context and content, both may be dissociated from each other. This is reflected in our empirical results with an influence of the brain implants on the personality whereas the personal identity remained unaffected. This, however, does not mean that personal identity remains principally unaffected, in general, by any kind of surgical interventions in the brain. One could imagine that surgery aiming at cutting the brain into two or several parts, like split brain surgery or hemispherectomy, may lead to changes in numerical i.e. diachronic identity and thus personal identity (see also Nagel 1979 and Northoff 2001). The exact kind of intervention within the brain should thus be considered with caution.

Accordingly, both the distinction between 'personal identity' and 'personality' and the exact kind of intervention within the brain should be considered as anthropological criteria in the ethical evaluation of brain surgery.

Secondly, the First-Person Perspective was revealed as one essential characteristic of personal identity (in Nagel's account) and described by qualia, centralization and "relation of mineness" (see above). While empirical results demonstrated that both centralization and qualia remained apparently unaffected by brain implants, they revealed the possibility of the development of a "relation of mineness". This is reflected in our patients' experience of "psychological integration" of the implant within their brain. This 'psychological integration' of the implant was apparently crucial in the subjective experience of our patients and is probably important too for 'physiological integration' within the brain.

Both theoretical-philosophical considerations and empirical-psychological results underline therefore the importance of the First-Person Perspective in general and the "relation of mineness" in particular. While in other kinds of brain surgery (for example, non-implantative procedures), qualia or centralization may be affected as can be observed in patients with frontal lobectomy (see Northoff 2001). These patients are no longer "centralized" and experience different or even absent qualia which is reflected in their altered or reduced consciousness.

Accordingly, the First-Person Perspective with its different characteristics should be considered as anthropological criteria in the ethical evaluation of brain surgery.

Thirdly, the two-fold nature of the relation between personal identity and the brain should be revealed in further detail. On the one hand, changes in the brain may affect personal identity via modifications in other functions, like motor or psychological functions – this would indicate a rather indirect relation. On the other hand, personal identity may be constituted by the brain itself. Many of us overtly or covertly believe in a kind of "neuroessentialism", that our brains define who we are and what we are (see Roskies 2002). In short, personal identity may be considered as a brain-based notion. Our subjective experience and the principal possibility of the concept of numerical i.e. diachronic identity and thus personal identity may be constituted by specific functions in the brain. Nevertheless, we are, at present, still far from understanding the exact empirical mechanisms underlying these functions.

The function of certain brain regions, like the frontal lobe, may be critical and essential for constitution of personal identity. Disease-induced alteration or therapeutic-related manipulation of these so-called "critical regions" may eventually lead to changes in both subjective experience and theoretical concept of personal identity (schizophrenic patients with ego-pathology who show frontal lobe changes and changes in their subjective experience of personal identity; see Northoff 2001). In contrast, these "critical regions" were in our case apparently neither affected by the disease i.e. Parkinson nor the implants.

Accordingly, the distinction between different kinds of brain regions and functions with regard to their importance and relevance for personal identity, like, "critical and non-critical" brain regions, should be considered as an anthropological criterion in ethical evaluation of brain surgery.

Fourthly, the exact kind of relation between personality and the brain should be revealed in further detail. Analogous to personal identity, the relation between personality and the brain may be two-fold. On the one hand, brain changes may affect the personality via some other functions. This could well be the case as revealed in our empirical results. Parkinson patients showed significant improvements in the personality dimension of 'social introversion' after surgery (see above). This may be related to their improvement in motor function which, relying on the subjective accounts by our patients, allow for better integration within the social world i.e. the environment as is reflected in the significant change in the dimension of 'social introversion'. The influence of the brain on the environment should thus be taken into account.

On the other hand, the specific dimensions of the personality may be constituted by particular brain regions and functions (see Northoff 2001). The exact functional mechanisms in the brain, which may underly the observed changes in the personality in our patients, however, remain unclear. Analogous to personal identity, one may nevertheless distinguish between "critical and non-critical regions" with respect to specific dimensions of the personality. Some of these regions must have been affected by the implants since otherwise there would have been no changes demonstrated in some of the dimensions of the personality. Moreover, since, in turn, the personality itself reflects the relation with the environment, these regions may be regarded as crucial for the interaction between brain and environment by means of which the latter may modulate the former.

Accordingly, the relation between brain, personality and environment should be considered as an anthropological criterion in the ethical evaluation of brain surgery.

Fifthly, the relation between psychological functions and the subjective experience of mental states should be considered. Parfit speaks of a "web of psychological functions" with "psychological connectedness and continuity" (see above). Subjective experience in First-Person Perspective may not be related with one particular psychological function (like, for example, working memory, attention, etc.). While the different characteristics of the First-Person Perspective (i.e. qualia, centralization and "relation of mineness") may eventually be accounted for by specific relations between the different psychological functions and thus with distinct "webs of psychological functions". This relation between subjective experience and "webs of psychological functions" may potentially reflect mental states and their particular characterization by qualia and centralization.

Moreover, these "webs of psychological functions" may be related to what Nagel calls "physico-mental intimacy" (see above). However, due to the intermediary role of psychological functions between the physical brain and the subjective experience of mental states, one should probably better speak of "psychophysiological-mental intimacy" than "physico-mental intimacy". Though "psychophysiological-mental intimacy" remained apparently intact in our case (no changes in either qualia or centralization), other diseases (for example, schizophrenia) and therapies (for example, frontal lobectomy) led to changes in qualia and centralization and thus in "psychophysiological-mental intimacy" (see Northoff 2001).

Accordingly, the relation between the subjective experience of mental states and the "web of psychological functions" with their consecutive "psychophysiological-mental intimacy" should be considered as an anthropological criterion in the ethical evaluation of brain surgery.

Sixthly, relying on Parfit criticism on Nagel (see above), one should distinguish between the "structural brain" (i.e. the "brain") and the "functional brain" (i.e. the "brain in certain states"). In our cases of brain surgery, the implants aimed at either "anatomical reconstruction" (i.e. the fetal cells) or "functional reconstruction" (i.e. the electrodes). Most important for the effect of the fetal cells is, however, not the anatomical reconstruction alone but the functional integration and connection with the other brain regions which then allows for "functional reconstruction" of motor function (Brundin et al. 2000, Northoff 2001).

The distinction between the structural-anatomical and the functional-psychophysiological level of the brain is further underlined by the possibility of their dissociation. Anatomical-structural lesions do not necessarily lead to changes in the functional-psychophysiological level and vice versa. The functional-psychophysiological level may be crucial for the "webs of psychological functions" and consecutively for the subjective experience of mental states. As a result it may account for what Nagel calls "organization and combination of matter" (see above).

Accordingly, the distinction between the structural-anatomical and the functional-psychophysiological level of the brain as well as their distinct impacts on the subjective experience of mental states should be considered as anthropological criteria in the ethical evaluation of brain surgery.

Conclusion

We investigated the relation between personal identity, personality and brain surgery by combining theoretical-philosophical and empirical-psychological methods. On the basis of the results from both kinds of investigation, we were able to develop anthropological criteria for the ethical evaluation of brain surgery. These included differentiation between 'personal identity' and 'personality', specification of surgical procedure, consideration of the First-Person Perspective including its distinct characteristics, distinction between "critical and non-critical regions" in the brain with regard to personal identity, specification of the complex interaction between brain, personality and environment, investigation of "psychophysiological-mental intimacy" and dissociation between the structural-anatomical and the functional-psychophysiological level of the brain (see above).

On the basis of these anthropological criteria, ethical problems may be discussed concerning the impact of either disease or therapy on the ability to give informed consent. For example, these anthropological criteria may be considered as the basis for the development of an operational model of "competence" (Wear 1993). This may not only include "thresholds" or "gates" with regard to the risk of the decision to be made (Buchanan and Brock 1989) but, in addition, "thresholds" and "gates" with regard to potential changes in personality and personal identity ("threshold concept" with several "gatekeeping functions"). As a result this operational model may account for the complex relation between 'personality'/'personal identity' and "competence" by including both subjective and objective components (see Rehbock 2002). The present investigation may therefore be regarded as a first step towards the development of a future "ethics of the brain" (Northoff 2001) or "neuroethics" (Roskies 2002) in the case of brain surgery.

Acknowledgements: The author is indebted to W. Oertel and A. Kupsch for cooperation in the empirical investigation of the Parkinson patients. Moreover, the author acknowledges and thanks D. Birnbacher for his support in theoretical-methodological questions. Finally, the author thanks all patients who revealed him more about personal identity, personality and the brain than any textbook could ever provide. The study was financially supported by grants from the German Research Foundation (Habilitationgrant, 304/1-1; Heisenberg grant 304/1-4).

References

Beauchamp, T.L., Childress, J.F. 1994. *Principles of Biomedical Ethics*. Oxford: Oxford Unviersity Press.

Birnbacher, D. 1995. "Identität der Persönlichkeit und Identität der Person: Philosophische Fragen im Zusammenhang mit der Transplantation von Hirngewebe", *Zentralblatt für Neurochirugie*, 56: 180-185.

Birnbacher, D. 1998. "Hirngewebstransplantationen und neurobionische Eingriffe – anthropologische und ethische Fragen", *Jahrbuch für Wissenschaft und Ethik*, 3: 79-96.

Birnbacher, D. 2002. "Der künstliche Mensch – ein Angriff auf die menschliche Wuerde?", *Aachener Studien zur Technikphilosophie*.

Brundin, P., Pogarell, O., Hagell, P., Piccini, P., Widner, H., Schrag, A., Kupsch, A., Crabb, L., Odin, P., Bjoerklund, A., Brooks, D., Marsden, C., Oertel, W., Quinn, N., Rehncrona, S., Lindvall, O. 2000. "Bilateral caudate and putamen grafts of embryonic mesenchephalic tissue treated with lazaroids in Parkinson's disease", *Brain*, 123: 1380-90.

Buchanan, A., Brock, D.W. 1989. *Deciding for others: The ethics of surrogate decision making*. Cambridge: Cambridge University Press.

Mayring, P. 1990. *Qualitative Untersuchung*. Heidelberg: Beltz Verlag.

Metzinger, T. 1993. *Subjekt und Selbstmodell*. Paderborn: Schoeningh Verlag.

Nagel, T. 1979. *Mortal questions*. New York: Cambridge University Press.

Nagel, T. 1986. *The view from nowhere*. New York: Oxford University Press.

Nagel, T. 1987. *What does it all mean?* New York: Oxford University Press.

Northoff, G. 1995. "Hirngewebstransplantationen: Medizinische und ethische Probleme", *Ethik in der Medizin*, 7: 87-92.

Northoff, G. 1995. "'Ethics of the brain' in brain tissue transplantation: Preservation or alteration of personal identity", *Bulletin of the ESPMH*, 3-4.

Northoff, G. 1996. "Brain identity in brain tissue transplantation: Preservation or alteration of personal identity?" *Journal of Medical Ethics*, 2, 5-18.

Northoff, G. 2001. *Personale Identität und operative Eingriffe in das Gehirn*. Paderborn: Mentis Publisher.

Northoff, G. 2002. "Are we our brains? A neurophilosophical account of personal identity", in: Kanzian, C., Quitterer, J., Rungaldier, E. (eds.) *Wittgenstein Proceedings. Personal identity.*

Northoff, G. 2004. *Philosophy of the brain – The Brain Problem*. John Benjamins Publisher.

Parfit, D. 1989. *Reasons and Persons*. Oxford: Oxford University Press.

Rehbock, T. 2002. "Autonomie – Fürsorge – Paternalismus", *Ethik in der Medizin*, 14: 131-150.

Roskies, A. 2002. "Neuroethics for the new millennium", *Neuron*, 35: 21-3.

Wear, S. 1993. *Informed Consent*. Dordrecht-Boston-London.

Appendix 1

Questions for the semistructured interview

1./ How do you define the terms 'personality' and 'personal identity'?

2./ Did your personal identity, personality and individuality change after surgery? Are you another i.e. different person?

3./ Did your relation to your brain and your body changed in the course of the disease and after surgery?

4./ Do you have the feeling that you have a personal relationship with the fetal cells/electrode? Is the implant 'part of yourself' and your brain/body?

5./ Do you think that the fetal cells/electrode need some kind of 'psychological integration'?

6./ Do you experience changes in your psychological functions after surgery?

7./ Do you experience changes in your motor functions after surgery?

8./ Has your relation to the environment changed during the disease and after surgery?

9./ Do you think that your mental states changed after surgery? Do you have a different consciousness of yourself and others after surgery?

10./ How do you compare the brain with other organs of the body? Do you attribute a special status to brain implants as compared to those in other organs?

Appendix 2

Visual-Analog Scale for subjective experience of personal identity and personality

1. My movements improved after surgery. -------------------- My movements did not improve after surgery
2. My perceptions did not change after surgery. ------------------------- My perceptions changed after surgery.
3. The experience of myself did not change after surgery. --------------------- The experience of myself changed after surgery.
4. My emotions and my mood did not change after surgery. ----------------------- My emotions and my mood changed after surgery.
5. My will did not change after surgery. --------------------- My will changed after surgery.
6. After surgery I can command my body according to my will. ------------- After surgery I cannot command my body according to my will.
7. I feel no longer locked within my own body after surgery. --------------------- I still feel locked within my own body after surgery.
8. My psyche did not change after surgery. ----------------------- My psyche changed after surgery.
9. My individuality did not change after surgery. --------------------- My individuality changed after surgery.
10. My personality did not change after surgery. ---------------------- My personality changed after surgery.
11. I did not become another person after surgery. ------------------ I became another person after surgery.
12. I do not have a different awareness of myself after surgery. ------------------ I have a different awareness of myself after surgery.

13. I do not have a different awareness of my body after surgery. ----------------- I have a different awareness of my body after surgery.

14. I do not feel isolated from the environment after surgery. ---------------------- I feel isolated from the environment after surgery.

15. Despite the surgical therapy I remain the same person. ------------------------ Due to surgical therapy I became a different person

Subjects had to make a cross on the line between the two contradictory statements according to the degree of the appropriateness of either statement.

Table 1

Results of scores in personality dimensions in the Minnesota Multiphasic Inventory (MMPI) in surgically- and drug-treated Parkinson patients and healthy controls before (t1) and six months (t3) after surgery/later

	Surgically-treated patients (n = 5)			Drug-treated patients (n = 5)			Healthy controls (n =5)			Variance analysis between groups (p)		
	t1	t3	t1-3	t1	t3	t1-3	t1	t3	t1-3	t1	t3	t1-3
Hypochondriasis	67.5b**	64.1b*	n.s.	77.4 c**	81.7c**	n.s.	50.8	50.3	n.s.	0.004**	0.003**	n.s.
Depression	66.8b**	63.8b*	n.s.	68.8c*	73.5c*	n.s.	48.3	48.0	n.s.	0.021*	0.018*	n.s.
Conversion Hysteria	67.0b*	63.4a*	n.s.	72.6c**	82.0c*	n.s.	53.3	52.0	n.s.	0.028*	0.031*	n.s.
Psychopathic deviate	54.0	55.3	n.s.	58.2	55.5	n.s.	51.8	50.2	n.s.	n.s.	n.s.	n.s.
Masculinity/ Feminity	50.8	48.2	n.s.	53.6	49.5	n.s.	53.4	50.7	n.s.	n.s.	n.s.	n.s.
Paranoia	51.0b*	52.6	n.s.	60.0c*	54.0c*	n.s.	44.1	45.3	n.s.	0.047	0.041	n.s.
Psychasthenia	60.6b**	52.9	n.s.	69.0c**	76.3	n.s.	48.1	48.2	n.s.	0.049*	n.s.	n.s.
Schizophrenia	59.9b*	53.9	0.042b*	64.8c*	68.7c*	n.s.	49.5	49.4	n.s.	0.042*	0.039*	0.039*
Hypomania	50.8	49.5	n.s.	53.9	49.5	n.s.	51.2	54.3	n.s.	n.s.	n.s.	n.s.
Social introversion	60.0b**	53.8	0.019ab*	58.2	52.5	n.s.	45.0	44.3	n.s.	0.015*	0.049*	0.029*

a = significant ($p < 0.05$) difference between surgically- and drug-treated patients
b = significant ($p < 0.05$) difference between surgically-treated patients and healthy controls
c = significant ($p < 0.05$) difference drug-treated patients and healthy controls

* = $p < 0.05$ (corrected)
** = $p < 0.005$ (corrected)

Figure 1

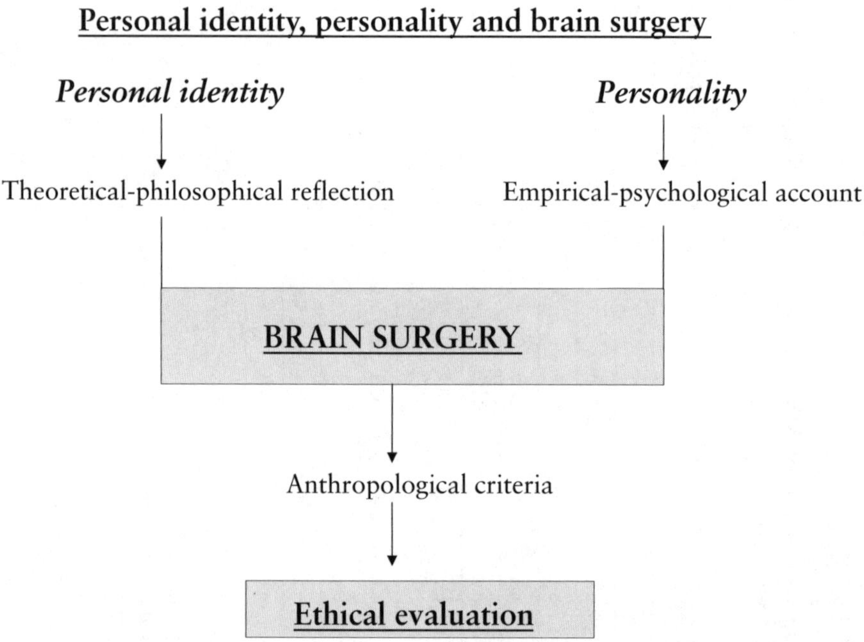
Personal identity, personality and brain surgery
Personal identity
Personality
Theoretical-philosophical reflection
Empirical-psychological account
BRAIN SURGERY
Anthropological criteria
Ethical evaluation

Psychiatric Ethics

Ethics as a Focus of Controversy in Postmodern Antagonisms*

Hanfried Helmchen

Ethical implications of the scientific development of medicine have become much clearer during the past two decades, even for the psychiatrist, not least due to public debates in which strong emotions have sometimes overshadowed arguments. Examples include aspects of eugenics or of data protection in genetics, research with patients unable to give informed consent, or the revived discussion about euthanasia triggered by demographic change. But what is the context of these debates?

A basic topic of mankind is the relationship between the individual and the society. At different times and in different regions various ideas have developed to become ethical principles, which, in turn, have determined the actual reality of life through morals and law. Both in the historical long-term view and the global cross-section these differences are demonstrated by the different weighting of the individual in relation to society. Each of these relationships has its own difficulties. They become extremely obvious if the one or the other side gains strong preponderance and finally results in excesses of a socially unattached individualistic freedom or a collectivistic and totalitarian society.

The relations are deeply influenced by the tremendous social consequences of modern scientific and technical development. One need only consider the desire of each individual to obtain the best possible medical treatment versus its costs for the community. Thus the progress of knowledge calls continuously for new solutions that serve the balance between individual (autonomy, dignity, welfare) and social (justice, responsibility) principles. Such solutions are made more difficult by the antagonism between the rapidity of scientific and technological progress and, in contrast, the slowness of the moral development of the human being. And yet the rapidity seems as inevitable as the slowness is necessary, because both ethical and legal rules will determine behaviour only if they have been generally recognized and internalized by members of the (respective) community. This, however, needs time. Furthermore, they can take effect only if they are sufficiently stable over a period of time. The discrepancy to the acceleration of progress is evident. Günter Anders understood this discrepancy as a "promethean drop" and characterized it as the "old-fashioned condition of the human being" (Anders 1956) almost 50 years ago.

* Appeared first in German as "Ethik im Spannungsfeld postmoderner Antagonismen", *Der Nervenarzt* 74 (3), 2003: 201-203.

Solutions must also be developed for the task of bringing these principles, e.g. human rights declared by the United Nations, which come from an enlightened rationality and claim to be globally valid, into accordance with regional culturally bound customs of living (Payer 1989). In order to make solutions acceptable and to define them as a mode of behaviour in society, it is necessary not to underestimate traditional regional customs of every-day living that have been handed down emotionally. The latter are particularly emphasized by postmodern multicultural critics who often view the universality of human rights as a product of the European enlightenment and condemn their world-wide implementation as cultural imperialism (Baker 1997, Macklin 1999).[1] [2]

However, a solution seems conceivable if one proceeds on the assumption that the transtemporal, transnational, and transcultural weight of an ethics codex is based not on the commonly accepted values but on the "mutuality of problems and conflicts" and the "related demand for solutions that lead to a culture adopting the conflict-solving norm of another culture" (Baker 1997). With the globalization of medical science, the related ethical dilemmas and its efforts to solve them according to the respective developmental stage of scientific medicine will also spread into different cultures. This is the reason for the world-wide importance of the Declaration of Helsinki to date (1964 to 2000) (Taupitz 2001) and the recently raised question whether the Convention on Human Rights and Biomedicine (CHRB) of the Council of Europe could be a suitable model for world-wide regulation (Taupitz 2002).

However, the efficacy of rules is bound to the societal structures of every-day life. These are expressed in myths, religions, and traditions (Engelhardt 1997), are part of the identity of a society, and thus determine the specific features of a region. To relinquish these rules would incur for many people a threat to the guidelines of their lives, to their moral stability. They resist therefore to renounce the specific regional features that they experience as being threatened by globalization. For example, the practice of informed consent is more widely established in the northern hemisphere with its more

---

1 We cannot deal here with the enormous discrepancies of the global distribution of resources that may influence such judgements (Macklin 2001). It can only be mentioned, for example, that the right of every human being to the best available psychiatric care declared by UN declaration 46/119 in 1991 is opposed to a serious lack of medical care in the majority of countries in the world. For example: countries without their own production of medical drugs depend on imports, e.g. Ethiopia, which, in 1997, had to spend all of its meagre funds for antibiotics alone, leaving no funds for psychotropic drugs, or in Somalia, where for the same reason, i.e. the lack of antipsychotic drugs, psychiatrists are forced to chain psychotically aggressive patients.

2 In 2003, the German Research Foundation (Deutsche Forschungsgemeinschaft) established a research group on "Kulturübergreifende Bioethik" in Bochum. (http://www.ruhr-uni-bochum.de/kbe/)

individualistic life style, whereas, in the more strongly family-oriented Mediterranean societies it is more susceptible for misunderstanding, and, in the more commonly organized Asian societies, met with incomprehension or, at best, only poor acceptance (Blackhall et al. 1995) e.g. in the traditional Japanese society (Baker 1997) where the physician will inform the family of the patient only in order to alleviate the anxiety of the patient who has already to contend with the burden of his illness. But even within large regions such as Europe with a more or less common cultural identity there are significant regional differences as is shown by the basically different handling of euthanasia in the Netherlands and in Germany, or the non-signing of the CHRB by the United Kingdom and Germany for opposing reasons.

To balance such antagonisms requires that each position be seriously considered. Furthermore, it requires time. As, for instance, the initially very heated and emotional public controversy at the so-called bio-ethics convention of the European Council resulted that Germany has still not signed the CHRB, due to the concern that national standards could be eroded, whereas Great Britain refused to sign because it expected a restriction of the freedom of research. In the meantime, the German discussion has become more factual and more differentiated and it has been shown that some standards of the CHRB are superior to the German ones (Taupitz 1998), and that other stricter German standards can be maintained. Of course not only ethical but also political considerations have played a role here. Public pressure may have prevented the government from signing the CHRB. The disadvantage of this is that Germany, because it is not a signatory power, cannot sign the supplementary protocol on banning human cloning although it is strongly in favour of it. Furthermore, Germany is in danger of losing its equally strong voice in the decisional processes of the further development of the CHRB.

However, time is relevant not only for a rational argumentation but also for the discussion in every-day life, i.e. experience and habit. The latter indicates that the concept of informed consent (which developed originally from the Kantian tradition in Prussia but has been practised most frequently in the particularly individualistically structured Anglo-American societies) needed generations in order to replace the paternalistic behaviour of the physician who concealed bad news but conveyed hope. But recently even in Asian societies this concept seems to be gaining importance as is shown by its place in the Japanese language as "informed(o) consent(o)". Is this a necessary adaptation to the changing world or a surrender of inalienable human values?

Such mechanisms of cultural identity, that are essential for the stability of a society, will be effective in a similar way for every single person. They will determine his position and decision in the case of specific ethical dilemmas and their solution also needs time. Thus, for example, just a generation ago, many physicians refused to expose patients to the burden of a controlled clinical trial of therapeutic measures, e.g. psychotherapeutic or social interventions, because it was considered as ethically questionable. On the other hand, the opinion arose that it is also unethical to introduce a therapy onto the market or to implement it in practice without proof of its efficacy and safety (Helmchen and Müller-Oerlinghausen 1975). Nowadays, despite many reservations, this "ethical paradox" appears to be solved (Helmchen 2002), and medical practice is being governed as evidence-based medicine. The former reservations have been curtailed by differentiation of ethical arguments and complex methodological developments.

However, the task remains to find solutions that do justice to such patient-oriented ethical reservations as well as to the immediate demands of hopeful patients. Thus, placebo control is accepted as the golden standard for many controlled clinical trials. Its use is seen as compelling for evidence of clinically relevant efficacy because the proof "is ethically acceptable only if it uses the optimal methods according to the state of the art" (Fritze et al. 2000). But the use of a placebo is opposed by ethical reservations (Taupitz 2002). These are based on withholding an effective (standard) therapy from the placebo-treated control group, and, even more so, if this only serves the introduction of another drug that may be truly superior to a placebo (and in this way fulfils the demands of the licensing authorities) but does not improve significantly the standard therapy or is no "more than insignificantly" effective than the level of the standard therapy (as stated in § 33a of the SGB V (German Social Law) from the year 2000) (Helmchen 2001). On the other hand, it is also ethically dubious to draw too far-reaching conclusions from placebo-controlled trials that cannot be generalized because of flaws of randomization due to difficulties in informing the patients (Lavori 2000). The efforts of an ethically flawless further development of placebo-controlled studies cost not only money but also the time and capacity of many researchers (and, not least, the patience of hopeful patients). This expenditure could slow down (real) progress but, on a positive note, speed up the further development of ethically impeccable research and the ethical competence of researching physicians.

References

Anders, G. 1956. *Die Antiquiertheit des Menschen. Über die Seele im Zeitalter der zweiten industriellen Revolution*. München 2.Aufl.: C.H.Beck.

Baker, R. 1997. "Transkulturelle Medizinethik und Menschenrechte", in: Tröhler, U., Reiter-Theil, S. (eds.) *Ethik und Medizin 1947–1997*. Göttingen: Wallstein, 433–459.

Blackhall, L.J., Murphy, S.T., Frank, F., Michel, V., Azen, S. 1995. "Ethnicity and Attitudes Toward Patient Autonomy", *JAMA* 274: 820–825.

von Engelhardt, D. 1997. "Wissenschaftlicher Fortschritt im sozialkulturellen Kontext", in: Tröhler, U., Reiter-Theil, S. (eds.) *Ethik und Medizin 1947–1997. Was leistet die Kodifizierung von Ethik?* Göttingen: Wallstein, 147–159.

Fritze, J., Gastpar, M., Möller, H.J. 2000. "Relevanz von Plazebo zur Kontrolle von Fehlerquellen beim Wirksamkeitsnachweis", in: Maier, W., Engel, R.R., Möller, H.J. (eds.) *Methodik von Verlaufs- und Therapiestudien in Psychiatrie und Psychotherapie.* Göttingen Bern Toronto Seattle: Hogrefe, 70–82.

Greaves, D. 1991. "Lessons from Victorian medical ethics", *Bull Med Ethics*, 65: 23–24.

Helmchen, H. 2001. "Therapeutische Wirksamkeit. Wirkungen, Wirksamkeit und Wertigkeit therapeutischer Maßnahmen", *Nervenarzt*, 72: 56–60.

Helmchen, H. 2002. "Evidenz der Evidenzbasierten Medizin?", *Nervenarzt* 73: 1–2.

Helmchen, H., Müller-Oerlinghausen, B. 1975. "The inherent paradox of clinical trials in psychiatry", *J Med Ethics* 1: 168–173.

Lavori, P.W. 2000. "Placebo control groups in randomized treatment trials: a statistician's perspective", *Biol Psychiatry*, 47(8): 717–723.

Macklin, R. 1999. "International research: ethical imperialism or ethical pluralism?" *Account Res*, 7 (1): 59–83.

Macklin, R. 2001. "Bioethics and public policy in the next millennium: presidential address", *Bioethics*, 15 (5–6): 373–381.

Payer, L. 1989. *Andere Länder, andere Leiden. Ärzte und Patienten in England, Frankreich, den USA und hierzulande.* Frankfurt/M.-New York: Campus.

Taupitz, J. 1998. "Die Menschenrechtskonvention zur Biomedizin-akzeptabel, notwendig oder unannehmbar für die Bundesrepublik Deutschland?", *VersR*, 542–546.

Taupitz, J. 2001. "Forschung am Menschen. Die neue Deklaration von Helsinki. Vergleich mit der bisherigen Fassung", *Dtsch Ärztebl* 98 (38): C1933–C1940.

Taupitz, J. 2002. "Note of Clarification. Kaum zu verantworten", *Dtsch Ärztebl* 99 (7): A 411.

Taupitz, J. (ed.) 2002. *Das Menschenrechtsübereinkommen zur Biomedizin des Europarates – taugliches Vorbild für eine weltweit geltende Regelung?* Berlin-Heidelberg-New York: Springer.

Compulsory Admission and Compulsory Treatment in Psychiatry

Harald Dreßing

Introduction

Mentally ill patients are sometimes not in the position to understand the nature of treatment or admission. As a consequence, psychiatric patients are occasionally compulsorily admitted to psychiatric hospitals and, under certain circumstances, also treated against their will. The necessity to apply coercive measures in certain cases distinguishes psychiatry from most other medical disciplines as psychiatry plays a central role in the custody and control of the mentally ill. Insofar compulsory admission and compulsory treatment have become central topics of psychiatric ethics and practice. Legal and ethical standards of compulsory admission and compulsory treatment have to take into consideration three contradictory interests: 1. Personal freedom of the mentally ill patient. 2. Public safety. 3. Need for treatment.

Changing patterns of attitude towards psychiatry have stressed these aspects very differently and the problem still remains unresolved.

In the following sections a short historical overview is given and the fundamental ethical and philosophical aspects are discussed.

History

Mental hospitals are of recent origin and it was not until the nineteenth century that the need of asylums was realized. The increase in number of these psychiatric asylums called for a specific legislation regulating admission and discharge. Involuntary admission on judicial order was the original and only method employed in the beginning. It was not until 1838, in France, that voluntary admission to mental hospitals was provided for the first time.

Nevertheless, there were always legal regulations allowing society the possibility of committing mentally ill patients, against their will, to mental hospitals. The justification for an involuntary hospitalization is that there is always a group of psychiatric patients who lack insight into their illness and, therefore, unwilling to undergo treatment. In the middle of the last century medical aspects were applied primarily when a mentally ill patient was committed compulsorily. The central motive for a compulsory admission was the need for treatment. With the arising of the civil rights movement in the United

States at the beginning of the 1960's, there emerged a restrictive attitude towards compulsory admission. There were strong claims to refrain from infringement of the fundamental civil rights of the mentally ill, accompanied by an almost total abandonment of the "need for treatment" principle that previously governed compulsory admission of the mentally ill in favour of reliance upon the determinations of danger. This led to rigorous civil commitment standards and procedures implementing multiple legal safeguards against improper commitment.

Ethical and Philosophical Aspects of Compulsory Admission and Compulsory Treatment

As autonomy, non-maleficence, beneficence and justice are central points of biomedical ethics (Helmchen and Okasha 2000), compulsory admission and compulsory treatment in psychiatry have to be justified in every instance because they constitute a breach of personal autonomy. Generally, most of the mentally ill patients are treated on a voluntary basis in psychiatric hospitals, however, a varying proportion of mentally ill patients world-wide is also hospitalized involuntarily. A recent study in this field showed that compulsory admission rates (episodes of compulsory admissions/100000 inhabitants) and compulsory admission quotas (percentage of involuntary placements of all inpatient episodes) in the European Union Member States differ considerably. Compulsory admission rates range from 6/100000 in Portugal to 218/100000 in Finland. Compulsory admission quotas amount to 3,2 % in Portugal to 30 % in Sweden (Dreßing and Salize 2002, Salize and Dreßing 2002). Experience in the former USSR (Fulford et al. 1993), and in Japan (Salzberg 1991), show that there is also a risk of abuse of involuntary hospitalization due to political or economical reasons. Even when the current legal and moral standards are followed rigidly abuse can not be wholly excluded (Rachlin et al. 1975).

What are the arguments for the far-reaching infringement of personal freedom in the case of involuntary hospitalization?

A medical model approach is based on the assumption that severe mental illness can substantially interfere with the capacity to make free decisions (Roth 1977). Mental illness affects the soundness of the mind and, therefore, also the legal competence of this person in question. If a mental illness renders the patients unable to make a free and informed decision to hospitalize themselves, their need for treatment in a hospital can not be ignored (APA 1983). Patients in this condition have a right to treatment, which has been affirmed as a constitutional right (Rachlin et al. 1975).

This medical viewpoint can be called in terms of moral philosophy a utilitarian approach (Mill 1871, Chodoff 1984, Appelbaum 1994). Utilitarian thinkers stress the point that the morality of an action is defined by its result with regard to the individual's benefit. If mental illness renders the individual unable to make a competent decision, then an involuntary hospitalization can be accepted as a last resort.

The contrary position can be called a legalistic approach (Forster 1997) or civil liberties approach (Appelbaum 1997). From this point of view compulsory admission is an assault on individual freedom, an act which can not be justified. This position is partly influenced by an antipsychiatric ideology, which calls in question the existence of psychiatric diseases and describes involuntary hospitalization as a means of social control (Szasz 1961).

Deontological theories may support this negative position towards compulsory admission and compulsory treatment:

> Deontological theories deny what teleological theories affirm. They deny that the right, the obligatory, and the morally good are wholly, whether directly or indirectly, a function of what is nonmorally good or of what promotes the greatest balance of good over evil for self, one's society, or the world as a whole. They assert that there are other considerations that may make an action or rule right or obligatory besides the goodness or badness of its consequences – certain features of the act itself other than the *value* it brings into existence, for example, the fact it keeps a promise, is just, or is commanded by God or by the state. (Frankena 1973, p. 15)

Since the 1960's, far-reaching changes in the delivery of mental health care, coupled with achievements of the human rights movement, have shifted the public focus from a paternalistic emphasis upon the need to treat patients who are not able to take care of themselves to the rights of the mentally ill patients. Alongside this development, the legal framework or commitment laws for the involuntary placement and treatment of the mentally ill have been reformed in many countries. A basic objective of many of these reforms had been to reduce the frequency of compulsory admission to mental health care (Curran 1978). In sharp contrast to these intentions, increasing rates of compulsory admission have been reported (Wall et al. 1999, Darsow-Schütte and Müller 2001). Additionally, it was criticized that over-emphasizing the human rights of patients would stress autonomy at the expense of treatment, thus neglecting the need for appropriate care, so that in extreme cases patients might even "die with their rights on" (Treffert 1973). The increasing number of homeless, mentally ill people in the United States is one consequence of this development (Torrey and Zdanowicz 2001). Involuntary detention of severely mentally disordered people is often not possible due to legislation that prohibits compulsory admission of such people when not judged as being a danger to themselves or to the society. A growing number of mentally ill persons among the prison and forensic population seems to be another consequence of rigid criteria for civil commitment (Lamb and Weinberger 1998). A decreasing number of beds in general psychiatry and a forced deinstitutionalization is accompanied by a growing number of beds in forensic psychiatry. This means that overemphasizing the aspects of human rights and patients' autonomy may lead to negative consequences (Schanda and Knecht 1997). Some of the seriously mentally ill, in the name of personal freedom, end up on the street, in prisons or in forensic psychiatric hospitals.

Conclusions

In the future, the application of coercive measures or compulsory interventions to mentally ill people will still be inevitable under specific circumstances, in order to avoid harm to the patients themselves as well as to the public. Compulsory admission and compulsory treatment, however, infringe fundamentally upon human rights. Therefore, appropriate legal regulations will be even more crucial in the future. It will be an ongoing task to adapt legal frameworks in all countries on a continual basis to keep pace with developments and new achievements in mental health care, and to balance patients' rights and interests against their need and right for treatment, and public safety.

References

American Psychiatric Association 1983. "Guidelines for Legislation on the Psychiatric Hospitalization of Adults", *American Journal of Psychiatry*, 140: 672-679.

Appelbaum, P.S. 1994. *Almost a Revolution.* New York/Oxford: Oxford University Press.

Appelbaum, P.S. 1997. "Almost a Revolution: An International Perspective on the Law of Involuntary Commitment", *Journal of the American Academy of Psychiatry and Law*, 25: 135-147.

Chodoff, P. 1984. "Involuntary Hospitalization of the Mentally Ill as a Moral Issue", *American Journal of Psychiatry*, 141: 384-389.

Curran, W.J. 1978. "Comparative Analysis of Mental Health Legislation in Forty-Three Countries: A Discussion of Historical Trends", *International Journal of Law and Psychiatry*, 1: 79-92.

Darsow-Schütte, K.I., Müller, P, 2001. "Zahl der Einweisungen nach PsychKG in 10 Jahren verdoppelt", *Psychiatrische Praxis*, 28: 226-229.

Dreßing, H., Peitz, M., Salize, H.J. 2002. "Involuntary placement of mentally ill in the European Union – Legislation and practice", *European Psychiatry*, 17 (Suppl 1): 141s.

Forster, R. 1997. *Psychiatrische Macht und rechtliche Kontrolle.* Wien: Döcker.

Frankena, W.K. 1973. *Ethics. Second Edition.* Englewood Cliffs, New Jersey: Prentice Hall.

Fulford, K.W., Smirnov, A.Y., Snow, E. 1993. "Concepts of Disease and the Abuse of Psychiatry in the USSR", *British Journal of Psychiatry*, 162: 801-810.

Helmchen, H., Okasha, A. 2000. "From the Hawaii Declaration to the Declaration of Madrid", *Acta Psychiatrica Scandinavica*, 101: 20-23.

Lamb, H.R., Weinberger, L.E. 1998. "Persons With Severe Mental Illness in Jails and Prisons: A review", *Psychiatric Services*, 49: 483-492.
Mill, J.S. 1871. *Utilitarianism.* (ed. Roger Crisp). Oxford: Oxford University Press 1998.
Rachlin, S., Pam, A., Milton, J. 1975. "Civil Liberties Versus Involuntary Hospitalization", *American Journal of Psychiatry*, 132: 189-192.
Roth, L.H., Meisel, A., Lidz, C.W. 1977. "Test of Competency to Consent to Treatment" *American Journal of Psychiatry*, 134: 279-284.
Salzberg, S.M. 1991. "Japan's New Mental Health Law: More Light Shed on Dark Place", *International Journal of Law and Psychiatry*, 14: 137-168.
Szasz, T.S. 1961. *The Myth of Mental Illness: Foundations of a Theory of Personal Conduct*. New York: Dell.
Salize, H.J., Peitz, M., Dreßing, H. 2002. "Involuntary placement of mentally ill in the European Union – admission rates and epidemiology", *European Psychiatry*, 17 (Suppl 1): 142s.
Schanda, H., Knecht, G. 1997. "Strafrechtliche Folgewirkungen des Unterbringungsgesetzes", *Neuropsychiatrie*, 11: 154-160.
Torrey, E.F., Zdanowicz, M. 2001. "Outpatient Commitment; What, Why and for Whom", *Psychiatric Services*, 52: 337-341.
Treffert, D.A. 1973. "Dying with Their Rights On", *American Journal of Psychiatry*, 130: 1041.
Wall, S., Hotopf, M., Wessely, S., Churchill, R. 1999. "Trends in the use of the Mental Health Act: England 1984-96", *British Medical Journal*, 318: 1520-1521.

Coercive Threats and Offers in Psychiatry

Thomas Schramme

As is generally the case in medicine, an important condition of a justified psychiatric intervention is the informed consent of a patient. The proper respect of autonomy is a basic moral and not just a medical duty, hence coercive treatment is a *prima facie* moral wrong and is in need of justification. In this paper, I would like to emphasize that there are a lot more cases where more justification would be necessary than is actually given. If a patient complies voluntarily with a certain proposal, we generally regard the treatment as legitimate. But a competent patient may also assent to a certain treatment only because he was compelled to do so. Influences on the formation of his decision may render his choice contrary to his will. It is my aim to focus on these particular forms of coercion which are often neglected in discussions of informed consent. Although the paper deals with an ethical problem which applies to each field of medicine, I am of the view that it is particularly common in psychiatry for reasons which will become more obvious later in the text. The reasons stem from the particular vulnerability and volitional indecisiveness of psychiatric patients and the asymmetrical relationship between the mentally ill and the psychiatrists or psychotherapists.

The kind of coercion I am concerned with is not identical to the well-known problem of medical paternalism, i.e. treatment against the stated will or without consent. Instead, it deals with an influence on the *genesis* of a patient's will. Obviously, not all influences on the deliberation and will-formation of a patient are coercive, e.g. facts and circumstances. But patients can be coerced into doing something or giving consent to a certain treatment by means of threats. In addition, some offers might be coercive too. This might appear dubious because offers – unlike threats – are predictions to better the situation of a person if she does what she is asked but without sanction if she does not. Nevertheless, I believe that offers are coercive when they are irresistible. In psychiatry especially this may be experienced quite often.

The doctrine of informed consent consists of several elements (Beauchamp 1997, pp. 185ff., VanDeVeer 1986, pp. 164ff.). In order to give valid consent to a proposed treatment a patient needs to be competent, well informed and understand the necessary facts and his assent the result of an autonomous choice. In this paper, I am exclusively concerned with the last condition, which cannot be fulfilled in case of threats and arguably some offers.

There are three main possible scenarios where an informed consent is lacking: Firstly, the patient may not be able to give or withhold informed consent. If so, one may be hesitant to call the treatment 'compulsory'. After all, it is assumed that coercive intervention involves treatment against the will of a person but one may argue that a person who is not competent to reason as to the proposed treatment is not able to state her own will – hence medical intervention would not be an instance of coercive treatment. Although it is a delicate question, especially in psychiatry, exactly where competence ends and incompetence begins, it seems obvious that in general, psychiatric patients are not incompetent (Brock 1987, pp. 98ff., Kopelman 1997, pp. 275ff.). They may be unable to perform certain tasks but that does not mean they are globally impaired. The abilities to consent are relative to certain tasks, in our case, to evaluate proposed treatments. Most mentally ill people are certainly capable to give their informed consent or refusal under the usual circumstances.

Secondly, the patient may autonomously disagree with a proposed medical intervention, and therefore, withhold informed consent. Here we find some well-known cases of coercion in medicine. They involve treatment against the competent will of a person in order to serve his best interest. When we think of morally problematic interventions in psychiatry we usually imagine these cases of compulsory treatment, e.g. where people are fixated or physically forced to take some form of medicine. These medical interventions are called strong (or hard) paternalistic interventions (Feinberg 1971). Of course, medical paternalism may be justified, after all, there may be a conflict between the patient's will and the opinion of what the doctor (and most other people) would see as best for the patient. Doctors are not merely obliged to respect the autonomy of a patient but also to ensure his well-being. In addition, in cases where the grounds for a psychiatric intervention concern danger of the patient to others, coercive treatment is arguably justified even if he is competent.

The third scenario occurs when the patient complies with a certain treatment but not because of an autonomous decision. As stated before, on the surface, this seems to be an instance of informed consent, hence non-coercive treatment. When consent to a certain intervention is given by a patient we would normally not see the treatment as being coercive. But this indeed depends on whether the consent was given freely or not. Not only the result – the assent itself – is taken into account when we evaluate medical interventions but also the genesis of the stated will of a patient. As is true to say, people can be manipulated and even forced into appearing compliant with a proposed course of treatment.

To give an example, when I hand over my wallet because you would otherwise threaten to shoot me, I am acting voluntarily to a certain degree, i.e. I could have done otherwise if I had chosen to do so.[1] But we could not say that my handing over the wallet was an autonomous, let alone a consenting act, since I was, after all, under threat. I had no other "real", i.e. reasonable, alternative.

Similarly, a psychiatric patient who consents to pharmaceutical experiments may also have been placed under threat to comply. If so, the treatment is coercive because it prevented the formation of an autonomous will. Thus, coercion does not merely consist of actions that ignore the actual choices of a person but also of threats which determine the free formation of his will and are, therefore, against the autonomous will of the person. As stated before, I am concerned here only with this type of coercion. To distinguish it from cases where the focus is usually placed on, i.e. paternalism, I will call it "interactive coercion". It is interactive because the patient is not just the object of medical intervention, as in the case of paternalism, but also an acting part in an interpersonal relationship. After all, the aim of coercion is to bring the person himself to do something (e.g. give his consent) and not merely to do something on him.

Threats and Warnings

The situations I have in mind when I refer to interactive coercion involve threats that influence the will and, thereby, the actions of a person. They can be defined as follows:

> Def. (interactive coercion): Q does/does not A because P predicts that a detrimental consequence R will follow if Q does not /does do A; (and that R will not follow if Q does/does not A[2]).

Since Q *ex hypothesis* does not want R – otherwise it would not constitute a threat –, P predicts a worse situation (damage or harm) for Q if he does not do A. Therefore, he threatens Q. An example of a possible threat in psychiatry would entail P (a member of the staff in a psychiatric hospital) asking Q (a patient) to stop smoking and threatening to take away his supply of cigarettes

---

1 This raises some controversy about freedom of the will and freedom of action that, for obvious reasons, will not be discussed here. For my claim it suffices to state that the threatened person must have a choice and act intentionally in order to be coerced in the way I am interested in. If I were physically forced to hand over my wallet or if I were under hypnosis, then things would be interpreted differently. That people sometimes, like in the example, do not have a "real" – i.e. a reasonable – choice constitutes the main grounds for the claim that coercion is *prima facie* immoral.

2 The second conditional is sometimes left implicit.

if he does not.[3] Also, when a psychiatrist asks a patient to give consent to a proposed treatment and threatens to write a bad report if he refuses, this may constitute an instance of interactive coercion. As I mentioned before, the formal acquiescence of a patient is not a sufficient criterion of informed consent.

However, it seems that the formula is not satisfactory in every case because there are examples, where harm for Q is predicted as a consequence of his non-compliance, but without involving a threat. Not every interaction with the deliberation and not every influence on the will of a patient is coercive. They can be non-coercive even when a limitation of all alternative ways but one is reached and the freedom of someone is delimited (Wertheimer 1987, p. 197). A psychiatrist should, for example, lay down all significant facts about the risks of a proposed treatment, the possible outcomes and alternatives that may also predict a worse situation for the patient. This may leave the patient without any alternatives apart from one (reasonable) choice. Nevertheless, these facts are essential for an autonomous choice. But when does an interaction become coercive?

Consider the following case: Doctor P says to patient Q, who refuses to take his medication: "Look, if you do not take these pills, you will become depressed." P predicts a worse situation for Q if he does not do what P advises him to do. Nevertheless, it obviously does not constitute a threat and we would rather refer to P's statement as a warning. The prediction is based merely on future causal events, hence the difference between a warning and a threat seems to be that the latter involves the intentional realization of a consequence R by P if Q does not A.

But the condition of intentional consequences instead of causal results is only a necessary, not a sufficient, condition of threats. Consider the slightly changed example: Doctor P says to patient Q: "Look, if you do not take these pills you will become agitated and we shall then have to put you on medication by force. It is better you take them voluntarily now." The second consequence, namely Q's being forced to take the pills would clearly form an intentional action, and not a mere causal chain of events. But does it constitute a threat?

Not all predicted intentional harm constitutes a threat. If a teacher promises to fail a student if she does not write an essay by the end of the month, this would be something he intentionally brings about. Nevertheless, it would not constitute a threat because the proposed action of the teacher would be entirely consistent with the institutional rules of a school.

Accordingly, the doctor in the given example may only warn the patient about a common and expected course of events. Both the fact that Q will

---

3 A psychiatric patient may also threaten a doctor but it seems that these cases are more rare for reasons of different power. I will stick to examples where patients are coerced.

become agitated if he does not take the pills and the following compulsory treatment seem to be the normal and common results of Q's choice. One might argue about the normative status of the second consequence, i.e. the justification of the enforced treatment in the case of his becoming agitated. But whether or not it is justified is independent of it being a reasonably expected course of events (Nozick 1969, pp. 31ff.).[4]

Of course I do not wish to deny that these kinds of cases, where Q obviously has no real alternatives, are especially problematic in psychiatry, because they are often felt like a threat by the warned person. The report of a woman illustrates this point: "I didn't want to go into hospital, but Graham [the consultant psychiatrist] said he was going to call for an ambulance and if I didn't go voluntarily then he would get my GP and I would be sectioned under Section 3 under the Mental Health Act." (Hart 1996, p. 100.) Still, I would not regard the statement of Graham as a threat but merely a warning about possible and expected courses of events. But of course, other things are not always equal.

Compare the example above with the following statement of P: "If you do not take the pills you will become agitated and then we will have to give you ECT." This obviously poses a threat and we might infer that this is because ECT is such a grave intervention. But the difference between a threat and a warning does not consist in the severity of the predicted harm, e.g. that ECT is much worse than compulsory medication, but whether the outcome can be expected by Q or not. In the second case P is threatening Q with an outcome, which would not only worsen his situation but also in a way that is quite unusual and unexpected. Needless to say, the notion of what is expected or usual and its contrasts are not only value-laden but also depend on the context, since they involve considerations of legitimate claims and use of power.

So far, we have identified two conditions for predicted harm to constitute a threat. The consequence needs to be intentional and unusual. Therefore, the formula at the beginning of the paragraph can be reformulated as follows:

> Def. (interactive coercion): Q does/does not A because P proposes that he will bring about a detrimental unusual consequence R if Q does not/does do A; (and that P will not bring about R if Q does/does not A.)

---

4 There are some problems with this criterion when used – as in Nozick's account – to distinguish between threats and offers. For this see Frankfurt 1973, pp. 29ff. One may also argue that P is nevertheless threatening Q because he does not leave him with a real choice. The alternatives for Q seem to involve his taking the pills voluntarily but against his own will or else be put on medication by compulsory measures. There does not seem to be a real choice for Q just as in the example of the robber at the beginning. But of course to have no real choice is hardly a *sufficient* condition of coercion. See also Feinberg 1986, pp. 143ff.

The formula above implies that in order to be coerced, Q must comply with P's proposal, i.e. do what P wants him to do (Nozick 1969, p. 17, Bayles 1972, p. 17, Wertheimer 1987, p. 204). Therefore, only effective threats constitute instances of coercion. Admittedly, we may suppose that threats are coercive in any case because they are against the will of the threatened person, either by realization of R or by Q doing A/not-A, both of which are *ex hypothesis* against the will of Q. I nevertheless think that we would not refer to the inconsequential threats or the sanctions by P, which are followed by non-compliance of Q, instances of 'coercion'. But, of course, attempted coercion by posing a threat is also prima facie morally wrong and, in any case, results in a worsened situation for Q.

It is clear that there is no rigid line between a threat and a warning. After all, what is to be expected is often not easy to say. One may maintain that it depends on explicit and implicit rules, but it is sometimes hard to define exactly what the rules entail. This raises ethical problems in psychiatry, which I can only hint at here. Obviously psychiatric personnel can exploit the situation by hiding what a patient could reasonably expect in a psychiatric ward. The following report of a patient illustrates fairly significantly the problem: "A nurse came to me and said 'Go to supper'. I said 'No'. She growled at me for not making an effort, but all my effort is going into making these thoughts and writing them down. The nurse punished me, saying, 'Well, I'm not bringing you any supper, you know." (O'Hagan 1996, p. 47.) Was the nurse stating a threat or a warning? Maybe one can expect a nurse to bring supper to a depressed patient but maybe not.

Threats and Offers

Threats are paradigm cases of interactive coercion since they pose a strong influence on the decision-making process and often succeed in influencing people to do things they would normally not do. This is because threats involve a predicted sanction. If instances of coercion involve threats of a worsened situation for Q if he does not do A, then it seems that an offer cannot be coercive. After all, an offer promises exactly the opposite of a threat, namely, to better the situation of Q if he does A. But is this true, are offers never coercive?

First of all, it is of course true that threats can be stated as if they were offers. For example, a psychiatrist may say: "I offer to refrain from taking away your cigarettes if you stop smoking now." From a linguistic view, this merely appears like an offer but is a threat after all. It becomes more obvious when the missing element of the bi-conditional is made explicit. It states that the patient will lose his cigarettes if he does not stop smoking now.

No promise of *bettering* the situation of Q is involved in the example, although that seems to be the defining criterion of an offer. But again, it is an important issue whether the predicted consequence is unexpected or not. An offer not to harm a patient can be a real offer when harm is usually to be expected. For example, P can spare Q from being punished for his bad conduct. If a sanction would be the normal result of Q's behaviour, then it could be an offer not to harm him.

P may also offer Q a certain benefit, e.g. cigarettes. This clearly seems to be an instance of an offer. But again it depends on the circumstances, namely, whether it is to be expected or not. If Q has a claim to a certain number of cigarettes then to offer him just these does not promise to better his situation.

So far we have only talked about the difference between "real" and "faked" offers. But can real offers be coercive? Again, since they would better the overall situation of Q it seems evident that this is impossible (Gorr 1986, Bayles 1972, Rhodes 2000). Nevertheless, I wish to maintain that offers can indeed be coercive, especially in psychiatry. Some of them fit the offered definition of interactive coercion:

> Def. (interactive coercion by offer): Q does/does not A because P proposes that he will bring about a beneficial unusual consequence R if Q does/does not A; (and that P will not bring about R if Q does not/does A.)

It seems that at least one decisive element is missing in this definition. After all, many offers are clearly not coercive. For example, when a doctor offers a patient an additional, i.e. unusual or unexpected, box of cigarettes for taking pills then there is usually no coercion involved, although one may tend to speak of manipulation. But often psychiatric contexts are more complex.

Consider an example, which is a slightly changed version of the above quote: Nurse P offers patient Q a bar of chocolate if she goes to supper. This looks like a clear case of a non-coercive offer. One conditional – not going to supper and not getting chocolate – seems to be neutral; the other – going to supper and getting chocolate – appears to be beneficial.

But now we should discuss a complication: There is often a price Q has to pay in order to get the chocolate, i.e. doing what P asked her to do. The price a patient has to pay for going to supper can vary, hence the overall value of the conditionals may vary, too. For example, if Q is depressed and does not want to go to supper, the first conditional is not really neutral to her, because it concerns something she desperately does not want to do, hence she cares about this alternative.[5] The other conditional would be mixed, because it would involve a benefit and a detriment. If Q goes to supper because of an offer, she nevertheless acts against her own (pre-offer) will, i.e. her will *not* to go to supper.

5 Although there may be good reasons for a nurse to try to persuade a depressed patient to go to supper.

This illustrates a difference – which is sometimes neglected – between cases where Q explicitly does not want to do A but does it anyway because of an offer, and cases where Q merely would not do A without the offer, but doing A is not directed *against* a want of Q, i.e. when Q is neutral about doing A. Only the first cases involve offers that are directed *against* the will of Q. We would expect that in psychiatric hospitals offers are often posed in order to get someone to do something against his own will, e.g. comply with, and give consent to a proposed treatment he does not want.

Still, since *ex hypothesis* Q wants R *more* than not-A, and she will not be harmed if she does not comply with the proposal of P, to claim that offers can be coercive seems unreasonable. Q has a choice not to do A, hence perform what is her own will. If she nevertheless does A because of the offer, then her reason presumably is that she thinks she will, on the whole, be better off with R. In a way she does what she wants because she chooses to do A. How can she be coerced?

Irresistible Offers

I think that we get a clearer picture if we make use of an analogy between threats and offers according to Harry Frankfurt. Both threats and offers can be *irresistible*. As I pointed out at the beginning, the prima facie wrong of coercion is based on it being directed against the autonomous will of a person. Frankfurt also maintains that both threats and offers are coercive when they "violate its victim's autonomy" (Frankfurt 1973, p. 42, Feinberg 1986, pp. 189ff.).[6] This fits in with the psychiatric cases quite well, a point I wish to emphasize. When Q does A because of P's irresistible offer, she is not merely doing something she did not want prior to the offer – as in the case of non-coercive offers. When an offer is irresistible, Q could not have chosen otherwise in the sense that P did not leave her with any *real* alternative. Again, this does not mean that Q did not act voluntarily or that she – in a strong sense – was compelled to make a certain choice. Alternatives or options have not been made impossible in any strong sense of the word but ineligible or unthinkable.[7]

It seems paradoxical to claim that a choice can be simultaneously voluntary and against one's own will. But Frankfurt's account solves this seeming paradox by introducing a hierarchical analysis of freedom of the will (Frankfurt

6 Virginia Held (1972, p. 58) made a similar point before: "A person unable to spurn an offer may act as unwillingly as a person unable to resist a threat."

7 Hence, this is not to be taken as a metaphysical point. "She could not have chosen otherwise" is meant in the same way as in the case where someone threats you with "money or life!"

1971). He distinguishes between first- and second-order desires. A person is able to evaluate his own motivating desires (i.e. his first-order volitions). Even if someone is not physically forced to choose to act in a certain way and is motivated by his desires, he may nevertheless not actually wish to act in this way, because he does not want to desire to act in this way. Hence, he may or may not identify with his choice. For example, a person addicted to drugs may choose to take the drug but, at the same time, not want to be motivated by the desire for drugs. He does not act on the desire he wants to act on. According to Frankfurt, the motivating desire, i.e. his will, is not in harmony with his second-order volitions. We may derive from this account that someone whose first- and second-order volitions are in conflict does not act from his *own* will, because he does not act from the desires he wants to be motivated by. If we apply this analysis to the question whether or not offers can be coercive, we may claim that they can indeed, if they irresistibly alienate the choices of a person from what he actually wants.

Offers are regarded as unlikely instances of coercion because the promised result R is beneficial to Q. But, as stated before, one should not forget that Q often has to pay a price for R, namely to do A. To be sure, Q prefers R to not-A, i.e. non-compliance, otherwise the offer would be ineffectual.[8] Nevertheless, he would not have done A without the offer. He does not act on his own free will. Because of an offer he does something he does not identify with. I suspect that this is the reason why many offers – at least in some contexts like psychiatry – can be regarded as morally dubious. Of course, I do not wish to claim that all offers are bad. If they are not directed against the will of a person they do not seem to pose any problem at all. For example, if a psychiatrist asks a patient to help him carry a heavy desk and offers him a box of cigarettes for making the effort, then this is hardly an instance of coercion. But offers that are directed against the will, even non-coercive offers, which – as I said before – we may refer to as cases of manipulation, have to be considered with suspicion.

It needs to be emphasized that the decision whether an offer is coercive or not depends on the subjective preferences of Q in two ways. Firstly, we would not call an offer coercive, unless Q does something he does not want (second-order) to do because of the offer. In short, he does something he does not identify with because of the offer. Secondly, whether an offer is coercive or not depends on its seductive force which is a function of the preferences of Q. An offer may be easily rejected by one person but irresistible for another.

---

8 So an offer has to be sufficiently seductive in order to be coercive. That of course is grist to my mill, because I claim that offers are coercive when they are irresistible.

Both of these features are shared by coercive threats and coercive offers. It makes no difference that offers are proposals to better the situation of Q and threats proposals to harm Q. Therefore, it seems more likely that the essential characteristic of coercion is based on its influence on the autonomous will and not on the welfare of a person. This supports my claim that offers can be especially problematic in the context of psychiatry. Psychiatric patients are more liable to be unable to resist an offer because they are usually in a less powerful position and, in addition, because their will is often precarious and vulnerable.

Especially in psychiatric wards, a patient has to pay a high price for compliance with a proposed treatment he does not really want, namely, he is losing a precious space of autonomous choice. For psychiatric patients there are already limited opportunities for doing what they really want to do. If a patient complies with a treatment which he objected to in the first place because of the offer of some form of benefit, he may then feel regrets afterwards even if it was allegedly the best thing for him to do. Does that merely constitute a psychological problem?

Consider this statement of an in-patient: "We are encouraged to be victims, to look vertically to experts for the solutions to problems they have defined (...). Our restricted role in our own treatment is of fundamental importance. The 'good' patient is usually the one who does what he is told." (Campbell 1996, p. 60) In addition, inequality of power may lead to a situation where the personnel has several ways to deal with "bad" patients. In fact, patients often comply with a proposed treatment for good autonomous reasons. But this is not always so.

I am of the opinion that manipulation and coercion – at least in psychiatric hospitals – do not only stem from the predicted consequences which bring people to do A, namely, that they want to prevent bad things from happening. This view naturally leads to the claim that only threats and not offers can be coercive. But if we add that manipulation and coercion also involve bringing a person to do something against her own autonomous will, we are presented with a different picture concerning offers. By adding our previous claim that coercive offers are irresistible offers, we gain the revised version of the definition of interactive coercion which now applies to offers.

Def. (interactive coercion by offer): Q does/does not A because P proposes that he will bring about a beneficial unexpected consequence R – which is irresistible to Q – if Q does/does not A; (and that P will not bring about R if Q does not/does A); and Q cares about not doing/doing A.

Exploiting Dependencies

I maintain that irresistible offers – as compared to manipulative offers, which are resistible – are coercive. For an offer to be irresistible it has to have certain characteristics. I would like to suggest here, slightly changing Frankfurt's account, that an offer is irresistible when it exploits a dependency.[9]

Psychiatry is an institution where dependencies play an important role. First of all, many patients are dependent on certain objects. Some of them are addicted to cigarettes, coffee or sweets. Patients are also dependent on the psychiatric staff in many ways. The relation is not merely unequal, but one, where the situation of the patients, in several respects, is determined by others. Both kinds of dependencies can constitute grounds for irresistible offers.

For example, when a psychiatrist offers a box of cigarettes to a patient – who is craving for a smoke and has no other sources to get hold of any – if he takes certain pills, then in my view it can become an irresistible offer, hence an instance of coercion. Admittedly, this sounds a bit exaggerated, since smoking does not constitute a basic need like eating or drinking, so the patient may do without cigarettes. But this, of course, is not true for people who are addicted, and especially not for people who are in a psychiatric hospital. Smoking has an entirely different significance in a psychiatric ward than it does in everyday life.

Offers, which are based on an interpersonal relationship of dependency, can also be irresistible. When a nurse tells an intimidated patient that if he joins the occupational therapy group, she will write him a good report, then he will be more than prone to accept, especially if the report is important for his release. In addition, he might think that the nurse will write a bad report if he doesn't comply, although she did not actually threaten to do that. The nurse may also offer to tell the mother of Q, whose affection is very important for him, how well behaved he is. Again, this may leave Q without a real choice.

There is at least one important objection to the argument so far, namely, that there is a difference between exploiting a dependency one is responsible for, and merely exploiting an existing dependency. According to the objection, only the first, if any, represent an instance of coercion. To use a rather hackneyed example: A department chairman offers a graduate student an assistantship if she goes to bed with him. She desperately needs the job and, we might add, it

9 Frankfurt (1973, p. 33) introduces exploitation of dependency and need as conditions of refused benefits becoming threats. I use his account in a slightly different context for I do not discuss whether refused benefits – or offers, for that matter – can ever become *threats*, but only claim that some offers can be coercive.

is for reasons of age her last chance to gain an assistantship. Some theorists assert that the offer can only be coercive if the chairman was responsible for placing the student in a position of dependency (cf. Gorr 1986, p. 399, Rhodes 2000, pp. 373f.).

I am not sure quite how to reply to this objection. It probably adds up merely to a linguistic point, although I would still think that the chairman *coerced* the student into going to bed with him on the assumption that she would be unable to resist the offer. This is not due to the question whether or not he is or is not responsible for her being dependent on the job, but rather to the fact that she is dependent on *him* to get what she desperately wants. And similarly, a psychiatric patient may be dependent on the personnel to get what he needs, e.g. a good report. Anyway, however we wish to call these instances, both to take advantage of a dependency one is responsible for, and to take advantage of a dependency one is not responsible for, are in fact morally dubious – though the latter case may be less so. Of course, it is not clear from the outset that coercive offers are morally wrong in *all* instances. After all, on some occasions it might be good to sacrifice the freedom of a patient for the sake of his well-being.

To conclude: My main aim here was to raise the consciousness for cases in psychiatry where a supposed consent is invalid because a coercive threat or offer was involved. Although I mainly used examples from psychiatric wards, the conclusions I drew also apply to other psychiatric and psychotherapeutic settings. I do not wish to claim that I have introduced clear-cut definitions. In real life, it is hard to tell when offers become irresistible. But it seems conclusive that there are more cases, which are indeed coercive, than are generally expected, because they involve offers that are irresistible to psychiatric patients. Even while aiming at the autonomous consent of a patient, hence supposedly acting non-coercively, members of the psychiatric staff need to be aware of their responsibility not to exploit a dependency by making irresistible offers that will manipulate his own free will.

References

Bayles, M. 1972. "A Concept of Coercion", in: Pennock J.R. and Chapman, J.W. (eds.) *Coercion. Nomos XIV*. Chicago: Aldine Press, 16-29.

Beauchamp, T. 1997. "Informed Consent", in: Veatch, R. (ed.) *Medical Ethics. 2nd Edition*. Sudbury, Mass.: Jones & Bartlett, 185-208.

Brock, D.W. 1987. "Informed Consent", in: VanDeVeer, D. and Regan, T. (eds.) *Health Care Ethics*. Philadelphia: Temple University Press, 98-126.

Campbell, P. 1996. "Challenging Loss of Power", Read, J., Reynolds, J. (eds.) *Speaking Our Minds. An Anthology of Personal Experiences of Mental Distress and its Consequences*. Hampshire and London: MacMillan, 56-62.

Feinberg, J. 1971. "Legal Paternalism", *Canadian Journal of Philosophy*, 1: 105-124.
Feinberg, J. 1986. *Harm to Self*, Oxford: Oxford University Press.
Frankfurt, H.G. 1971. "Freedom of the Will and the Concept of a Person", reprinted in Frankfurt, H.G. *The Importance of What We Care About*, Cambridge: Cambridge University Press 1988, 11-25.
Frankfurt, H.G. 1973. "Coercion and Moral Responsibility", reprinted in Frankfurt, H.G. *The Importance of What We Care About*. Cambridge: Cambridge University Press 1988, 26-46.
Gorr, M. 1986. "Toward a Theory of Coercion", *Canadian Journal of Philosophy,* 16: 383-406.
Hart, L. 1996. "Stay Calm and Charm Them", in: Read, J., Reynolds, J. (eds.) *Speaking Our Minds. An Anthology of Personal Experiences of Mental Distress and its Consequences.* Hampshire and London: MacMillan, 100-104.
Held, V. 1972. "Coercion and Coercive Offers", in: Pennock J.R., Chapman, J.W. (eds.) *Coercion. Nomos XIV*. Chicago: Aldine Press, 49-62.
Kopelman, L.M. 1997. "Moral Problems in Psychiatry", in: Veatch, R. (ed.) *Medical Ethics. 2nd Edition*. Sudbury, Mass.: Jones & Bartlett, 275-320.
Nozick, R. 1969. "Coercion", reprinted in Nozick, R. *Socratic Puzzles*, Harvard: Harvard University Press 1997, 15-44.
O'Hagan, M. 1996. "Two Accounts of Mental Distress", in: Read, J., Reynolds, J. (eds.) *Speaking Our Minds. An Anthology of Personal Experiences of Mental Distress and its Consequences*. Hampshire and London: MacMillan, 44-50.
Rhodes, M.R. 2000. "The Nature of Coercion", *The Journal of Value Inquiry*, 34: 369-381.
VanDeVeer, D. 1986. *Paternalistic Intervention*. Princeton: Princeton University Press.
Wertheimer, A. 1987. *Coercion*, Princeton: Princeton. University Press.

The Moral Economics of Psychotherapy

Markus Pawelzik and Aloys Prinz

Healthcare is a moral enterprise. It is the mission as well as the aim of medicine to heal patients or, at least, to alleviate their suffering as far as possible. Although this explication of the task of medicine is universally acclaimed, one has to concede that this statement is too general and unspecific to determine the concrete medical proceedings in a modern health care system.

Many people would disagree with this last statement and purport that any compromise of the moral good inevitably leads to the moral bad. Budgetary restrictions which imply allocation decisions based on economic rationality appear to be regarded as an evil, an evil that compromises the core of medical ethics – the physician's duty to offer the most optimal form of treatment to the patients. The result is that ill people in need of medical treatment do not get the treatment they might well obtain in a morally sound health care system. Compromises between ethics and economic rationality therefore undermine the very essence of medicine.

The idea that economic rationality inevitably jeopardizes the moral good is obviously mistaken, as shown in the following two arguments: (i) Medical interventions should be effective. *In*effective measures are morally problematic because they imply a waste of money and resources that could be used more favourably to help others in need. An additional problem concerns the violation of the moral premises of valid informed consent. Patients who accept ineffective treatment are either irrational or misinformed. Both cases violate the moral requirements of informed consent (Faden and Beauchamp 1986). (ii) Any kind of inefficient use of resources is morally troublesome as well. Since *all* patients are entitled to effective treatment, this means that any kind of wasting, misallocation and exorbitantly expensive treatments will lead to a violation of the principle of justice (under conditions of a budgetary restriction).

Both arguments can be determined as moral ones although they make use of the economic concepts of "effectiveness" and "efficiency". They suggest that any feasible specification of the moral mission of medicine has to rely on economic and econometric concepts and data. This idea is an anathema to the public, the media and important opinion leaders in Germany. Ethics and economics are widely regarded as antipodes; it is assumed that any compromise between moral imperatives and economic rationality will lead to a violation of the morally right and good.[1]

---

1 'Signs' and 'symptoms' supporting this 'diagnosis' can be found in "Deutsches Ärzteblatt",

We believe that this attitude is dangerously naïve; it depends on obviously false beliefs and alone jeopardizes the moral foundations of medicine. By criticizing this attitude we wish to show that health care ethics and economic rationality should rather constitute a complementary relationship; one is dependent on the other. To establish this thesis we shall argue in favour of the following points: (i) Moral imperatives per se are insufficient to steer our health care system effectively. (ii) One reason is that the conduct of health care workers is determined by economic incentives more so than by moral reasons. (iii) This fact does not automatically lead to an opposition of morality and economic rationality. (iv) In order to test our thesis we shall take a closer look at psychotherapy as practised in private practice.

1. Health Care Management: Will the Principle of Beneficence do the Job?

Medicine constitutes a highly regarded profession. The functional role of medical professionalism is based on a balanced system of privileges and moral obligations. The most important privileges are a monopoly in health care, collective self-organization, self-employment and self-determined work, social prestige and high income (Freidson 1970). The moral obligations concern the well-being of the public, i.e. actual and potential patients. They take the form of a public promise, as the etymology of the term "profession" has it:[2] "We, as physicians, shall do everything we can to cure the (individual) patient. Our knowledge and our skills shall serve the patient's good. Doing otherwise violates the destination of our vocation. Doctors who violate our moral rules are to be expelled from our profession. They are unworthy to join our ranks."[3]

The core of medicine's altruism is the obligation to treat every patient with maximum beneficence. This point may be exemplified by the special contractual relationship of doctors and patients: The doctor-patient relationship differs from the common fee-for-service-contract. It is a "healing relation" which is strongly determined by the obligation to take care of the well-being of the patient. The moral demands on a fee-for-service-contract are satisfied when the conditions of a fairly negotiated contract are fulfilled by both sides, a medical

---

the official organ of the German physicians, in most of the German daily newspapers and in many political pronouncements. A very trenchant actual example were the presentations on the huge congress "Psychosoziale Versorgung in der Medizin", Hamburg, September 2003, where virtually every speaker condemned economic rationality and its consequences.

2 "Profession" derives from the Latin *profession* which means "public confession"; the Latin verb *profiteri* means "to confess in public"; see Dosdowski 1989, pp. 551f.

3 This is our explication of the core of medicine's professional ethos. Cf. e.g. Freidson 1999.

'healing contract' compensates for the fact that illness is an unfortunate fate that may cause great misery. To compensate for this misfortune, the doctor takes over the role of a trustworthy fiduciary who does what he can in his power to cure the illness (Pawelzik 1999).

The prominent philosophers of medicine, Pellegrino and Thomasma, explicated the overall mission of medicine in their influential book *A Philosophical Basis of Medical Practice* as follows:

> The end of medicine, formally considered, is therefore a right and good healing action taken in the interest of a particular patient. All the science and art of the physician converge on the choice: among the many things that can be done, that which should be done for the person in this particular situation of life. It is a choice of what is right in the sense of what conforms scientifically, logically, and technically to the patient's needs, and a choice of what is good, what is worthwhile for this patient. (...) This culmination in a right and good healing action is what *constitutes medicine qua medicine*. (Pellegrino and Thomasma 1981, p. 211; emphasizes added).

Following this line of reasoning on can say: Any kind of medical practice that does *not* realize the good of medicine is ethically flawed. Such practices jeopardize the professional status of medicine. In the long run, doctors would lose their privileges for the benefit of a bureaucratically controlled health care system (Freidson 2002).

For most commentators in this country it takes but a small inferential step from the undisputable moral role of medicine to accept the idea that ethics is the most effective steering instrument of our health care system: "Doctors do what they should do, morally. Moral medicine is the best for the individual patient as well as for the society as a whole. The costs of medicine should be borne by a just, i.e. collectively financed, health care system. That these costs are steadily rising underlines the fact that our society is becoming a better one, i.e. a society that looks after the well-being of each individual."

That this beneficence-dominated perspective will run into all kinds of practical problems is to be expected. It is crucial that such problems, including controversial allocation problems, should be solved in a moral manner. Following this line of reasoning, Pellegrino and Thomasma argue:

> Each medical decision involves the complicated interplay of several value sets – those of the physician, of the patient, and of society. In a pluralistic society, these value sets may differ sharply from each other. The possibilities of conflict in the conception of the good between physician and patient are many. A very special problem in medical decision making is how to resolve these conflicts in a *morally defensible way*. (Op. cit., p. 212; emphasizes added).

Moral principles and rules should play an important role in medical decision making. They are general signposts to direct the medical endeavours. But these signposts are worthless if the actual context is not taken into account – the context determines the significance of the signpost – or if different signposts point in different directions, as they mostly do. To make effective use of moral rules one needs further information, especially econometric information about effect sizes, expectable outcomes, de facto outcomes, costs, etc. and economic concepts that allow specification and balance of the relevant principles (Beauchamp and Childress 2001).

We believe that ethics alone never has and never will succeed in effectively steering a health care system. The traditional beneficence-dominated medical ethic with its almost exclusive focus on the individual clinical encounter is insufficient to deal with a situation of limited resources.

Let us take a look at a few well known 'anomalies' which demonstrate that the primacy of medical beneficence would lead to inadequate or paradox results:

Medical altruism. Doctors in private practices as well as owners of hospitals are entrepreneurs. Bankruptcy is unavoidable if their income does not cover their costs. With this fact in mind one should not be astonished to learn that economic incentives strongly determine the way in which patients are treated. Medically unnecessary diagnostic as well as therapeutic procedures, prolonged treatments etc. increase the income of the doctor or the clinic, thereby wasting resources that might be needed elsewhere.

Endless health care needs. Medical treatment shall confine itself to "medical necessary" interventions, as stated by the German health care laws. But where are the boundaries of medical necessity? Who defines them? And what impact do medical innovations have? We have to concede that not every patient receives the treatment he needs these days due to budgetary restrictions. There is widespread non-disclosed rationing of benefits. Offering "state-of-the-art"-treatments that conform to established treatment guidelines would increase costs at a relevant magnitude. Furthermore, scientific and technical innovations permanently relocate the limits of optimal treatments. But even if one is offered what is available nowadays: the remaining suffering constitutes health care needs that should be satisfied, as laid down by the beneficence-dominated ethics of medicine. As long as illness, suffering and premature death persist, health care needs are, in principle, without restriction (Callahan 1990).

Conflicting societal priorities. Germany spends more than 10% of its Gross Domestic Product (GDP) on health care; the US health care system – the most expensive (though pretty ineffective) health care system in the world – consumes 13% of its GDP (OECD 2002). Why should we not be prepared to spend even more, given the obligations of a beneficence-dominated health care ethics? The answer is that higher expenditures would compromise other important social causes, such as education, culture or social security. The resulting conflicts concerning the question which societal task should be given priority cannot be solved by medical beneficence alone.

Demographic development. The demographic pyramid of our population stands up-side down. The higher the percentage of elderly individuals, the higher the medical expenditures. This trend, as is well known, jeopardizes the social security and welfare systems of the industrialized societies all over the world. This is an especially grave problem since it leads to an unsolvable paradox: More money for more medicine does not necessarily lead to less morbidity. On the contrary: Due to the achievements of modern medicine people live longer to experience more illness during their lifetime. It is a side effect of the success of medicine that brings about an indefinite increase in the costs until the 'final solution of the illness-problem' is achieved (Pawelzik 1999).

Scientific and technical innovation. Progress and improvement in medicine is certainly a good thing because it allows to help those people in need, as we followers of the Enlightenment tend to believe. But progress is costly, especially in the field of medicine. Scientific innovation may be the most important cost driver, as shown by econometric analysis (e.g. Breyer and Ulrich 2000).

Taken together, the mentioned facts constitute a vicious circle of ever increasing costs: Medical progress, a disproportional high percentage of elderly patients, endless health care needs, the economic interests of the caregivers and the virtual inability to solve priority conflicts in our consensus oriented society will inevitably lead to a crisis in the case that change is postponed.

One should keep in mind that the logic of this beneficence-motivated development – health care needs must be covered sufficiently and treatments should be implemented more effectively – is not a sound one, as the following facts may demonstrate:

- The history of medicine shows that the health of a population depends on more than just advanced medicine. Non-medical conditions such as food, sanitary conditions, housing, income, general conditions of living, social justice and changes in life style proved to be more effective in granting general health (Wolinsky 1988).
- The effectiveness of a medical procedure in several proven cases does not guarantee the same results for the society as a whole. Nor does valid information about clinical effectiveness allow inferences to its efficiency when generally applied.
- Progress increases the range of applicable procedures, thereby increasing the pressure on drawing decisions. Since many procedures do not differ in clinical effectiveness, one has to rely on economic decision criteria, e.g. costs.

- In the near future molecular medicine will supply new, highly effective bio-technological treatments at extremely high costs. Since budgetary restrictions will limit the use of these technologies, this will lead to difficult allocation decisions.

Taking these facts into account, three conclusions seem inevitable: (i) The general premise of a beneficence-dominated medical ethics – every patient should be given optimal treatment – will lead to a breakdown of the health care system and is, therefore, not sustainable. (ii) The individual claim for optimal treatment must therefore be restricted. The obligations that derive from the principle of beneficence have to be balanced with the obligations that follow from the principle of justice. (iii) The management priorities of a just health care system, a health care system that is based on solidarity agreement, should conform to the public health idea. Focus should be set on the overall health of the society.

2. Health Care Management: Economics versus Morality

The result of the preceding section can be described briefly as follows: The moral concept of a 'good' health care system has almost nothing in common with the real health care system. Obviously the health care system is based rather on the self-interest of the service providers than on their beneficence. In a sense, the economic nature of the system dominates the moral obligations of the individual participants. This seems to be true for the providers of the services as well as for the patients. As a consequence, it is inappropriate and misleading to ignore the economic incentives of the participants in the discussion of a functional health system. As shown in the following, integration of economic rationality into the concept of a good health care system is, to a certain extent, inevitable. Economics, thus, may be called the maid of morality.

A precondition for economic problems in the health care system is that the costs incurred for useful medical diagnostic and therapeutic procedures exceed by far the financial means of a society. Nowadays, this precondition is given and the medical-technical progress increases greatly the number of available procedures. Consequently, the number of illnesses that become treatable is increasing, likewise, the number of effective procedures. This creates a genuine economic problem that may only be solved with economic instruments. The reason is that procedures of similar effectiveness differ in their costs. Choosing among such procedures is an economic problem. Even the question to determine to which point a treatment should be extended is not only a medical question of effectiveness, but also an economic question of efficiency. Accepting the shortage of resources and, consequently, a budget restriction for the health care system, creates the necessity of economic analysis and instruments. Hence, running a modern health care system is a medico-moral-economic business.

In addition, the organization of a health care system implies also a wide range of economic questions – with far reaching consequences if the economics of the systems are not fully comprehended. To a large extent, the economic questions concern the incentives for the participants in the system. Because it is in the favour of all service providers to earn a living, they are responsive to the economic incentives of the system. Since it is not possible to construct a health care system without (at least implicit) incentives, a careful analysis of these incentives is required. The objectives of the system as well as of the incentives will be based on ethics or medicine, however, the selection among incentives is again a genuine economic task.

Neither the organization nor the running of the health care system is possible using moral principles only. The reason is that the moral obligation of beneficence is solely based on the clinical effectiveness of the procedures at hand, i.e. the efficiency of procedures is generally neglected. This is relevant because it indicates that the general shortage of resources has not been taken into account. Measures that ignore the shortage of resources are not sustainable.[4] Hence they violate the rules of the rational use of resources and not only harm contemporary but also future generations. In order to understand this, consider the extent of treatments with the beneficence rule only. If the beneficence-based rule requires to extend the treatment of an illness up to the point where the utility of the treatment equals its costs, this would be a contradiction to economic rationality. Economic rationality – i.e. the rational use of scarce resources[5] – requires that the treatment is extended until the *marginal* utility equals *marginal* costs of the treatment.[6] With increasing marginal costs, taken into account the scarcity of resources, the *optimal* treatment will be shorter than with the beneficence rule which prescribes the *maximal* treatment.[7]

---

4 The notion of 'sustainability' originates from forestry and was in 1987 eventually introduced into the ecological discussion with the so-called Brundtland Report; see Wissenschaftlicher Beirat beim Bundesministerium der Finanzen 2001, p. 5. The central statement of the Report is: "Sustainable development is development that meets the needs of present generations without compromising the ability of future generations to meet their own needs."

5 In economic terms, this is called 'allocation' or 'allocative efficiency'. It describes the fact that a rational use of scarce resources requires that the resources have to be employed ('allocated') to their most productive use. See e.g. Black 1997, pp. 10 and 139.

6 See, for instance, Szucs 1997, p. 64 and the literature quoted there.

7 See also the critique of Elster: "On the other hand, efficiency is undermined by doctors' professional norms, which lead them to concentrate on critically ill patients even when the very acuteness of their condition makes treatment unlikely to succeed", Elster 1989, p. 116.

So far, the micro level (running a health care system) and the meso level (organizing and designing a health care system) have been considered. However, also the *macro level* of a health care system poses genuine economic questions. On the macro level, it is up to the society to decide how much of its scarce resources are allocated to certain purposes. This decision may be explicit or implicit: the size of the sector of car manufacturing, for instance, is implicitly decided via the sum of individual decisions to buy cars. These decisions are based on the individual household's willingness and ability to pay for a car. In a purely private health care system, the same principle would apply. Each household would privately decide whether or not and to what extent to buy health insurances or medical services. Aggregating over the expenditures for medical services of all households and health insurances would determine the size of the health care sector. As is well known, a purely private solution for the determination of the size of the health care sector is, from a moral point of view, not acceptable. If a person falls ill, she *should* be entitled to medical help and treatment. This means that access to the health care services cannot be based solely on the willingness and ability to pay. Hence, the size of the health care sector must be determined in another way. In a democratic society, the political system is legitimized to choose an adequate amount of resources to furnish this sector.

However, free access to the health care system triggers an economic problem if the use of medical treatment is not restricted. Free access in combination with free use would eliminate the budget restriction of the sector and contradict the scarcity of resources. Because the needs for treatment are essentially without limits, the resources constraint on the macro level would be permanently violated. Hence, sustainability requires that free access to the health care system is to be supplemented by economic tools to enforce the budget restriction of the sector on the meso and the micro level of the system. For this purpose, morality is not an adequate instrument since the problems are of an economic nature. However, morality may provide additional constraints for the design of economic tools. Some tools for the restriction of the use of medical resources are e.g. co-payments, medical guidelines as well as general or specific budget restrictions. As a result, we have a division of labour between morals and economics: Objectives and priorities for the health care sector are to be defined by using moral principles, whereas the implementation of the necessary restrictions and incentives are to be carried out by using economic principles and tools. In other words, since free access to the health care system is based on moral considerations, the instruments to enforce the budget constraint(s) for the use of medical resources are based on economics.

The restriction of the use of medical resources by economic tools is not new. It provides empirical evidence for the conclusion that a dominantly or even purely moral control of the health care sector has been abandoned a long time ago. Applying the reasoning of the theory of systems makes quite clear why this is necessarily so. The subsystems of modern societies (e.g.

medicine, arts, courts) are governed by a genuine logic that separates and immunizes one particular system from another. According to Niklas Luhmann, there is no chance to integrate the subsystems into the system of the society, as a whole, with morals (Luhmann 1990, pp. 23f.): The autonomy of the subsystems originates from the specific functions the subsystems provide for society and a special binary code (as e.g. 'true' and 'false' for the subsystem 'science'). These individual codes of the subsystems are not equivalent to the binary code of morality ('right' and 'wrong'). On the contrary, the subsystems require codes of 'higher amorality' since the values of the specific codes enter into the operations of the system in its entirety. In other words, the moral code is not appropriate to connect and coordinate the operations of the different subsystems. In a sense, functionality is superior to morality. Luhmann's conclusion is that a society that is functionally differentiated into subsystems has to abandon the idea of moral integration. Nevertheless, the inclusion or exclusion of persons in a society happens via the moral concept of respect and disregard (Luhmann 1990, p. 25; Cf. Luhmann 1997, pp. 1043f.).

In conclusion, it is crucial to understand that the subsystems of a modern society cannot be governed and coordinated with morality. This also holds true for the medical subsystem. This subsystem as such must solve moral, medical and economic problems. Morality is neither the sole nor the dominant principle required to guarantee the functionality of the subsystem. The medical-technical progress extends the potential effectiveness of the health care system, but, at the same time, threatens the financial basis of the system. Without economic backup the health care system is at risk to waste to a large extent the resources and to reduce in this way the beneficial procedures for the sick and suffering persons.

3. Health Care Management: Moral Economics

Economic incentives play a significant role in the sense that they are not based on the benevolence or altruism of people. Economists do not deny that persons are benevolent or altruistic at some time, but they deny that it is feasible to base the economic incentives in a society on altruism or benevolence. Assuming a rather immoral *homo oeconomicus* prevents the exploitation of moral persons by immoral ones because the incentive system is designed for immoral persons. Moral persons may deviate from the incentive system by deliberately applying a different incentive system that may be based on mutual altruism. However, the interaction with immoral persons will be based on incentive schemes which assume selfishness. This protects moral people from becoming exploited by immoral ones who could otherwise free ride on an incentive system based on altruism.

One of the most renowned passages in *The Wealth of Nations* by Adam Smith says exactly this with unmistakable clarity:

> It is not from the benevolence of the butcher, the brewer, or the baker that we expect our dinner, but from their regard to their own interest. We address ourselves, not to their humanity but to their self-love, and never talk to them of our own necessities but of their advantages. Nobody but a beggar chooses to depend chiefly upon the benevolence of his fellow-citizens. (Smith 1998, p. 16)

Even physicians have self-interests. That is the reason why economics designs incentive tools that provide personal advantages for the participants in market transactions. Obviously this does not exclude morality-based actions and arguments in the health care sector.[8] The crucial point is, however, that the central incentive systems cannot be based mainly on morality, but also on economics.[9] The moral principles of 'good' and 'right' as well as 'evil' and 'wrong' are *de facto* inadequate to allocate scarce resources to best support a system that is as large and as complex as the health care system.

A different question is, however, whether certain medical procedures should be applied *at all*. Whether it should be allowed to clone human beings or to practise euthanasia cannot be answered with economic reasoning. These are genuine moral questions that are to be answered in collective decision making processes in the society as a whole. The domain of medical ethics may, then, be delimited as follows:

1. Medical ethics defines those medical procedures that should not in any way be permitted for the treatment of human beings.
2. Medical ethics determines the code of conduct for medical service providers with respect to patients as persons.

That means that the task of medical ethics is to ensure that medical service providers commit themselves to a code of conduct. It emphasizes the collective judgement that not all procedures that are medically feasible should

---

8 Adam Smith himself, too, does not recognize a conflict between 'self-interest' (dominating in his *The Wealth of Nations*) and 'sympathy' (dominating in his *The Theory of Moral Sentiments*): "Smith believed that every man had a basic desire to be accepted by others. To obtain this sympathy, people would act in a manner that would gain respect and admiration. In economic life, this meant enlightened self-interest, wherein both seller and buyer mutually benefit in their transactions. Moreover, Smith contended that economic progress and surplus wealth were a prerequisite for sympathy and charity. In short, Smith desired to integrate economics and moral behaviour", Skousen 2001, p. 23 (quoting Fitzgibbons 1995, pp. 3-4 and Tvede 1997, p. 29).

9 "The great advantage of the market is that it is able to use the strength of self-interest to offset the weakness and partiality of benevolence, so that those who are unknown, unattractive, and unimportant will have their wants served", Coase 1976, p. 544.

also be approved. In this way, medical ethics as a sub-subject of collective moral judgements supports decision making health care workers insofar as it relieves them from moral dilemmas as it simply interdicts or disregards *a priori* certain actions.[10]

The crucial question is whether these ethical guidelines for health care workers based on the principle of beneficence for patients may come into conflict with the economic rationality of a 'good' health care system. We intend to prove that the allegation is not justified, namely, that economizing the health care system would imply injustice and mercilessness. We believe that a lack of knowledge with regard the working of economic rationality is the main reason for this judgement. Together with the majority of other people, economists too share the characteristics of 'hard heads and soft hearts' (Blinder 1987).

Economic rationality (which is also called *efficiency*) can be defined in two ways (Black 1997, p. 139):

1. Attaining a fixed amount of output with the smallest amount of input. Applied to psychotherapy this means e.g. curing a phobia with the lowest possible input of hours of therapy.
2. Attaining a maximal output with a given amount of input. This means in the example above: reduction of the phobia as far as possible with a fixed input of, say, 20 hours of therapy.

The implication of these definitions is that the rationale of economics is to bring about the best outcome for the input of resources. That sums up exactly the meaning of efficiency. Better said, efficiency requires that there be no wastage of input resources. Economics can be understood as the pursuit for a waste-free society. In the health care sector, the patients are primarily the winners of economic rationality. Hence, from this viewpoint, there is no contradiction between medical morality and economic rationality. The ultimate objective of both is the well-being of the patient with respect to her health, given the scarce resources and the structure of the health care system. The sustainability of the performance of the health care system with scarce resources requires that moral principles are supplemented by economic ones. Insofar, economic efficiency is a moral business. Our central thesis is therefore:[11]

There is no fundamental contradiction between medical morality and economic rationality in the health care sector. The implementation of economic rationality into the health care system is not only an economic but also a moral necessity.

---

10 This deliberate restriction of the set of actions, ('precommitment') is also analysed in economics; see e.g. Glazer and Weiss 1992, Maital 1986 as well as Schelling 1984; for a philosophical analysis see Elster 1984.

11 For a more general analysis of the ethical relevance of economic efficiency see Pies 2000.

The main effect of applying economic rationality to the health care sector is to increase its efficiency and to extend in this way the means for the treatment of illnesses. The waste of resources reduces the means for treatment. Hence, inefficiencies harm the patients.

One could argue that it is a special aspect of medical morality to provide for all patients and, especially for the poor and socially weak patients, an equal supply of medical procedures. That would imply that the distribution of the resources of the health care system should be concentrated on those who cannot help themselves. It is feared that economic rationality favours the wealthy and harms the poor.

The crucial point here is that in addition to efficiency a second economic problem is to be considered, i.e. the distribution of resources among patients of a different wealth status. A health care system based purely on individual decisions and on market principles would harm the poor and sick people because they are not in the position to afford the medical insurances they need to protect themselves against the costs of falling ill and of medical treatment. However, as already mentioned, the health care system is supposed to be a *publicly* organized system that uses both moral and economic principles to solve the problems of efficiency and the distribution of resources among patients. Hence the critique of a purely private health care system is, as a consequence, not applicable. Our 'good' health care system integrates the moral principle of justice with the economic principle of efficiency. This combination creates a win-win situation: economic efficiency provides a 'cake' (medical resources) that is as large as possible, given that its distribution to patients is independent of their ability to pay. In other words, a high degree of efficiency is the precondition for providing the best possible medical treatment for the poor, weak and sick people. Note, however, that the just distribution of the medical resources is a restriction for the implementation of economic efficiency. In a sense, moral principles dominate and economic tools are applied up to the point that they do not violate the objective of justice. This dominance principle prevents a conflict between economics and ethics. This is the reason that we call this approach *moral economics*. If a conflict between morality and economics arises, morality is put first. Economics is then the maid of morals.[12]

Last but not least, it should be emphasized that there are not only moral, but also economic limits for the control of the health care sector. Economic incentives cannot be designed to eliminate each and every inefficient action and waste. There will, due to necessity, remain some areas for individual actions that may be misused for wasteful and indecent conduct. We suppose, however, that the application of moral economics will enable the society to

---

12 Historically, economics is even the child of moral philosophy. See, for instance, Langholm 1992 for a comprehensive analysis of economics in medieval times.

prevent the self-destruction of the system itself. Without a certain moral-economic conscience of all actors within the system a just and efficient health care system will never be established.

4. Psychotherapy and Moral Economics

In our view, health care ethics and economic rationality have to form a complementary relationship to effectively regulate our health care system. Let us now take a closer look at a concrete example, the field of psychotherapy, to exemplify our thesis.

Psychotherapy is a rather Janus-faced part of health care: on the one hand, there are highly effective methods of therapy that allow optimal treatment of a broad range of mental as well as physical disorders (Nathan and Gorman 2003, Ehlert 2003, Creer et al. 2004). On the other hand, we have to face the fact that practicing psychotherapists do not make use of these evidence-based therapies (Beutler 2000). The practice of psychotherapy is quite heterogeneous (the therapy market offers more than 400 different methods of psychotherapy), intransparent (psychotherapists avoid objectifying quality assurance measures) and arbitrary (therapist do what they think best; Garb 1998). This situation may explain why psychotherapy is regarded as a dubious craft with a rather marginal standing in our health care system (Pawelzik forthcoming).

Let us discuss the situation based on the simple scenario of three parties that interact in out-patient psychotherapy: the therapist, the patient and the cost-covering institution, i.e. the collectively financed health insurance system in Germany.

The *patient* suffers from a certain psychic problem and decides to look for psychotherapeutic help. His situation is characterized by little knowledge of the available therapies and little means for a comparative evaluation of the given options. His ignorance concerns the best option (*what should be done in therapy?*) as well as the possible quality of this option (*how should it be done?*).

The patient, in general, is looking for a quick, easy and simple solution for his problem. He wants to feel accepted by his therapist, expects effortless progress and tries to avoid pain and costs. Unfortunately, miracle cures of this kind are seldom available. Successful psychotherapy is characterized by painstaking effort, difficult insights and behaviour changes and the intentional activation of aversive affects. The sustainability of therapeutic success depends decisively on the fact that the patient *himself* changes things actively and takes care that these changes continue to persist. Although it is objectively rational for the patient to choose this route to health, he depends on the fiduciary role and morality of his therapist. Why should the therapist offer a rather difficult, but potentially effective route, if it would be much easier for her and her patient to choose a more effortless, but also less successful way to proceed?

The answer to this question has two issues to consider – a moral one and an economic one: (i) The therapist has to respect the autonomy of the patient. This obligation is generally realized by the informed consent procedure. If the therapist offers an 'easy way'-therapy without withholding relevant information concerning alternatives, success rates etc. and without manipulating the patient, we are faced with a dilemma: there is no violation of the moral rules of informed consent; i.e. the patient-therapist interaction is morally sound. But the patient may choose the 'easy way'-therapy, which offers little chance for success – a likely waste of resources and a disadvantage for the collective of insured persons. This would violate the principle of justice. (ii) In terms of economic psychology, the problem may be called a *double moral hazard problem* on the side of the patient:[13] The patient takes advantage of the therapy sessions as long as he gains a positive net effect without paying for it in form of monetary and psychic costs. For a short-run gain the patient sacrifices, at the same time, his own long-run mental health and the resources of the health insurance system avoiding a promising 'hard way'-therapy.

Our solution of the dilemma focuses on the incentives of the involved parties. It is in the interests of the *health insurance system* to offer effective treatments that deliver sustainable success. Ineffective 'easy way'-therapies compromise this premise by wasting money and resources. The health insurance system should therefore contract only therapists who are able to guarantee an adequate level of quality and success. This entails the use of evidence-based therapies, conformity with treatment guidelines, quality assurance routines and participation in benchmarking and peer review procedures. To gain effective results in psychotherapy as well as in medicine generally, it is necessary to reduce the variance of therapeutic interventions. Therapy is neither an art based on intuition nor a bare sample of scientifically established techniques; therapy is an elaborate craft that induces functional change processes, processes whose essential ingredients are already well established.

The contract between therapist and the health insurance system narrows the range of options that may be chosen by the patient and his therapist. It is

13 In the context of health care, moral hazard means generally that a patient demands quantitatively and qualitatively more medical services than he would demand according to his own willingness to pay because the costs of the services are borne by the health insurance system. (For the standard definition of moral hazard see e.g. Folland et al. 2001, pp. 152-155.) Here, we add a further component: Since the patient irrationally ignores the future costs of not solving his problem, he chooses the 'easy way'-therapy. In addition to that, he may anticipate that the future costs of an additional psychotherapy will also be borne by the health insurance system.

the task of the therapist to inform his patient about the available options. It is up to the *patient* to decide which way to proceed. If an 'easy way'-therapy is desired, he may contract another therapist, paying the costs of the therapy himself. In the case that he consents to the suggested treatment plan, he should none the less be charged an affordable co-payment to cover the moral hazard problem that might exist even in this case.

The *therapist* has the most exacting and responsible position concerning treatment plan and therapy – morally as well as economically, since she has the greatest influence on the ensuing process. She is the guide of the intended change process. Despite the quality assuring contract with the health insurance system, there is still a broad range of options the therapist may choose; her temperament, interactive style and talents strongly determine the therapeutic alliance, the patient's motivation for change and the implementation of definite procedures. Last but not least, it is her commitment to the well-being of the patient that has a decisive influence on the outcome. With this in mind, we ask: Which incentives are most effective to ensure that the therapist performs a good job?

Our answer is based on three premises: (i) Money is not the strongest incentive for highly qualified professionals. Professionals try to gain the recognition of their peers, as Parsons (Latham 2002) realized long ago. The main reason is that only qualified professionals have the knowledge to estimate the performance of a colleague. Professionals work hard to increase their self-esteem by demonstrating good professional performances, performances whose recognition depends on the estimation of professional authorities. For this reason professional standards play an important role in the *lingua franca* of expert discussions. (ii) Psychotherapy is a very peculiar profession. The therapist herself is the instrument of the craft. This causes specific mental strains that the therapist has to endure. A further source of stress results from the fact that the object of one's work is less transparent than in other domains of health care and even expert therapists often experience little control and success. To cope with these combined stress factors, the therapists engage in a certain kind of 'identity politics': they immunize themselves against failure, rationalize the patient's 'dysfunctional' behaviour and look for support from their peers. Psychotherapists are strongly in need of support by their peers in order to stabilize their own personal identity. The local representatives of the profession take an important but little reflected responsibility for colleagues in need (Pawelzik forthcoming). (iii) Last but not least, also therapists have to earn a living. That their average income is located at the lower end of all health care professions underlines the fact that psychotherapy (undeservedly) has no strong standing in the health care system.

Based on these premises we come to the conclusion that it is of utmost importance that psychotherapists develop a strong professional identity as members of a morally reflected, scientifically educated, well trained und supervised 'collective of healers'. Professional socialization, strong personal identity and fair job opportunities are essential prerequisites to promote good and motivated therapists.

Although the individual motivation plays an important role, it seems necessary to implement further checks and balances to watch out for potential black sheep. One example of effective measures the health insurance system should look for are collective benchmarking procedures: Every contracted therapist should participate in quality assurance routines, e.g. by using standardized outcome measures that allow for evaluation of her performance in relation to the average. Therapists who attain substandard results should be guided by peer review procedures of professional organizations. The difficulty of a scientifically informed craft that deals with the indetermination of individual situations could thereby be held in a morally and economically adequate balance.

References

Beutler, L.E. 2000. "Empirically based decision making in clinical practice", in: *Prevention & Treatment*, Vol. 3, Article 27, http://www.journals.apa.org/prevention/volume3.html.

Black, J. 1997. *A dictionary of economics*, Oxford and New York.

Blinder, A.S. 1987. *Hard heads, soft hearts: tough-minded economics for a just society*, Reading/Mass., 2nd printing.

Beauchamp, T. L., Childress, J.F. 2001. *Principles of biomedical ethics*, 5th ed., New York.

Breyer, F., Ulrich, V. 2000. "Gesundheitsausgaben, Alter und medizinischer Fortschritt: Eine Regressionsanalyse", in: *Jahrbücher für Nationalökonomie und Statistik*, Vol. 220, pp. 1-17.

Brundtland Report. 1987. *Our common future*. Oxford.

Callahan, D. 1990. *What kind of life: The limits of medical progress*, New York.

Coase, R.H. 1976. "Adam Smith's view of man", in: *Journal of Law and Economics*, Vol. 19, pp. 529-546.

Creer, T.L., Holroyd, K.A., Glasgow, R.E., Smith, T.W. 2004. "Health psychology", in: Lambert, M.J. (ed.) *Bergin and Garfield's handbook of psychotherapy and behavior change*, New York.

Dosdowski, G. 1989. "Profession", in: *Duden Etymologie. Herkunftswörterbuch der deutschen Sprache*, (Der Duden Vol. 7), 2nd ed., Mannheim, Wien, Zürich, pp. 551 f.

Ehlert, U. (ed.) 2003. *Verhaltensmedizin*, Berlin.

Elster, J. 1989. *The cement of society. A study of social order*, Cambridge.

Elster, J. 1984. *Ulysses and the sirens*, rev. ed., Cambridge.

Faden, R.R., Beauchamp, T.L. 1986. *A history and theory of informed consent*, New York.

Fitzgibbons, A. 1995. *Adam Smith's system of liberty, wealth, and virtue,* New York.

Folland, S., Goodman, A.C., Stano, M. 2001. *The economics of health and health care*, 3rd ed., Upper Saddle River, N.J.
Freidson, E. 1970. *Profession of medicine: a study of the sociology of applied knowledge*, Chicago.
Freidson, E. 1999. "Professionalism and institutional ethics", in: Baker, R., Caplan, A., Emanuel, L., Latham, S. (eds.) *The American medical ethics revolution*, Baltimore.
Freidson, E. 2001. *Professionalism: the third logic*, Chicago.
Garb, H. 1998. *Studiying the clinician*, Washington, D.C.
Glazer, J., Weiss, A. 1992. "Conflicting preferences and voluntary restrictions on choices", *Discussion Paper* Tel Aviv University and Boston University.
Langholm, O. 1992. *Economics in the medieval schools*, Leiden et al.
Latham, S.R. 2002. "Medical professionalism: a Parsonian view", in: *The Mount Sinai Journal of Medicine*, Vol. 69, 363-369.
Luhmann, N. 1997. *Die Gesellschaft der Gesellschaft*, Vol. 2, Frankfurt a.M.
Luhmann, N. 1990. "Paradigm lost: Über die ethische Reflexion der Moral", in: Luhmann, *Paradigm lost: Über die ethische Reflexion der Moral*, Frankfurt a.M., pp 9-48.
Maital, S. 1986. "Prometheus rebound: On welfare-improving constraints", in: *Eastern Economic Journal*, Vol. 12, pp. 337-344.
Nathan, P.E., Gorman, K.M. 2003. *A guide to treatments that work*, 2nd ed., New York.
OECD. 2002. *OECD Health Data 2002*.
Pawelzik, M. 1999. *Krankheit, das gute Leben und die Krise der Medizin*, Münster.
Pawelzik, M. forthcoming. "Psychotherapie als Profession", in: Pawelzik, M., Mauler, B. (eds.) *Zehn Jahre Christoph-Dornier-Klinik für Psychotherapie*, Münster.
Pellegrino, E.D., Thomasma, D.C. 1981. *A philosophical basis of medical practice*, New York.
Pies, I. 2000. "Wirtschaftsethik als ökonomische Theorie der Moral – zur fundamentalen Bedeutung der Anreizanalyse für ein modernes Ethikparadigma", in: *Wirtschaftsethische Perspektiven*, Vol. 5, pp. 11-33.
Schelling, T.C. 1984. "Ethics, law, and the exercise of self-command", in: Schelling, T.C. *Choice and consequence*, Cambridge/Mass. and London, pp. 83-112.
Skousen, M. 2001. *The making of modern economics. The lives and ideas of the great thinkers*, Armonk, New York and London, England.
Smith, A. 1998. *Plain texts from key thinkers* (ed. by A. Kellbrook), London.
Smith, A. 1776. *An inquiry into the nature and causes of the wealth of nations*, London.
Smith, A. 1759. *The theory of moral sentiments*, London.
Szucs, T. 1997. *Medizinische Ökonomie*, München.
Tvede, L. 1997. *Business cycles: From John Law to chaos theory,* Amsterdam.
Wissenschaftlicher Beirat beim Bundesministerium der Finanzen. 2001. *Nachhaltigkeit in der Finanzpolitik*, Berlin.
Wolinsky, F.D. 1988. *The sociology of health*, 2nd ed., Belmont, California.

Index